Seventh Edition

HEALTH PROMOTION IN NURSING PRACTICE

Nola J. Pender, PhD, RN, FAAN
Professor Emerita
University of Michigan
School of Nursing
Ann Arbor, Michigan

Carolyn L. Murdaugh, PhD, RN, FAAN
Professor Emerita and Adjunct Professor
University of Arizona
College of Nursing
Tucson, Arizona

Mary Ann Parsons, PhD, RN, FAAN
Professor Emerita and Dean Emerita
University of South Carolina
College of Nursing
Columbia, South Carolina

PEARSON

Boston   Columbus   Indianapolis   New York   San Francisco   Upper Saddle River
Amsterdam   Cape Town   Dubai   London   Madrid   Milan   Munich   Paris   Montréal   Toronto
Delhi   Mexico City   São Paulo   Sydney   Hong Kong   Seoul   Singapore   Taipei   Tokyo

Publisher: Julie Levin Alexander
Product Manager: Katrin Beacom
Program Manager: Erin Rafferty
Editorial Assistant: Erin Sullivan
Director of Marketing: David Gesell
Senior Marketing Manager: Phoenix Harvey
Marketing Specialist: Michael Sirinides
Pearson Project Manager: Patrick Walsh
Manufacturing Manager: Maura Zaldivar-Garcia
Art Director: Maria Guglielmo
Cover Design: Cenveo Publisher Services
Cover Art: Elena Rudyk/Fotolia
Full-Service Project Management: Mansi Negi/Aptara®, Inc.
Composition: Aptara®, Inc.
Printer/Binder: RR Donnelley/Harrisonburg
Cover Printer: RR Donnelley/Harrisonburg

Library of Congress Cataloging-in-Publication Data
Pender, Nola J. – author.
  Health promotion in nursing practice/Nola J. Pender, PhD, RN, FAAN, Professor Emerita University of Michigan School of Nursing, Ann Arbor, Michigan Carolyn L. Murdaugh, PhD, RN, FAAN, Professor Emerita University of Arizona College of Nursing, Tucson, Arizona, Visiting Professor, University of Alabama at Birmingham, Mary Ann Parsons, PhD, RN, FAAN, Professor Emerita and Dean Emerita University of South Carolina College of Nursing Columbia, South Carolina.—Seventh edition.
    pages cm
  Includes bibliographical references and index.
  ISBN 978-0-13-310876-7—ISBN 0-13-310876-7
  1. Health promotion.   2. Preventive health services.   3. Nursing.
I. Murdaugh, Carolyn L., author.   II. Parsons, Mary Ann, author.   III. Title.
  RT67.P56 2015
  610.73—dc23
                                                                                    2014012119

10 9 8 7 6 5 4 3

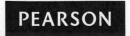

ISBN 13: 978-0-13-310876-7
ISBN 10:   0-13-310876-7

Dedication

To all nurses who practice and promote health, I wish you success as you strive to promote a healthier society.

—C. Murdaugh

To my grandsons Blake, Andrew, Sterling, Campbell, Graham, and Jennings for whom I wish a happy and healthy life.

—M. A. Parsons

CONTENTS

Part 2 Planning for Health Promotion and Prevention

Part 5   Health Promotion in Diverse Populations

Chapter 11   Self-Care for Health Promotion Across the Life Span   234

FOREWORD

This seventh edition of *Health Promotion in Nursing Practice* is an essential tool for nurses as they develop and deliver evidence-based health promotion services to diverse populations. *Health promotion is for everyone*. Becoming healthier improves the quality of life for all individuals, including cancer survivors, persons with disabilities, those with chronic diseases, and those of advanced age. The American Heart Association (AHA) recently issued an advisory statement that nurses should routinely assess health behaviors, just like vital signs, and provide behavior change counseling as an integral part of services to all patients (Spring, Ockene, Gidding, Mozaffarian, Moore, Rosal, et al., 2013). Nurses, the largest health workforce in the nation, are strategic to the provision of health promotion services in diverse care settings such as primary care clinics, emergency rooms, school clinics, work sites, community health programs, and nursing homes. According to the AHA, unhealthy behaviors must be treated as aggressively as other risk factors. Nurses need to fully embrace this exciting challenge of leading the way to healthier lifestyles in our nation and around the globe.

In late 2013, the U.S. Preventive Services Task Force convened an invitational forum of behavioral counseling and primary care research experts, agencies that fund health promotion research, and experts that develop guidelines on behavioral counseling interventions (S. Curry, personal communication, September 24, 2013). The goal of the meeting was to seek recommendations about how to optimize the development and dissemination of prevention and health promotion evidence-based guidelines and to identify research opportunities and gaps in knowledge about how to improve public health and well-being. Another task force, the Community Preventive Services Task Force, provides evidence-based recommendations on programs and policies to advance environmental/community health. Together, the guidelines of both task forces are intended to assist nurses and other health care personnel to reach the goals of *Healthy People 2020*. However, dissemination of guidelines is only the first step. Nurses need to be a part of the leadership team that integrates health promotion and prevention research findings and guidelines from all sources into policies and practices in key health care settings. Further, nurses can capitalize on the rapidly growing use of electronic media, particularly among the younger generation, to create innovative programs for self-monitoring and decisional support for healthy choices. Nurses must be bold and creative in health promotion programming, modeling healthy lifestyles as they shape health promotion strategies and provide care.

Although progress in health promotion is evident in improved outcomes in some domains, many challenges remain. For example, the current U.S. population still has a high percentage of obese adults and children. This trend presents major challenges to improving health and quality of life. Further, poverty and cultural differences create inequalities in the health and safety of living and working environments. In order to flourish, diverse populations need environments free from crime and other health threats, as well as adequate access to quality care. An additional concern is the plight of women in many countries where they are suppressed and victimized. A transition in values and policies is needed to provide freedom of choice and opportunities for women to experience their full health and human potential.

Health policies and programs should be evidence-based. Research findings must continue to enlighten our approaches to health promotion and prevention. For example, in the October 6, 2013, issue of the *Chicago Tribune* (Section 6, Page 11), new research regarding the "world of the newborn" indicated that predisposition toward a healthy diet may start before birth. Taste and smell filter through the amniotic fluid so that a mother's diet may shape the food preferences of the newborn. According to research conducted in France, when women were given a designated spice during their pregnancy, infants turned toward the odor after birth, showing preference. Infants of mothers not given the spice turned away from the odor. If these findings are replicated, food aromas experienced *in utero* may influence food preferences throughout life. This makes promoting healthy diets for pregnant women of even greater importance due to the direct influence of their diets on the emerging lifestyles of their infants.

Nurses are exemplary in addressing the health and well-being of the whole person: physical, psychological, social, and spiritual. This text provides valuable information to help nurses carry out this mission. Commendable features of this new edition include a greater emphasis on practice, new information about emerging technology to support health promotion, presentation of new research to undergird evidence-based practice, expanded discussion of culturally competent interventions, and new learning activities and websites to support nurses in their health promotion efforts. Drs. Murdaugh and Parsons have a rich background of experience in promoting health among diverse populations. Their exceptional work in crafting this seventh edition is highly commendable. I trust that this text will inspire nurses to lead the way to a health care system that places health promotion at the forefront of health services provided throughout the life span.

Nola J. Pender, PhD, RN, FAAN
Distinguished Professor
Marcella Niehoff School of Nursing
Loyola University Chicago
Professor Emerita
School of Nursing
University of Michigan

Reference

Spring, B., Ockene, J. K., Gidding, S. S., Mozaffarian, D., Moore, S., Rosal, M. C., et al; on behalf of the American Heart Association Behavior Change Committee of the Council on Epidemiology and Prevention, Council on Lifestyle and Cardiometabolic Health, Council for High Blood Pressure Research, and Council on Cardiovascular and Stroke Nursing. Better population health through behavior change in adults: a call to action. *Circulation*. 2013 Nov; 128. DOI: 10.1161/01. cir.0000435173.25936.e1. [Epub ahead of print].

PREFACE

Major challenges continue to influence health promotion and health care reform as we complete the seventh edition. Health care disparities are ongoing barriers to promoting the health of a large segment of our population. The expanding "obesogenic" environment promotes unhealthy foods and inactive lifestyles across the life span. Health promoting lifestyles must begin in early childhood to reverse the devastating trend toward increasing chronic illnesses, escalating health care costs, and shorter life spans for the first time in many generations.

The purpose of the text is to (1) present an overview of the major individual and community models and theories to guide health promotion programs and interventions; (2) offer evidence-based strategies to implement and evaluate health promotion programs for diverse populations across the life span; and (3) encourage critical thinking about the most effective interventions and methods for health promotion practice. We believe information in the text helps provide the foundation on which to build the practice of health promotion.

The content of the text is organized into six sections. In Part I, The Human Quest for Health, health and health promotion are defined, and individual and community models to guide health promotion programs and research are described. In Part II, Planning for Health Promotion and Prevention, strategies are described to assess health, health beliefs, and health behaviors and develop a health promotion plan. In Part III, Interventions for Health Promotion and Prevention, four core areas are targeted to promote health: physical activity, nutrition, stress management, and social support. In Part IV, Evaluating the Effectiveness of Health Promotion, models for program evaluation are addressed. Part V, Health Promotion in Diverse Populations, addresses strategies for self-care across the life span and culturally sensitive approaches to promote health and health literacy in vulnerable populations. In Part VI, Approaches for Promoting a Healthier Society, community partnerships for health promotion and policies to promote social and environmental changes for a healthier society are described.

Each chapter contains considerations for practice, opportunities for research, and learning activities. The content in all chapters has been updated, based on published research evidence. The *Healthy People 2020* goals, an ecological approach to health promotion, and the role of technology in promoting health have been integrated throughout the text. The text is ideally suited for undergraduate students in nursing and health promotion programs, graduate students in nurse practitioner and doctor of nursing practice programs, and health promotion practitioners.

The term *client* is used rather than *patient* throughout the text to refer to individuals, families, and communities who are active participants in health promotion. *Health* and *wellness* are used interchangeably. *Health protection* and *prevention* also are used interchangeably throughout the text.

Our sincere appreciation is extended to Michael Giacobbe, Maria Reyes, and Patrick Walsh at Pearson Health Science, who have worked with us in the preparation of the text, and to Mansi Negi at Aptara and Bret Workman who worked with us on production. We are very appreciative of Patrick's expertise in the final stages of preparation and Bret's and Mansi's attention to detail in the production phase. We are also deeply indebted to Alice Pasvogel, PhD, Research Specialist, College of Nursing, University of Arizona, who spent countless hours editing, formatting, and preparing the tables and figures. Her willingness to step in and take over the editorial work, attention to detail, and expert editorial assistance enabled us to finish the text in a timely manner.

Carolyn Murdaugh
Mary Ann Parsons

Reviewers

Terese Blakeslee, MSN Ed, RN
Nursing Instructor
UW Oshkosh College of Nursing
Oshkosh, WI

Mary Brown, MSN, MEd, RN, CNE
Nursing Program Director
Yavapai College
Prescott, AZ

Ann Denney, MSN, RN
Associate Professor of Nursing
Thomas More College
Crestview Hills, KY

Michele Dickens, MSN, RN
RN to BSN Program Instructor
Campbellsville University
Campbellsville, KY

Susan England, MSN, RN
Professor
Texas State Universty
Round Rock, TX

Janice Johnson-Umezulike, RN, BSN, MN, CNS, ANP, DNS
Professor
Lee College
Baytown, TX

Sherry Lovan, PhD, RN
Associate Professor, BSN Program
Coordinator
Western Kentucky University School of
Nursing
Bowling Green, KY

Margaret McAllister, PhD, FNP-BC, FAANP
Dir. Post Master's Certificate Program
and Co Dir. DNP Program
Clinical Associate Professor
University of Massachusetts Boston
College of Nursing and Health Sciences
Boston, MA

Vicki Moran, MSN/MPH, CNE, RN
Instructor
Saint Louis University
St. Louis, MO

Jean Rodgers, RN, MN
Course Coordinator
Hesston College
Hesston, KS

Ira Scott-Sewell, RN, MSN, MHA, MS
Professor
Alcorn State University School of Nursing
Natchez, MS

Nancy Simpson, MSN, RN-BC, CNE
Professor
University of New England
Portland, ME

Pamela Wendall RN, MSN
Instructor
Gila Community College
Payson, AZ

Rhonda M. White, MSN, RN
Associate Professor, Nursing Program
Clinical Coordinator
BridgeValley Community & Technical
College
South Charleston, WV

The Changing Context of Health Promotion

The major goals of health promotion are to help people of all ages stay healthy, optimize health in cases of chronic disease or disability, and create healthy environments. These goals require strategies that not only improve the health of individuals within the context of their families and communities, but also address the environments in which they live, work, and play.

Even though the United States is one of the wealthiest nations in the world, it lags behind other high-income nations in life expectancy and health for all its citizens. Likely explanations for these differences include the following:

- *Health systems.* Americans have more limited access to primary care, report lapses in quality of care outside of hospitals, and are more likely to be uninsured than people in peer nations.
- *Social and economic conditions.* The United States has higher levels of poverty and income inequality, lower rates of social mobility, and lack of a safety net for the poor and disadvantaged as compared to peer nations.
- *Physical environments.* Americans are more likely to live in environments that discourage physical activity and contribute to obesity compared to other high-income nations.
- *Health behaviors.* While Americans are less likely to smoke, and consume less alcohol than people of peer countries, they consume more calories per person, are less likely to use seat belts, and have higher rates of drug abuse, alcohol-related traffic accidents, and gun violence.

Upper-income, advantaged Americans' health also lags behind that of their counterparts in other high-income nations (Institute of Medicine, 2013).

The current health disadvantages experienced by Americans will have even greater health and economic consequences unless the United States takes action. To build a healthier America, health promotion and prevention must become priorities using innovative approaches, partnerships, and capacity building. If we are to move the health care system from *sick* care to *health* care, we must develop effective solutions that result in better health for *all* stakeholders: individuals, families, schools, and communities (Levi, Segal, Miller, & Lang, 2013). In addition, the solutions must enable individuals and communities to take control over the personal, socioeconomic, and environmental factors that affect their health, including the physical, mental, social/cultural, and spiritual dimensions (Bauman, Finegood, & Matsudo, 2009).

Health professionals recognize the need to change the context of health promotion and prevention and have started to engage in promising new strategies to help people of all ages stay healthy. Factors that are changing the context of health promotion to decrease disparities and inequities in health include the following:

- Multilevel interventions and strategies
- Mobile wireless computer technologies
- Community/sociopolitical partnerships

MULTILEVEL INTERVENTIONS AND STRATEGIES

Given the magnitude of the challenges in health promotion, the multilevel, comprehensive interventions and strategies that are more likely to succeed address a health issue(s) across all levels, individuals, families, schools, communities, worksites, and populations, and incorporate personal, socioeconomic, and environmental factors. Critical to the success of health promotion is consideration of multiple social and environmental factors, whether the focus is on the actions of individuals, families, schools, communities, or governments.

Each of these levels requires an evidence base that accounts for the contextual factors that influence outcomes. For example, successful individual-level, evidence-based interventions provide guidance to practitioners in providing direct health promotion activities. Interventions and programs targeting the school or community level provide evidence of adoption of positive health behaviors by students and families. While there are efforts to ensure coherence and coordination across these levels, the success of these efforts in terms of effecting sustained behavior change is not evident. Long-term maintenance of health behavior change is difficult without concomitant support from the social and built environments.

Population level change is critical to improve health across all ages. This is difficult, as "active living" approaches are expensive and have a limited evidence base. Population-level behavior change may require structural solutions over evidence generation to have the kind of sustainable impact on health behaviors that is vital for a healthier America (Bauman, Finegood, & Matsudo, 2009).

MOBILE WIRELESS COMPUTER TECHNOLOGIES

The expansion of mobile wireless computer technologies and social media applications, including telemedicine and telecare, has had a major influence on health promotion and prevention, unlike any in recent history. E-health (electronic health) or m-health (mobile health) includes a diverse set of informatics tools that have been embraced as a promising new way to prevent health problems and promote healthy behaviors at all levels, with particular enthusiasm for addressing population-level change.

Traditionally, health promotion has been a low-tech area in comparison with innovations in medical technologies used in health care settings. The expansion of the Internet for personal and professional use has increased its application for health promotion strategies, program delivery, and research. Social media, such as YouTube, Twitter, Facebook, and blogs, and smartphones and tablet computers promote the "personalizing" of health messages—"reaching into individuals' everyday lives" by sending, for example, tailored messages about individual health concerns or problems, or a "happy note" to acknowledge a positive change in "step counts" delivered by an accelerometer. With geographical applications, individuals can be located and body movements can be recorded. Because m-health devices can be taken almost everywhere, the user is usually connected and accessible (Lupton, 2012).

The use of m-health represents a significant change in health promotion strategies and research methodologies. Health and nursing journals now report the importance of e-health in health promotion research. Researchers have described using m-health to access, recruit, and deliver health interventions to adolescents and young adults as well as hard-to-reach minority and underserved populations (Lori, Munro, Boyd, & Andreatta, 2012; Park & Calamaro, 2013). The benefits of text messaging include improvements in self-care outcomes. The use of auto-mated telephone monitoring has been shown to improve chronic disease management outcomes in low- and middle-income countries (Piette, Lun, Moura, Fraser, Mechael, Powell, & Khoja, 2012). Web-based, self-administered questionnaires and the ability to access wide and diversified populations with quick returns have resulted in cost advantages (Hercberg, 2012). The use of m-health has also been linked to greater acceptance of individual responsibility for healthy life-styles (Lupton, 2012).

Nevertheless, concerns about promoting m-health to shift the responsibility of health from health care professionals to individuals require careful examination. Some e-health advocates view client empowerment as a positive outcome of m-health. Unfortunately, there is limited evidence that all clients are willing, or capable of, assuming this level of health responsibility. The focus on individualized health messages reduces health problems to a micro level rather than attending to the broader sociocultural/political dimension. In addition, home monitoring–based telecare has the potential to coerce older people into isolation, unless redesigned systems promote creative engagement with technology (Mort, Roberts, & Callen, 2012). Also of significance is the digital divide, which demonstrates limited adoption of these technologies based on socioeconomic group and health literacy level. Other moral, ethical, and privacy issues signal caution to the health pro-motion community concerning an immediate total buy-in of m-health. However, e-health, when used appropriately, will play a significant role in improving the health of the public.

COMMUNITY/SOCIOPOLITICAL PARTNERSHIPS

Two 2013 global conferences, the World Health Organization's (WHO) Eighth Global Confer-ence on Health Promotion and the 21st International Union for Health Promotion and Education World Conference (IUHPE), highlighted key challenges confronting health promotion. The WHO conference focused on "Health in All Policies" to encourage governments to adopt an approach that considers the health impact of *all* policies, regardless of where in the system the policy originates. This approach allows considerations of the contextual influences of policy to move from a sole focus on the health sector to all government sectors.

The theme of the IUPE conference was "Best Investments for Health." Concepts of suffi-ciency, efficiency, effectiveness, and equity were all included in the concept of "best," while financing, capacity building of human resources, systems, and interventions were included in the concept of "investments." Outcomes of this conference support a framework for governments to build healthy public policies (Sparks, 2013). Some countries have committed to one or more of the concepts, while others are lagging behind. However, many countries are forming partnerships to examine their public health policies.

Community/socioeconomic/political partnerships have the human capacity and political power to bring national attention to the many promising strategies that address the public's health. *Healthy People in Healthy Communities*, a national partnership initiated by the U.S. Department of Health and Human Services, involves the federal government, the states, local communities, and many public and private sector groups. This partnership guides national health promotion and disease prevention efforts to improve the health of all people in the United States. Each decade, *Healthy People* sets objectives and provides science-based benchmarks to track and monitor progress in order to motivate and focus action on identified health issues. *Healthy People 2020* represents the fourth generation of this partnership, building on a foundation of three decades of work.

Healthy People 2020 is committed to a vision of a society in which all people live long, healthy lives. New features in the 2020 initiative, noted below, will help make this vision a reality.

- Health equity is emphasized by addressing social determinants of health and promoting health across all stages of life.
- Traditional print publications have been replaced with an interactive website as the main vehicle for dissemination.
- A website is maintained to enable users to tailor information to their needs and explore evidence-based resources for implementation However, real progress depends on whether the public and political communities are willing to make a social commitment of effort and resources to improve the overall health of Americans.

NURSING AND HEALTH PROMOTION: A NATURAL PARTNERSHIP

Nurses, the largest segment of health care professionals, are in a key position to take a leadership role to meet the national health promotion goals, which are to:

- help people of all ages to stay healthy.
- optimize health in cases of chronic disease or disability.
- create healthy environments.

Many disciplines contribute to meeting these goals. However, nursing, which is grounded in a holistic approach, offers a bridge between individual health promotion and promoting the health of families, communities, and populations. Nurses are educated to care for all persons within the context of the individual's culture and community. Four key elements of the nurse's role promote and support health promotion:

- *An individual perspective.* Nurses facilitate individuals and families in their health decisions and support their health promotion activities.
- *A philosophy of empowerment.* Nurses collaborate with individuals, groups, and communities to enable them to increase control over their health.
- *Knowledge of social and health policy.* Nurses advocate for and support local, state, national, and international policies to promote health equity.
- *A community orientation.* Nurses collaborate with all health professionals and community leaders to promote healthy communities.

Nurses need advanced skills and knowledge to implement health promotion activities, including (1) interprofessional knowledge; (2) communication, collaboration, and political skills; and (3) an advocacy orientation. In addition, nurses need to practice health behaviors and role model a healthy lifestyle (Kemppainen, Tossavainen, & Turunen, 2012). Health promotion activities should occur in all practice settings. In every client encounter, nurses can both model and teach positive health promotion and prevention practices. Nurses need not only to be knowledgeable of the importance of individual-level health promotion, but also to demonstrate their political knowledge to help change the socioeconomic and physical environments. Nurses, collaborating with colleagues, should champion a culture where health promotion principles are integrated, valued, and practiced in all settings (Savage & Kub, 2009). Nurses are essential to shaping the future of health promotion. As new challenges warrant new approaches, nurses should be prepared to take leadership roles in promoting the health of all.

References

Bauman, A., Finegood, D., & Matsudo, V. (2009). International perspectives on the physical inactivity crisis-Structural solutions over evidence generation? *Preventive Medicine, 49*, 309–312.

Hercberg, S. (2012). Web-based studies: The future in nutritional epidemiology (and overarching epidemiology) for the benefit of public health? *Preventive Medicine, 55*, 544–545.

Institute of Medicine. (2013). *U.S. Health in International Perspective.* Washington, DC: National Academy of Sciences.

Kemppainen, V., Tossavainen, K., & Turunen, H. (2012). Nurses' roles in health promotion practice: An integrative review. *Health Promotion International Advance*, 1–12. doi:10.1093/heapro/das034

Levi, J., Segal, L., Miller, A., & Lang, A. (2013). *A Healthier America 2013*. Princeton, NJ: Trust for America's Health.

Lori, J., Munro, M., Boyd, C., & Andreatta, P. (2012). Cell phones to collect pregnancy data from remote areas in Liberia. *Journal of Nursing Scholarship, 44*(3), 294–310.

Lupton, D. (2012). M-health and health promotion: The digital cyborg and surveillance society. *Social Theory & Health, 10*, 229–244. doi:10.1057/sth.2012.6

Mort, M., Roberts, C., & Callen, B. (2012). Ageing with telecare: Care or coercion in austerity? *Sociology of Health & Illness, 35*(6), 799–812. doi:10.1111/shil.2013.35

Park, B., & Calamaro, C. (2013). A systematic review of social networking sites: Innovative platforms for health research targeting adolescents and young adults. *Journal of Nursing Scholarship, 45*(3), 256–264.

Piette, J., Lun, K., Moura, L., Fraser, H., Mechael, P., Powell, J., & Khoja, S. (2012). Impacts of e-health on the outcomes of care in low- and middle-income countries: Where do we go from here? *Bulletin of the World Health Organization, 90*(5), 365–372. doi:10.2471/BLT.11.099069

Savage, C., & Kub, J. (2009). Public health and nursing: A natural partnership. *International Journal of Environmental Research and Public Health, 6*, 2843–2848. doi:10.3390/ijerph6112843

Sparks, M. (2013). The changing context of health promotion. *Health Promotion International, 28*(2) Editorial. doi:10.1093/heapro/dat034

CHAPTER 1

Toward a Definition of Health

OBJECTIVES

This chapter will enable the reader to:

1. Compare traditional and holistic definitions of health.

2. Contrast conceptions of individual health.

3. Describe conceptions of health by nurse theorists.

4. Discuss family and community definitions of health.

5. Describe the social determinants of health.

6. Discuss the significance of global health.

7. Describe the changing conceptions of health promotion.

Health, person, environment, and nursing constitute the commonly accepted metaparadigm of the discipline of nursing (American Nurses Association, 2010; Fawcett & Desanto-Madeva, 2012). Although health is the frequently articulated goal of nursing, different conceptions about the meaning of health are common. These differences result from the increasingly diverse social values and norms that shape conceptualizations of health in societies with many distinct ethnic, religious, or cultural groups. What many health professionals once assumed was a universally accepted definition of health—the absence of diagnosable disease—is actually only one of many views of health held today. All people who are free of disease are not equally healthy. Furthermore, health can exist without illness, but illness does not exist without health as its context.

The emergence of health promotion as the central strategy for improving health has shifted the paradigm from defining health in traditional medical terms (the curative model within a biologic perspective) to a multidimensional definition of health with social, economic, cultural, and environmental dimensions. In a multidimensional model, health benefits can potentially be achieved from positive changes in any one of the health dimensions.

This expanded perspective of health opens up multiple options for improving health and no longer places the responsibility for poor health entirely on the individual. During the course of human development, the definition of health changes over the life span. As children mature and move into adolescence, their definition of health becomes more inclusive and more abstract. Health definitions of adolescents show a trend toward greater thematic diversity (physical, mental, social, and emotional health) and less emphasis on the absence of illness with increasing age. As children mature, the focus on health also changes. Young adults ages 16 to 24 years report a lower priority on health and less engagement in health behaviors than do adolescents 12 to 15 years and adults 25 years and older (Goddings, James, & Hargreaves, 2012). Older adults hold a more holistic definition of health that integrates physical, mental, spiritual, and social aspects, reflecting how health is embedded in everyday life experiences and surroundings (Goins, Spencer, & Williams, 2011).

In addition, gender is a critical sociocultural determinant of health throughout the life course (Gelb, Pederson, & Greves, 2011). Gender differences in health are due to genetic and biologic factors, as well as social and behavioral factors such as risk-taking behaviors, health-seeking behaviors, and coping styles (Eriksson, Dellve, Eklof, & Hagberg, 2007; Evans, Frank, Oliffe, & Gregory, 2011). The social structural context of men and women has been documented to be a major determinant of gender differences in health. The promotion of gender equality and empowerment interventions is crucial to improving women's health. In addition it is vital to increase understanding of the influence of masculinity in shaping men's health and health behaviors (Gelb, Pederson, & Greaves, 2011). Nursing can play a significant role in provision of education and knowledge sharing to increase the health and well-being of women and men.

In a positive model of health, emphasis is placed on strengths, resiliencies, resources, potentials, and capabilities rather than on existing pathology (resilience reference). Despite a philosophic and conceptual shift in thinking about health, the nature of health as a positive life process is less understood empirically, as attention continues to focus on forces that undermine health and lead to disease, rather than factors that lead to health. Morbidity (prevalence of illness) and mortality (death) are still commonly used to define the health of a population. These indicators more accurately reflect disease burden and the need for health care, not health. A focus on disease morbidity and mortality frames health within a biologic definition: the body without disease. However, evidence indicates that complex interwoven forces embedded in the social and environmental context of people's lives determine health. Health cannot be separated from one's life conditions, as neighborhood, social relationships, food, work, and leisure, which lie outside the realm of health practice, positively or negatively influence health long before morbid states are evident (Reutter & Kushner, 2010).

HEALTH AS AN EVOLVING CONCEPT

A brief review of the historical development of the concept of health provides a background for examining definitions of health found in the professional literature. The ancient Greeks were the first to write that health could not be separated from physical and social environments and human behavior (Tountas, 2009). Their philosophy maintained that harmony, equilibrium, and balance were the key elements to health, and illness resulted when this balance was upset. This led to Plato defining health as a state of being in complete harmony with the universe. Hippocrates went on to define health as a balance between environmental forces and individual habits. Illness was considered an upset of this equilibrium (Tountas, 2009).

The word *health* as it is commonly used did not appear in writing until approximately 1000 AD. It is derived from the Old English word *health,* meaning being safe or sound and whole of body (Sorochan, 1970). Historically, physical wholeness was of major importance for acceptance in social groups. Persons suffering from disfiguring diseases, like leprosy, or congenital malformations were ostracized from society. Not only was there fear of contagion of physically obvious disease, but also repulsion at the grotesque appearance. Being healthy was construed as natural or in harmony with nature, while being unhealthy was thought of as unnatural or contrary to nature.

With the advent of the scientific era and the resultant increase in medical discoveries, society became concerned about helping individuals escape the catastrophic effects of illness. *Health* was defined as "freedom from disease." Because disease could be traced to a specific cause, often microbial, it could be diagnosed. The notion of health as a disease-free state was extremely popular into the first half of the twentieth century and continues to be recognized by some in the medical community as *the* definition of health (Miller & Foster, 2010). Health and illness were viewed as extremes on a continuum—the absence of one indicated the presence of the other. This gave rise to "ruling out disease" to assess health, an approach still prevalent in the medical community today. The underlying erroneous assumption is that a disease-free population is a healthy population.

The concept of mental health as we now know it did not exist until the latter part of the nineteenth century. Individuals who exhibited unpredictable or hostile behavior were labeled "lunatics" and ostracized in much the same way as those with disfiguring physical ailments. Being put away with little or no human care was considered their "just due," because mental illness was often ascribed to evil spirits or satanic powers. The visibility of the ill only served as a reminder of personal vulnerability and mortality, aspects of human existence that society wished to ignore.

For several decades, the importance of mental health became obscured in the rapid barrage of medical discoveries for treatment of physical disorders. However, the psychologic trauma resulting from the high-stress situations of combat during World War II expanded the scope of health as a concept to include consideration of the mental status of the individual. Mental health was manifest in the ability of an individual to withstand stresses imposed by the environment. When individuals succumbed to the rigors of life around them and could no longer carry out the functions of daily living, they were declared to be mentally ill. Despite efforts to develop a more holistic definition of health, the dichotomy between individuals suffering from physical illness and those suffering from mental illness persisted for many years. In 2011, the World Health Organization (WHO) defined mental health as a state of well-being in which individuals realize their potential, can manage usual life stresses, work effectively, and participate in their community (World Health Organization, 2011). This definition is consistent with the WHO definition of health.

In 1946, the WHO proposed a landmark definition of health that emphasized "wholeness" and the positive qualities of health: "Health is a state of complete physical, mental, and social well-being and not merely the absence of disease and infirmity" (World Health Organization, 2005). The definition was revolutionary in that it (1) reflected concern for the individual as a total person, (2) placed health in the context of the social environment, and (3) overcame the reductionist definition of health as the absence of disease. The breadth of this historical definition mandated a comprehensive approach to health promotion, and inherently, created an imperative for health equity (Friel & Marmot, 2011).

The WHO definition continues to be criticized by many who think that it is utopian and too broad, and that the absoluteness of the term "complete" makes health impossible to achieve (Huber et al., 2011). The definition was formulated when acute disease presented the major burden to society. However, people living with chronic diseases for decades are increasing worldwide, and this is not accounted for in the definition. Despite the criticisms and calls for reformulation, the WHO definition continues to be the most popular and comprehensive definition of health worldwide and was reaffirmed at the 2005 assembly (World Health Organization, 2005). In spite of its universal recognition, recommendations continue to revise the definition and to view the WHO definition only as a historical document. Many authors think that more current, less utopian, measurable definitions are needed (Bok, 2008; Huber et al., 2011). It is now accepted that individual health cannot be separated from the health of society and that individuals are interdependent with the totality of the world. Moreover, the relationship of human health to the health of the earth's ecosystem is also recognized as an important dimension. In other words, one cannot be healthy in an unhealthy society or world. Within these dimensions health has been defined as the ability to adapt to one's environment. Health is not a fixed state, as it varies depending on an individual's life state. This conception, originally proposed by Georges Canguilhem in 1943, enables the changing context to be taken into consideration to understand the meaning of health (Huber et al., 2011).

In the following sections, definitions of health are discussed that focus on the individual, the family, and the community. In the past, defining health for individuals received more attention than defining health for families and communities. However, it has become clear that individual health is almost inseparable from the health of the larger community, and the health of every community influences the overall health status of the nation.

HEALTH AND ILLNESS: DISTINCT ENTITIES, OR OPPOSITE ENDS OF A CONTINUUM?

Health and illness have been presented as a continuum with reference points such as (1) optimum health, (2) suboptimal health or incipient illness, (3) overt illness and disability, and (4) very serious illness or approaching death (Niebroj, 2006). These descriptors have only one point representing health, whereas multiple points on the scale represent varying states of suboptimum health or illness. Dunn, the first author to provide a definition of wellness, maintains that health and illness are separate concepts, and continua must allow the differentiation of varying levels of health as well as varying levels of illness (Dunn, 1977; Roscoe, 2009).

When health and illness are assumed to represent a single continuum, it is difficult to discuss healthy aspects of the ill individual. The presence of illness ascribes the "sick role," and the individual is expected to direct all energies toward finding the cause of the illness and engage in behaviors that will result in a return to health as soon as possible. However, health can be manifested in the presence of illness. Poor health can exist even if disease is not present, and good health can be present in spite of disease.

The authors of this text believe that health and illness are qualitatively different, interrelated concepts that may coexist. In Figure 1–1, multiple levels of health are depicted in interaction with episodes of illness. Illness, which may have a short (acute) or long (chronic) duration, is represented as discrete events within the life span. Health can still be an aspiration to those with a chronic illness or disability, and health can be achieved despite being diagnosed with a disease or living with a disability (Institute of Medicine, 2012). Illness experiences can either hinder or facilitate one's continuing quest for health. Thus, good health or poor health may exist with or without overt illness.

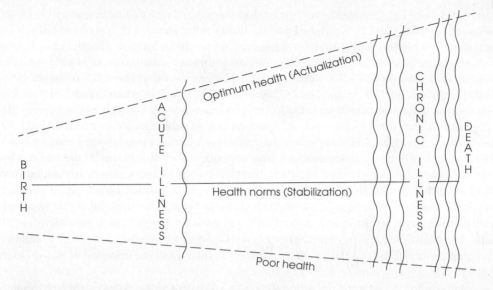

FIGURE 1-1 The Health Continuum Throughout the Life Span

DEFINITIONS OF HEALTH THAT FOCUS ON INDIVIDUALS

Health as Stability

Stability-based definitions of health are based on the physiologic concepts of homeostasis (internal stability) and adaptation. Dubos (1965), an early advocate of the stability position, defines health as a state that enables the individual to adapt to the environment. The degree of health experienced is dependent on one's ability to adapt to the various internal and external tensions that one faces. Dubos considered optimum health to be a mirage because in the real world individuals must face physical and social forces that are forever changing, frequently unpredictable, and often unsafe. Some authors continue to believe in this position (Flannery, 2009), As an early scientist who viewed the environment as a major influence on health, Dubos considered the closest approach to optimum or high-level health to be a physical and mental state that permits one to function effectively within the environment (Flannery, 2009).

Definitions of health based on normality can be described as stability-oriented. Norms represent average effectiveness states rather than excellence or exceptional effectiveness in human functioning (Ereshefsky, 2009). Health is considered a normal function (a statistical average), and disease represents an impairment of normal function (below the statistical average). A major issue with normative definitions of health is that they predict "what could be" based on "what is," leaving little room for incorporating growth, maturation, and evolutionary emergence into a definition of health. Environmentally focused models of health can be described as stability oriented, as the essence of these models is adaptation of individuals to their environment. Health is determined by the ability of individuals to maintain a balance with the environment. Health exists when one is able to adapt to the environment successfully and is able to grow, function, and thrive. In contrast, lack of adaptation is seen as a gap between one's ability to adapt and the demands of the environment.

Parsons' conceptualization of health is compatible with an environmental model. More than 50 years ago Parsons defined health in terms of social norms rather than physiologic norms, describing health as individuals' effective performance of roles and tasks for which they have been socialized (Parsons, 1958). This definition remains relevant.

Health has also been defined in terms of functional norms. This conception of health is the ability to perform socially valued activities usual for a person's age and social roles with a minimum probability of change to less valued functional levels. The client's desired functional level, as well as the probability that their current condition or state will change to a higher or lower functional level, must be considered in assessing health when using this definition.

A number of nurse-theorists have proposed definitions of health emphasizing stability, beginning with Florence Nightingale. Nightingale viewed health as being the best that one could be at any point in time (Selanders, 2010). Levine, an early nurse theorist, defines health as a state in which there is balance between input and output of energy and in which structural, personal, and social integrity exists (Schaefer, 2010). Johnson, in her behavioral system model, does not explicitly define health. However, a conception of health that focuses on stability can be inferred from her conceptualization of internal homeostasis (Holiday, 2010). Health is balance and stability among the following behavioral systems: attachment or affiliative, dependency, ingestive, eliminative, sexual, aggressive, and achievement. Behavioral system stability is demonstrated by efficient and effective behavior that is purposeful, goal-directed, orderly, and predictable. Neuman has defined health as a condition in which all subsystems—physiologic, psychologic, and sociocultural—are in balance and in harmony with the whole of humankind. Health is a state of saturation, of inertness, free of disruptive needs. Disharmony is created when the individual cannot cope with disrupting forces or noxious stressors, reducing the level of health. In a health state, total needs are met, and more energy is generated and stored than expended to maintain a strong, flexible line of defense, providing the individual with considerable resistance to disequilibrium (Neuman & Fawcett, 2011, 2012).

Roy also subscribes to a stability definition of health (Roy, 2011). The central concept in Roy's model is adaptation. Health is a state and process of successful adaptation that promotes being and becoming an integrated whole person. The four adaptive modes through which coping energies are expressed are physiologic, self-concept, role performance, and interdependence modes. Adaptation promotes integrity, which implies soundness or an unimpaired condition that can lead to completeness and unity. The person in an adapted state is freed from ineffective coping attempts that deplete energy. Available energy can be used to enhance health.

Health as Actualization

When individual health is defined more broadly as actualization of human potential, it is called *wellness*. Wellness is considered to be less restricted than the concept of health. However, *health* and *wellness* tend to be used interchangeably in the health promotion literature, and so these terms are used interchangeably in this text.

Halbert Dunn, the creator of the modern-day definition of wellness, was an early advocate for emphasizing actualization in a definition of health. Dunn coined the term *high-level wellness*, which he described as integrated human functioning that is oriented toward maximizing an individual's potential. This requires that individuals maintain balance and purpose within the environment where they are functioning (Dunn, 1977). Although the definition identifies balance as a dimension of health, major emphasis is on the realization of human potential as individuals move toward their personal optimum level based on their capabilities and potential.

Definitions of wellness have evolved since Dunn initially defined the concept and launched the wellness movement. The dominant view is that wellness is holistic and includes multiple positive dimensions of health. These dimensions include social, emotional, physical, spiritual, and intellectual wellness (Roscoe, 2009). The definition includes building on one's strengths and optimizing one's potential (McMahon & Fleury, 2012). The terms *health*, *well-being*, and *wellness* are used interchangeably in the literature, although each concept is considered to have distinguishing features (Miller & Foster, 2010). Health is considered a stable physiological state, while wellness is the subjective experience or the state of well-being (Mackey, 2009). However, there are consistencies in the conceptualization of wellness, including (1) it is not merely the absence of disease; (2) it consists of multiple holistic and interrelated dimensions; (3) there is a dynamic balance among the dimensions of wellness; and (4) wellness represents optimal functioning (Roscoe, 2009).

Health is also considered a concept separate from well-being by some (Bok, 2008; World Health Organization, 2012). The concept of well-being includes health as well as other subjective and objective domains. An initiative by the WHO Regional Office in Europe has defined well-being and developed objective and subjective measures of the domains of well-being (World Health Organization, 2012).

Orem uses *health* and *well-being* to refer to two different but related human states (Orem & Taylor, 2011). She defines *health* as a state characterized by soundness or wholeness of human structures and bodily and mental functions. *Well-being* is defined as an ideal state characterized by experiences of contentment, pleasure, and happiness; spiritual experiences; movement toward fulfillment of one's self-ideal; and continuing personalization. Personalization is movement toward maturation and achievement of human potential. Engaging in responsible self-care and continuing development of self-care competency are facets of the process of personalization. Individuals can experience well-being even under conditions of adversity, including disorders of human structure and function. Parse (2011), in describing her man-living-health theory of nursing, presents five assumptions about health that essentially define the concept from her perspective:

1. Health is an open process of becoming, experienced by individuals.
2. Health is a rhythmically co-constituting process of the individual–environment relationship.
3. Health is an individual's patterns of relating value priorities.
4. Health is an intersubjective process of transcending with the possible.
5. Health is an individual's negentropic evolution, as it moves to increasing order.

Neuman, building on the grand theory of Martha Rogers, defines health as the totality of the life process, which is evolving toward expanded consciousness (Neuman & Fawcett, 2011; Phillips, 2010). This definition emphasizes the actualizing properties of individuals throughout their life span. Four dimensions of health are identified:

1. Health is a fusion of disease and nondisease.
2. Health is the manifestation of an individual's unique pattern.
3. Health is expansion of consciousness.
4. Health encompasses the entire life process, which evolves toward a higher and greater frequency of energy exchange.

Key life process phenomena include consciousness, movement, space, and time. Neuman's model of health addresses holistic characteristics of human beings. However, similar to Roy's theory, there is no intent to create empirical measures for many of the concepts, limiting potential testing and clinical applicability of the model.

Both Neuman and Parse build on Martha Rogers' theory of unitary person. Both represent early attempts to define health in terms of holism. The emergent nature or actualization potential of the healthy individual and the capacity for open energy exchange with the environment are characteristics of both Neuman's and Parse's definitions of health.

Actualization or wellness models have been criticized because of the difficulties in measuring subjective perceptions. In addition, perceptions of health and wellness vary according to age and sociocultural context. Another criticism is that the expanded definitions of health in some wellness models do not distinguish health from happiness, quality of life, and other global concepts. In spite of these criticisms, the wellness models provide a holistic focus and promote the positive aspects of health.

Health as Actualization and Stability

Models of individual health also incorporate both stability and actualization. In these models, health is defined as a feeling of well-being, a capacity to perform to the best of one's ability, and the flexibility to adapt and adjust to varying situations created by one's environments. King, an early nurse theorist, proposes a definition of health that emphasizes both stabilizing and actualizing tendencies. She identifies health as the goal of nursing. *Health* is a dynamic state in the life cycle of a person that implies adjustment to stressors in the environment through optimum use of resources to achieve maximum potential for daily living (Alligood, 2010; King, 2007). In King's model, a holistic health perspective relates to the way individuals handle stressors while functioning within their culture. King views health as a functional state in the life cycle; illness is considered to be interference in the life cycle. Nurse scholars have extended King's theory of goal attainment to the study of family health (Doornbos, 2007).

A definition of health must be applicable to everyone—to the well, to those with an acute illness, and to those with chronic disease or disability. The authors of this text believe that a definition of health should incorporate both actualizing and stabilizing tendencies, and define *health* as the realization of human potential through goal-directed behavior, competent self-care, and satisfying relationships with others, while adapting to meet the demands of everyday life and maintain harmony with the social and physical environments. This broad conceptual definition has led to a classification system that describes affective and behavioral expressions of health by individuals (Table 1–1). The major culture-free dimensions of health expression include affect, attitudes, activity, aspirations, and accomplishments. The physical, mental, social, and spiritual components of health that are now cited in expanded definitions of health, including the WHO definition, are encompassed in this classification. The dimensions are further divided into subcategories that may be culture specific. The system is based on the assumptions that health is a manifestation of person and environment interactional patterns that become increasingly complex throughout the life span. These interactional patterns are influenced by conditions of daily life as well as the economic, political, and sociocultural context. The classification system provides a framework for a comprehensive assessment of health that is consistent with a positive, unitary, humanistic view.

Health as an Asset

The conceptualization of health as a resource or asset was introduced in 1986 at the First International Conference on Health Promotion (World Health Organization, 1986), when health was defined as not an end in itself but a resource for daily living. This conception was further described as the capacity to engage in various activities, fulfill roles, and meet the demands of daily life. The definition expanded the WHO recognition of health as the strengths and capabilities inherent in individuals (Williamson & Carr, 2009). Health as an asset has also been described as the repertoire

TABLE 1–1   Classification System for Affective and Behavioral Expressions of Health

Affect

Serenity	Harmony	Vitality	Sensitivity
Calm	Spiritual	Energetic	Aware
Relaxed	Contemplative	Vigorous	Connected
Peaceful	At one with the universe	Zestful	Intimate
Content		Alert	Loving
Comfortable			Warm

Attitudes

Optimism	Relevancy	Competency
Hopeful	Useful	Purposive
Enthusiastic	Contributing	Initiating
Open	Valued	Self-motivating
Reverent	Committed	Self-affirming
Resilient	Involved	Innovative

Activity

Positive Life Patterns	Meaningful Work	Invigorating Play
Healthy eating	Realistic goals	Meaningful hobbies
Regular exercise	Varied activities	Satisfying leisure activities
Stress management	Challenging tasks	Energizing diversions
Adequate rest	Collaboration	
Positive relationships		
Health monitoring		
Constructive coping		

Aspirations

Self-Actualization	Social Contribution
Growth	Global harmony and interdependence enhancement
Personal mastery	Environmental preservation

Accomplishments

Enjoyment	Creativity	Transcendence
Pleasure from daily living	Maximum use of capacities	Freedom, harmony
Sense of achievement	Innovative contribution	Purpose in life

of internal and external attributes of the individual that mobilize positive health behaviors and optimum outcomes (Rotegard, Moore, Fagermoen, & Ruland, 2010). Health as an asset was noted in Schlotfeldt's model of nursing, which was developed over 40 years ago. She described health as an asset, as she stressed focusing on individual strengths rather than problems (Schlotfeldt, 1987). Internal attributes are characteristics inherent within individuals, such as personality, attitude, and motivation (Rotegard et al., 2010). Internal attributes are dependent on an individual's external attributes, which include the social and cultural contexts. Inclusion of external assets is consistent with the focus on the social determinants of health.

An Integrated View of Health

Health is a holistic experience; however, it may become fragmented in the minds of health professionals. Although the biological model provides technological excellence and sophisticated medical care, it has led to a narrow focus on disease. An expansive view of health goes beyond disease prevention and risk reduction. An expansive view emphasizes personal and social resources as well as physical capacities and can be integrated with traditional biomedical models (disease) and public health models (mortality, morbidity, risks) of health to provide a holistic biopsychosocial view (Williamson & Carr, 2009). The biopsychosocial view enables clinicians and researchers to promote health and manage illness and disease together, rather than separating the concepts. Therefore, understanding the relevance of a broad definition of health for individuals in their everyday experiences in different social contexts is critical.

DEFINITIONS OF HEALTH THAT FOCUS ON THE FAMILY

The complexity of the family and the diversity of family life in different ethnic, cultural, and geographic settings pose a challenge for defining and promoting family health. The traditional definition of family as two or more persons living together who are related by marriage, blood, or adoption is no longer adequate in American society. Families may be defined by biological, legal, or emotional ties, whether or not they are living together. Families may include nuclear families, single-parent families, blended families, same-sex partnerships, families without children, and sibling families. One broad definition of *family* now accepted is two or more persons who depend on one another for emotional, physical, or financial support. In this definition family members are self-defined and may include any individuals who make a significant commitment to each other outside of marriage. It is critical that variation in family structure be taken into consideration in defining and measuring family health.

Conceptual frameworks of family health have evolved with the changing definition of family. Family nursing conceptual models and theories are found in the family social science disciplines, family therapy theory, and nursing. Social science theories have provided direction for development of nursing knowledge in family health, including developmental theory, systems theory, structural functional theory, and interactional theory. In addition, transitions theory is important in understanding family health (Meleis, 2010).

Two relevant family theories are family systems theory (Skelton, Buehler, Irby, & Grzywacz, 2012) and family ecological theory (Davidson, Lawson, & Coatsworth, 2012). Family systems theory describes the family as an open, complex system in which all of the members are interconnected. Family ecological theory is an ecological model with a family system perspective. In these models, family health is shaped by factors proximal to family members as well as the context in which the family lives.

Several approaches have been proposed to promote family health. These include the family as context, client, system, and a component of society. A model of family reciprocal determinism takes into account the complexity of the family environment in promoting health (McAllister, Perry, & Parcel, 2008). Within this model, behavior is a function of the shared environment with other family members and their behavior and personal characteristics. The family plays an important role in health promotion because health information is shared and behaviors are learned, practiced, and reinforced in daily routines, which are facilitated or hindered by family values and beliefs. In this approach the interaction of the individual with other members of the family or other units in society is emphasized.

A biopsychosocial definition of *family health* describes family health as a dynamic, changing state of well-being, including biologic, psychologic, sociologic, spiritual, and cultural factors of the family system. In this definition an individual's health affects family functioning, and in turn, family functioning affects individual health. Thus, both the family system and the individual members must be part of the health assessment.

Characteristics of healthy families have been described and include affirmation and support for one another, shared sense of responsibility, shared leisure time, shared religious core, respect, trust, and family rituals and traditions. These qualities address stability of family functioning and balance in interaction among family members. Family typologies, such as traditional–nontraditional, have also been developed to identify a common profile that may be linked to health in families. Health promotion interventions must be implemented in ways that are compatible with family values, beliefs, and orientations. Additional research is needed to evaluate the effects of health-related interventions based on family type.

Many factors influence how family health is defined. Social, cultural, environmental, and religious/spiritual factors play a central role in determining how families view their health. Families' strengths, resources, and competencies also are an integral part of a positive conceptualization of health. Family health processes are receiving attention by scientists in nursing and other disciplines. Development and testing of models to describe family health will help health professionals identify determinants of family well-being to promote family health.

DEFINITIONS OF HEALTH THAT FOCUS ON THE COMMUNITY

Communities are usually defined within one of two frameworks: spatial or geographical area, or relational/functional. Geographical definitions are based on legal or geopolitical areas such as cities, towns, or census tracts. Relational definitions are based on how people interact to achieve common goals. The WHO defines community as a social group determined by both geographical area and common values, with members who know each other and interact within a social structure (World Health Organization, 1974). Community members create norms, values, and social institutions for its members. The WHO definition focuses on both spatial and relational/functional dimensions of a community.

Social ecological theories of community health emphasize the interaction and interdependence of individuals with their family, community, social structure, and physical environment (Richard, Gauvin, & Raine, 2011). A social ecology model described in the *Ottawa Charter for Health Promotion*, a landmark policy statement, outlines the essential dimensions of community health (World Health Organization, 1986). Fundamental to community health are peace, shelter, education, food, income, a stable ecosystem, sustainable resources, social justice, and equity. The Healthy Cities projects in the United States, Europe, and Australia were based on a social ecological view that the roots of ill health lie in social and economic factors.

The projects supported the premise that responsibility for health is widely shared in the community with collaborative decision making about health issues. Cultivating healthy communities is now a priority for the Centers for Disease Control and Prevention (CDC), which maintains that four key ingredients are essential: (1) There must be local investment in communities; (2) venues need to be provided for communities to learn about effective change strategies; (3) partners need to be mobilized for change; and (4) communities need tools for local health promotion (Giles, Holmes-Chavez, & Collins, 2009). Informed political action and healthy public policies are also essential to healthy communities.

Three major dimensions have been identified to develop a broad understanding of community health. The dimensions provide complementary information to assist in developing a clear picture of the health of the community (Stanhope & Lancaster, 2012):

1. *Status dimension:* Biological, emotional and social components, measured by morbidity, mortality, life expectancy, risk factors, consumer satisfaction, mental health, crime rates, functional levels, worker absenteeism, and infant mortality.
2. *Structural dimension:* Community health services and resources measured by utilization patterns, treatment data, and provider/population ratios; social indicators measured by socioeconomic and racial distributions and median education level.
3. *Process dimension:* Effective community functioning or problem solving that results in community competence observed by commitment, self–other awareness, effective communication, conflict containment and accommodation, participation, management of relations with larger society, and mechanisms to facilitate interaction and decision making.

Based on these dimensions, *community health* can be defined as meeting the collective needs of its members through identifying problems and managing interactions within the community and between the community and the larger society.

Community health is more than the sum of the health states of its individual members; it encompasses characteristics of the community as a whole. Individual, family, and community health are intimately related. The health of the community depends on individual health as well as whether the social, physical, and political aspects exist to enable individuals to live healthy lives. Community characteristics have an important influence on individual health and risk behaviors. The relationship between community social and economic conditions and individual health also has been documented. *Social capital* also has been described as a major determinant of health in communities. This term, which includes trust, reciprocity, and cooperation among families, neighborhoods, and entire communities, is discussed in more detail in Chapter 3. Healthy communities support healthy lifestyles. Likewise the collective attitudes, beliefs, and behaviors of individuals influence the health of their community. All social and physical environmental components that interact with individuals must be assessed before developing strategies to create healthier communities.

The traditional focus on an individual, curative model, while successful in chronic disease care, unintentionally relegates individual and community health to a position of secondary importance. The focus must go beyond the individual to include community-level factors. A body of evidence supports an expanded view of individual health that is inseparable from the community and larger society. Effective health-promotion interventions should be based on the assessment of a community's social environment as well as societal and physical environmental level factors, as recommended in the *Healthy People 2020* document (see Healthy People 2020 website).

SOCIAL DETERMINANTS OF HEALTH

More than 100 years ago, Florence Nightingale understood that the environments in which people live, as well as lifestyle behaviors, were major contributors to health and disease (Selanders, 2010). She also believed the environments could be altered to improve health. Her observations during the Crimean war and working in poor environments led to these observations. Of the four broad determinants of health (personal attributes, health care accessibility, acquired health behaviors, and social determinants), the social conditions in which people live are considered to be the most significant, as they influence health directly and indirectly (Reutter & Kushner, 2010). The social determinants of health are the social conditions in which people are born, live, work, and age, including the health care system (Marmot, Allen, Bell, Bloomer, & Goldblatt, 2012). The social determinants of health are responsible for inequities in health, or the differences in health seen within and between individuals, families, communities, and countries (World Health Organization, 2012). The social conditions under which people live—including poverty with its accompanying inadequate housing, poor sanitation, suboptimal food, lack of education, and social discrimination—have a dramatic impact on health. Differences in health can be attributed to socioeconomic, political, cultural, and geographic dimensions, as they are driven by inequities in power, money, and resources (Marmot et al., 2012). The influence of these factors is evident when comparing the health of individuals at the top of the social ladder with individuals at the bottom.

Both downstream and upstream determinants of health need to be addressed in health promotion. Individual factors, including knowledge, beliefs, attitudes, and behaviors, are downstream factors, which are shaped by upstream determinants, or living and working conditions, and economic and social opportunities and resources (Braveman, Egerter, & Williams, 2011). The Robert Wood Johnson Commission to Build a Healthier America conceptual framework depicts how downstream factors are shaped by an individual's upstream factors. This framework (see Figure 1–2) highlights the need to address downstream individual factors within one's socioenvironmental context.

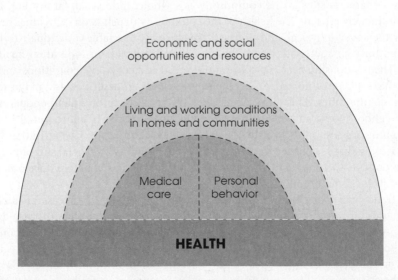

FIGURE 1–2   Upstream and Downstream Determinants of Health   *Source:* Adapted from Braveman, P., Egerter, S., & Williams, D. (2011). The social determinants of health: Coming of age. *Annual Review of Public Health, 32,* 381–398.

In *Healthy People 2020*, the national health agenda, one of the four major goals is to create social and physical environments that promote health (U.S. Department of Health and Human Services, 2013a). The *Healthy People 2020* agenda documents the multiple determinants of health and health behaviors, including personal, social, and physical environments and the interrelationships that exist among these different health determinants. The need for multilevel (individual, family, community) interventions is emphasized to promote health and well-being.

Some people have criticized the term *social determinant*, as they believe that the expanded focus results in a loss of individual identity. Still others believe that the term *social* should not be used. Rather, determinants of health should be the focus to avoid the politicized view of health. Regardless of the terms used, it is now understood that a broader view of health that takes into account the social, cultural, and physical environments, is necessary to improve the health of all. An understanding of the social determinants is important for nurses and other health care professionals to effectively intervene in neighborhoods, organizations, and communities to improve individual health. This is discussed in more detail in Chapter 14.

SOCIAL DETERMINANTS AND GLOBAL HEALTH

Global health has been defined as the transnational impact of globalization (interconnectedness) on the determinants of health and health problems, which are beyond the control of institutions or individual countries (Kaplan, Bond, Merson, Reddy, Rodriquez, Sewankambo, & Wasserheit, 2009). The definition has evolved over time and includes two elements: the level of analysis, which involves the world's population; and the relationship of interdependence, which binds together the units of social organization that make up the world's population (Frenk & Moon, 2013). The goal of global health is to improve health for all people in all nations by promoting wellness and eliminating avoidable diseases, disabilities, and deaths. In other words, global health is public health for the world. Global health issues include the vulnerability of refugee populations, the marketing of harmful products, the erosion of social and environmental conditions, and the exacerbation of income differences, pandemic epidemics, and global climate change.

Globalization is important, as it plays a crucial role in global security. Globalization has resulted in health threats extending across borders, bringing about health interdependence of nations in promoting health and reducing health threats (U.S. Department of Health and Human Services, 2013b). Solutions to global health include the development of new technologies, such as vaccines; improved capacities and resources, including workforce training; new health care systems to promote population health; and improved global governance and coordination (Friedman, Gostin, & Buse, 2013). Although the major drivers in global health are government and nongovernment agencies, health care providers need to be aware of the increasing importance of addressing community and population health, as international borders are increasingly becoming invisible (see Chapter 14).

CONCEPTIONS OF HEALTH PROMOTION

The changing, expanding definitions of health have led to changing views of health promotion. Early health promotion efforts focused on individual responsibility for health and emphasized behavioral determinants and educational approaches. However, evidence has shown that health promotion programs must also address social and physical environments, as these also contribute to poor health. This view was expressed in the *Ottawa Charter for Health Promotion*, the first document to focus on health promotion as a process to enable people to overcome challenges and increase control over their environments to improve their health (World Health Organization, 1986). This document laid the foundation for the theory and practice of health promotion and emphasized the role of social and personal resources as well as physical capabilities, and the need to achieve equity in health. The *Ottawa Charter* also documented the responsibility of nongovernment and government agencies in creating supportive environments and health public policy.

The *Bangkok Charter for Health Promotion* updated the Ottawa Charter to make health promotion central to the global development agenda and a core responsibility of all governments (World Health Organization, 2005). The Bangkok Charter addressed the changing context of health promotion that had occurred since the adoption of the Ottawa Charter. The document moved health promotion from an individual health lifestyle education model toward a socio-ecological model that addresses social determinants of health. In the Bangkok Charter many challenges are recognized due to the multiple determinants of health in a globalized world; health promotion is considered a core responsibility for all governments.

Health promotion and *health education* are often used interchangeably. Although the terms are closely linked, they are not the same. Health education focuses on learning activities and experiences for individuals and groups. As a component of health promotion it is considered an essential part of communication between health care providers and clients. Health education has progressed from health care professionals providing information they think the client should know to a shared decision-making process. The Ottawa Charter was the catalyst that moved health promotion beyond being defined as an educational activity to a broader concept that also focused on the social and political environment (McQueen & De Salazar, 2011). The expanded definition of health promotion is evident in the principles defined to guide health promotion programs (Tremblay, Richard, Brouselle, & Beaudet, 2013). These seven principles are summarized in Table 1–2.

The term *health protection* has been used interchangeably with *health promotion*. Tannahill defines health protection as legal or fiscal controls and other regulations to enhance health and prevent disease (Tannahill, 2009). His expanded definition of health promotion includes health fostering and ill health prevention policies; strategies and activities to address social, economic, and physical environments; cultural factors; equity and diversity; education and learning; services, amenities, and products; and community-led and community-based activities.

TABLE 1–2   Core Principles of Health Promotion

Principle	Explanation
Participation	Involve the stakeholders at all stages of the project.
Empowerment	Enable individuals and communities to take control over the personal, socioeconomic, and environmental factors that affect their health.
Holism	Consider all health components: physical, mental, social, and spiritual.
Intersectoral	Ensure collaboration from all the disciplines and areas concerned.
Equity	Seek fairness in health and social justice.
Sustainability	Implement changes that can be maintained after programs have ended.
Multiple strategies	Rely on several approaches in combination.

Source: Adapted from Rootman, I., Goodstadt, M., Hyndman, B., McQueen, D. V., Potvin, L., Springett, J., & Ziglio, E. (2001). *Evaluation in Health Promotion: Principles and Perspectives.* WHO Regional Publication, European Series No. 92. Denmark: World Health Organization.

Health promotion has moved from being considered a goal or desired end point to a process or tool to facilitate movement toward accomplishment of goals. It is both the art and science of helping people make lifestyle changes and is considered a combination of educational and ecological supports for actions and conditions of living conducive to health. A combination of health promotion strategies are needed to address the multiple determinants of health. Ecological strategies address the social, economic, and physical environments that influence health.

MEASUREMENT OF HEALTH

In general, most health status measures are derived from an illness or curative model. Many commonly used measures of health continue to focus primarily on mortality- or morbidity-related indices such as dysfunction, disability, or impairment. Such measures of health are really measures of illness. Measures of health need to encompass the complexity of health. They should (1) characterize health by conditions that define its presence rather than its absence, (2) identify a spectrum of health states, and (3) reflect a life-span developmental perspective. In addition, measures of the social determinants of the health of individuals and communities must be taken into consideration when measuring health.

On the basis of the WHO definition, Ware (1987) proposes five distinct dimensions as a minimum standard for a comprehensive health measure: physical health (functional and structural integrity), mental health (emotional and intellectual functioning), social functioning, role functioning, and general perceptions of well-being. These dimensions are now widely accepted measures of health status. Two views of self-rated health assessments include spontaneous assessment and enduring self-concept. In the spontaneous assessment view, self-rated assessments of health are considered responsive to observable indicators of illness and have been shown to take a wide range of factors into consideration, including functional ability, lifestyle and health practices, sociocultural constructions of health, physical symptoms, and positive vitality (Ballis, Segall, & Chipperfield, 2003). Individual ratings of health may be transitory, with respect to multiple dimensions of one's health. The enduring self-concept view characterizes self-rated health as a reflection of one's established beliefs about one's health. In this view, self-rated health is stable over time and is based on one's self-concept. Therefore, self-rated health may not reflect the objective indicators of health, as it is independent of one's physical status. This view is more congruent with an expansive definition of health, as an individual's self-evaluation of overall health is more related to an overall sense of well-being. However, if one takes the view that health depends on one's circumstances, then the individual's social and physical context must be taken into consideration in assessing one's view of health.

Measures of wellness that encompass a holistic assessment are available (Brown & Applegate, 2012). Most of these measures assess the major dimensions of wellness, including physical, social, emotional, spiritual, and intellectual. Some measures also assess occupational, environmental, and financial dimensions. Several questionnaires have over 100 items, and the psychometric properties (reliability and validity) are not reported for others. However, the holistic approach to the measurement of health is a major strength.

The focus on social determinants of health has generated the need to develop accurate, easy-to-use measures of the built environment as well as individual behaviors. Community assessment indexes have been designed to measure policies, programs, and practices in the community that affect healthy behaviors. An example of one effort is the Community Healthy Living Index. This assessment identifies the extent to which the community supports active living and healthy eating across a variety of venues (Kim, Adamson, Balfanz, Brownson, Wiecha, Shepard, &

Alles, 2010). Progress has also been made in measuring the food environment and walkability in communities using new technologies, such as Global Positioning Systems, smart phones, and web-based tools (Berrigan, 2012). Although major challenges remain and the technology is in the early stages of development, the measures will result in valuable health information for public policy.

The multilevel nature of health and its determinants points to the need for measureable personal, social, and physical environmental indicators. Standardized measures are needed to evaluate the effectiveness of multilevel health promotion interventions across individuals, families, and communities. In addition, both individual and aggregate measures are needed to assess and monitor health at the individual, family, and community levels. Measurement of health and its multiple determinants is complex; it becomes even more so when all perspectives are taken into account. This challenge poses multiple research opportunities.

CONSIDERATIONS FOR PRACTICE IN THE CONTEXT OF HOLISTIC HEALTH

The definition of *health* has evolved from traditional usage in a medical, curative model to a multidimensional phenomenon with physical, social, spiritual, environmental, and cultural dimensions. Nurses and other health care professionals need to understand and assess all dimensions. The assessment information can then be used to identify health needs and develop strategies to intervene. For example, a traditional biomedical assessment may be useful in guiding genetic counseling or screening interventions. Information gleaned from a spiritual and cultural assessment can provide valuable knowledge in developing health promotion interventions for diverse populations. An assessment of the social and physical environment will provide useful information about aspects of the environment that may be positively or negatively affecting the health of the individual or community. In a holistic view of health, an assessment is not complete unless it involves individuals, families, and communities in which individuals live and function. Nurses work in partnership with clients to provide the knowledge and skills needed to empower them to achieve their health goals or to adapt to their circumstances to move toward their health goals. Last, health should be viewed from a positive perspective when conducting an assessment or designing health promotion strategies. This means focusing on available resources, potentials, and capabilities. When health is viewed in a positive model, strategies can be developed that concentrate on strengthening resources as well as decreasing negative risks.

OPPORTUNITIES FOR RESEARCH ON HEALTH

The fundamental purpose of nursing research is to build knowledge to improve health. The power of nursing in health promotion depends, in part, on the way in which health knowledge is grounded in science. Nursing research has been active in knowledge development to improve the health of all. However, many questions remain unanswered. What are the gender, culture, and racial differences in the expressions of health? How does health differ at varying points of life span development? What interactive conditions between persons and their environment enhance or deplete health? Which health determinants are critical to assess the health of families? Which health determinants are key to improving the health of communities? How do issues related to globalization affect the health of individuals and communities? What dimensions need to be included in measuring family health? How can behavioral and social determinants be more accurately measured? Generating knowledge using both qualitative (ethnographic) and quantitative (descriptive) research will advance the scientific base to enable nurses to implement effective health-promoting interventions and begin policy discussions for change.

Multilevel models of health that incorporate ethnic, cultural, social, environmental, political, and global factors are needed to examine the determinants of health. Furthermore, longitudinal studies are needed to investigate the developmental variations in health perceptions and the role of social determinants across the life span in different racial and cultural groups. Multidisciplinary research teams are suggested to develop and test multilevel interventions to address the social determinants of health. Measures to assess the expanded conceptualizations of health should be constructed that will provide information needed to guide these interventions.

Summary

Varying definitions of *health* have been presented that provide the foundation on which health promotion programs for individuals, families, and communities can be based. To promote health, one must first assess how health is defined by the individual or family or community and identify realistic strategies to achieve desired health goals. Individual health cannot be separated from the health of the family, community, nation, and world. A shift to this broader perspective of health facilitates development of proactive policies to improve the health of all. The complexity of factors known to determine the health of individuals and communities also raises many challenges; however, increasingly great emphasis on these factors is occurring at both national and international levels.

Learning Activities

1. Based on the definitions provided in the chapter, write your own definition of *health*, and state the rationale for the factors you considered in developing the definition.
2. Interview three persons of various ages (adolescent, young adult, elderly person) to obtain their perspectives of their health and the health promotion strategies they perform to stay healthy. Ask them to identify the personal, social, and environmental barriers and facilitators to pursuing a healthy lifestyle.
3. Suggest health promotion strategies to realistically overcome the barriers stated by the interviewees.
4. Develop a plan to conduct an assessment to describe the health of a family or a community, using the social determinants of health.
5. Design a clinical experience that incorporates the principles of health for a student assigned to a community-based organization.

References

Alligood, M. R. (2010). Family health care with King's theory of goal attainment. *Nursing Science Quarterly* 23(2), 99–104.

American Nurses Association. (2010). *Nursing's Social Policy Statement: The essence of the profession* (3rd ed.). Washington, DC: Author.

Ballis, D. S., Segall, A., & Chipperfield, J. G. (2003). Two views of self-rated general health status. *Social Science and Medicine, 56*(2), 203–217.

Berrigan, D. (2012). Better measurement for healthier places. *Preventive Medicine, 55,* 567–568.

Bok, S. (2008). WHO definition of health, rethinking the. In *International Encyclopedia of Public Health,* 590–597.

Braveman, P., Egerter, S., & Williams, D. (2011). The social determinants of health: Coming of age. *Annual Review of Public Health, 32,* 381–398.

Brown, C., & Applegate, B. (2012). Holistic wellness assessment for young adults. *Journal of Holistic Nursing, 30*(4), 235–243.

Davidson, K. K., Lawson, H. A., & Coatsworth, J. D. (2012). The family-centered action model of intervention layout and implementation (FAMILI): The example of childhood obesity. *Health Promotion Practice, 12*(4), 454–461.

Doornbos, M. M. (2007). King's conceptual system and family health theory in the families of adults with persistent mental illnesses. In C. L. Sieloff & M. A. Frey (Eds.), *Middle range theory development using King's conceptual system* (pp. 31–49). New York, NY: Springer.

Dubos, R. (1965). *Man adapting*. New Haven, CT: Yale University Press.

Dunn, H. L. (1977). High-level wellness: A collection of twenty-nine short talks on different aspects of the term "High-level wellness for man and society." Thorofare, NJ: Charles B. Slace, Inc.

Ereshefsky, M. (2009). Defining "health" and "disease." *Studies in History and Philosophy of Biological and Biomedical Sciences, 40*(3), 221–227.

Erkisson, J., Dellve, L., Eklof, M., & Hagberg, M. (2007). Early inequities in excellent health and performance among young adult women and men in Sweden. *Gender Medicine, 4*(2), 170–177.

Evans, J., Frank, B., Oliffe, J., & Gregory, D. (2011). Health, illness, men and masculinities (HIMM): A theoretical framework for understanding men and their health. *Journal of Men's Health, 4*(1), 7–15.

Fawcett, J., & Desanto-Mediva, S. (2012). *Analysis and evaluation of contemporary nursing knowledge: Nursing models and theories*. Philadelphia, PA: FA Davis Co.

Flannery, M. C. (2009). The mirage of health. *The American Biology Teacher, 71*(9), 558–561.

Frenk, J., & Moon, S. (2013). Governance challenges in global health. *New England Journal of Medicine, 368*(10), 936–942.

Friedman, E. A., Gostin, L. O., & Buse, K. (2013). Advancing the right to health through global organizations: The potential role of a framework convention on global health. *Health and Human Rights, 15*(1), 71–86.

Friel, S., & Marmot, M. G. (2011). Action on the social determinants of health and health inequities goes global. *American Review of Public Health, 32*, 225–236.

Gelb, K., Pederson, A., & Greaves, L. (2011). How have health promotion frameworks considered gender? *Health Promotion International, 27*(4), 445–452.

Giles, W. H., Holmes-Chavez, A., & Collins, J. L. (2009). Cultivating healthy communities: The CDC perspective. *Health Promotion Practice, 10*(2), 86s–87s.

Goddings, A., James, D. R., & Hargreaves, D. S. (2012). Distinct patterns of health engagement in adolescents and young adults: Implications for health services. *The Lancet*, published online November 23, 2012.

Goins, R. T., Spencer, S. M., & Williams, K. (2011). Lay meanings of health among rural older adults in Appalachia. *The Journal of Rural Health, 27*(1), 13–20.

Holiday, B. (2010). Dorothy Johnson's behavioral systems model. In Alligood, M. R., & Tomey, A. M., *Nursing theorists and their work* (7th ed., pp. 366–391). Maryland, MO: Elsevier Mosby.

Huber, M., Knottnerus, J. A., Green, L., van der Horst, H., Jadad, A. R., Kromhout, D., . . . Smid, H. (2011). How should we define healthy? *British Medical Journal, 343*, 1–3.

Institute of Medicine. (2012). *Living well with chronic illness: A call for public health action*. Washington, DC: The National Academies Press.

Kaplan, J. P., Bond, T. C., Merson, M. H., Reddy, K. S., Rodriquez, M. H., Sewankambo, N. K., & Wasserheit, J. N. (2009). Towards a common definition of global health. *Lancet, 373*, 1993–1995.

Kim, S., Adamson, K. C., Balfanz, D. R., Brownson, R. C., Wiecha, J. L., Shepard, D., & Alles, W. F. (2010). Development of the Community Healthy Living Index: A tool to foster healthy environments for the prevention of obesity and chronic disease. *Preventive Medicine, 50*, S80–S85.

King, I. M. (2007). King's structure, process and outcome in the 21st century. In C. L. Sieloff and M. A. Frey (Eds.), *Middle range theory development using King's conceptual system* (pp. 3–11). New York, NY: Springer.

Mackey, S. (2009). Toward an ontological theory of wellness: a discussion of conceptual foundations and implications for nursing. *Nursing Philosophy, 10*, 103–112.

Marmot, M., Allen, J., Bell, R., Bloomer, E., & Goldblatt, P. (2012). WHO European review of social determinants of health and the health divide. *Lancet, 380*, 1011–1029.

McAllister, A. L., Perry, C. L., & Parcel, G. S. (2008). How individuals, environments and health behavior interact: Social cognitive theory. In K. Glanz, F. M. Lewis, & B. K. Rimer (Eds.), *Health behavior and health education* (4th ed., pp. 169–188). San Francisco, CA: John Wiley & Sons.

McMahon, S., & Fleury, J. (2012). Wellness in older adults: A concept analysis. *Nursing Forum, 47*(1), 39–51.

McQueen, D. V., & De Salazar, L. (2011). Health promotion, The Ottawa Charter and developing personal skills: A compact history of 25 years. *Health Promotion International, 26*(52), 194–201.

Meleis, A. (2010). *Transition theory: Middle range and situation specific in nursing research and practice*. New York, NY: Springer.

Miller, G., & Foster, L. T. (2010). Critical synthesis of the wellness literature. Accessed online at the British Columbia Atlas of Wellness, http://www.geog.uvic.ca/wellness.

Neuman, B., & Fawcett, J. (2011). *The Neuman systems model* (5th ed.). Upper Saddle River, NJ: Pearson.

Neuman, B., & Fawcett, J. (2012). Thoughts about the Neuman Systems model: A dialogue. *Nursing Science Quarterly, 25*(4), 374–376.

Niebroj, L. T. (2006). Defining health/illness: Societal and/or clinical medicine. *Journal of Physiology and Pharmacology, 57* (suppl 4), 251–262.

Orem, D. E., & Taylor, S. G. (2011). Reflections on nursing practice sciences: The nature, the structure, and the foundation of nursing sciences. *Nursing Science Quarterly, 24*(1), 35–41.

Parse, R. R. (2011). The human becoming modes of inquiry: Refinements. *Nursing Science Quarterly, 24*(1), 11–18.

Parsons, T. (1958). Definitions of health and illness in the light of American values and social structure. In E. G. Jaco (Ed.), *Patients, physicians and illness* (p. 176). New York, NY: Free Press.

Phillips, J. R. (2010). The universality of Rogers' science of unitary human beings. *Nursing Science Quarterly, 23*(1), 55–59.

Reutter, L., & Kushner, K. E. (2010). Health equity through action on the social determinants of health: Taking up the challenge in nursing. *Nursing Inquiry, 17*(3), 269–280.

Richard, L., Gauvin, L., & Raine, K. (2011). Ecological models revisited: Their uses and evolution in health promotion over two decades. *Annual Review of Public Health, 32*, 307–326.

Roscoe, L. J. (2009). Wellness: A review of theory and measurement for counselors. *Journal of Counseling and Development, 87*, 216–226.

Rotegard, A. K., Moore, S. M., Fagermoen, M. S., & Ruland, C. M. (2010). Health assess: A concept analysis. *International Journal of Nursing Studies, 47*, 513–525.

Roy, C. (2011). Research based on the Roy Adaptation model: Last 25 years. *Nursing Science Quarterly, 24*(4), 312–320.

Schaefer, K. M. (2010). Myra Estrin Levine: The conservation model. In M. R. Alligood & A. M. Tomey, *Nursing theorists and their work* (7th ed., pp. 225–241). Maryland, MO: Elsevier Mosby.

Schlotfeldt, R. M. (1987). Resolution of issues: An imperative for creating nursing's future. *Journal of Professional Nursing, 3*, 136–142.

Selanders, L. C. (2010). The power of environmental adaptation. Florence Nightingale's original theory for nursing practice. *Journal of Holistic Nursing, 28*(1), 81–88.

Skelton, J. A., Buehler, C., Irby, N. B., & Grzywacz, J. G. (2012). Where are family theories in family-based obesity treatment? Conceptualizing the study of families in pediatric weight management. *International Journal of Obesity, 36*(7), 891–900.

Sorochan, W. (1970). Health concepts as a basis for orthobiosis. In E. Hart & W. Sechrist (Eds.), *The dynamics of wellness.* Belmont, CA: Wadsworth Inc.

Stanhope, M., & Lancaster, J. (Eds.). (2012). *Public health nursing: Population centered health care in the community* (8th ed.). Maryland Heights, MO: Elsevier Mosby.

Tannahill, A. (2009). Health promotion: The Tannahill model revisited. *Public Health, 123*, 396–399.

Tountas, Y. (2009). The historical origins of the basic concepts of health promotion and education: The role of ancient Greek philosophy and medicine. *Health Promotion International, 24*(2), 185–192.

Tremblay, M. C., Richard, L., Brousselle, A., & Beaudet, N. (2013). How can both the intervention and its evaluation fulfill health promotion principles? An example from a professional development program. *Health Promotion Practice, 14*, 563–571.

U.S. Department of Health and Human Services. (2013a). *Healthy People 2020.* Washington, DC: U.S. Government Printing Office. Accessed at http://www.healthypeople.gov.

U.S. Department of Health and Human Services. (2013b). *Global health security.* Accessed at http://www.globalhealth.gov/global-health-topics/global-health-security/index.html.

Ware, J. E. (1987). Standards for validating health measures: Definition and content. *Journal of Chronic Diseases, 40*, 473–480.

Williamson, D. L., & Carr, J. (2009). Health as a resource for everyday life: Advancing the conceptualization. *Critical Public Health, 19*(1), 107–122.

World Health Organization. (1974). Community health nursing: Report of a WHO expert committee. *Technical Report Series No. 558.* Geneva, Switzerland: WHO.

World Health Organization. (1986). Ottawa Charter for Health Promotion. *Health Promotion, 1*(4), ii–v.

World Health Organization. (2005). Constitution of the World Health Organization (55th ed.). Suppl. Accessed at http://www.who.int/governance/eb/who_constitution_en.pdf

World Health Organization. (2011), *Mental health: A state of well-being.* Accessed at http://www.who.int/features/factfiles/mental_health/en

World Health Organization. (2012). Measurement of and target-setting for well-being: An initiative by the WHO regional Office for Europe. First meeting of the expert group, Copenhagen, Denmark.

CHAPTER 2

Individual Models to Promote Health Behavior

OBJECTIVES

This chapter will enable the reader to:

1. Discuss the rationale for using behavior change theory to structure interventions.

2. Describe commonalities and differences in the individual models of behavior change.

3. Apply the stages of change model to designing interventions to promote health behaviors.

4. Discuss the revised health promotion model and its usefulness in nursing practice.

5. Describe theory-based strategies for changing behavior.

6. Discuss the concept and application of tailoring behavior strategies to promote healthy behavior outcomes.

Health promotion activities provided by health professionals in the United States are aimed toward assisting individuals, families, and communities achieve their full health potential. Health promotion promotes lifestyles and behaviors that enable persons to maximize their potential through individual, organizational, and community change. Primary prevention focuses on persons who are at risk for disease, while secondary prevention aims to prevent further illness in persons who are already diagnosed with a disease. Secondary prevention is receiving more attention as the numbers of persons living with chronic illnesses continue to increase. While primary prevention strategies reduce the occurrence or prolong the onset of diseases, such as diabetes, heart disease, stroke, and cancer, secondary prevention activities promote health within the limits of the illness or disability. Health promotion (action to contribute to health) and primary prevention (action to avoid or forestall illness/disease) have been shown to have substantial benefits in improving quality of life and longevity. Both health promotion and primary prevention are based on behavioral or sociopolitical models of health care that recognize the effects of multiple systems on health outcomes.

Health protection refers to the use of regulatory measures to promote health. Historically, health protection has included measures to address public health issues such as safe drinking water. However, health protection measures have extended to other aspects of the environment, such as automobile safety and consumer product safety. Individuals do not need to take an active role to be protected, as health protection strategies are addressed by government regulations. The goal of improving population health is best served by emphasizing health promotion and primary prevention throughout the life span. Progress toward this goal requires an understanding of the motivational dynamics of actions that enhance health. This chapter focuses on models and theories useful in explaining and predicting individual health behaviors, or actions that are motivated by the desire to prevent disease or promote health. Interventions and programs that have been tested using the theories and models provide examples of successful strategies for changing behavior.

Health behavior may be motivated by a desire to protect one's health by avoiding illness or a desire to increase one's level of health in either the presence or absence of illness. *Health promotion* is directed toward increasing the level of well-being and self-actualization of an individual or group (see Chapter 1). Health promotion focuses on efforts to move toward a positive state of high-level wellness and well-being. In reality, for many health behaviors, both "approaching a positive state" and "avoiding a negative state" serve as sources of motivation for behavior. Health behaviors of middle age and older adults can be explained by approach and avoidance. In contrast, children are more likely to be motivated toward positive healthy behaviors. Avoidance lacks relevance because negative states (illness) are more likely to occur in the future.

HUMAN POTENTIAL FOR CHANGE

Individuals have tremendous potential for self-directed change due to their capacity for self-knowledge, self-regulation, decision making, and problem solving. Clients have the power and skill to change health behaviors or modify health-related lifestyles. The nurse's role is to promote a positive climate for change, serve as a catalyst for change, assist with various steps of the change process, and increase the individual's capacity to maintain change.

USE OF THEORIES AND MODELS FOR BEHAVIOR CHANGE

Theories and models of health behavior are systematic attempts to explain why individuals do or do not engage in health behaviors and how individuals change negative behaviors or implement new health behaviors. They specify the concepts that may determine the desired health behavior, and the relationship among these concepts provides direction for how to intervene to promote change and predict the expected outcomes. Understanding the mechanisms for behavior change and sustainability of these changes is necessary to develop effective health promotion and prevention interventions. To understand the possible mechanisms of change, the mediators, or intervening variables that describe the process responsible for the effect of the intervention on the health behavior, also must be examined. Mediators describe how the change occurs. The mediators, or mechanisms of behavior change, enable health care providers to develop and deliver effective, theoretically driven interventions based on the most powerful predictors of health behavior. The scientific knowledge gained from testing theories and models also informs public policy, as the research evidence is used to improve health care practice.

To date, no one theory or model completely predicts behavior or behavior change, so multiple theories are presented. The models and theories presented focus primarily on individual, intrapersonal, and interpersonal influences to promote health. These models originated in educational and social psychology and expectancy-value, social cognition, and decision-making theories. Cognitive processing of information is important in all the models because individuals' perceptions and interpretations of what they experience directly affect their behaviors. Knowledge of the elements and mechanisms of behavior-change theories enables health care professionals to optimize their counseling effectiveness and success in structuring behavioral interventions for clients.

SOCIAL COGNITION THEORIES AND MODELS

Social cognition models incorporate cognitive and affective factors as proximal determinants of behavior (Sutton, 2010). They are called social cognition models because of the focus on cognitive variables as the major determinant of individual health. Although other factors influence behavior, social cognition models assume that the effects of these factors are mediated by the proximal factors specified in the model. The proximal determinants are amenable to change and can be used as the basis for health promotion interventions. Social cognition models include the health belief model, the theory of reasoned action and planned behavior, social cognitive and self-efficacy theory, the wellness motivation model, and the health promotion model. These models are similar in their determinants of health behavior, although labeled differently in the models. The shared concepts of the theories are described in Table 2–1. Each model provides an understanding of the determinants of health behaviors and behavior change. However, in most cases they do not provide direction on how to change behavior. In addition, Bandura's social cognitive theory is the only one that accounts for environmental and social factors (Burke, Joseph, Pasick, & Barker, 2009).

TABLE 2–1   Shared Psychosocial Concepts in Five Individual Theories/Models of Health Behavior

	Psychosocial Concepts			
Theories/Models	**Self-Efficacy**	**Outcome Expectations**	**Evaluation of Benefits and Barriers**	**Health Behavior Goals**
Health Belief Model (Revised)	+	+	+	−
Theory of Reasoned Action	−	+	+	+
Theory of Planned Behavior	+	+	+	+
Health Promotion Model	+	+	+	+
Social Cognitive Model	+	+	+	+

Key: + Concept present; − Concept absent in Theory/Model

The Health Belief Model

The health belief model (HBM) was proposed in the 1950s to describe why some people who are free of illness will take actions to prevent illness, whereas others fail to do so (Carpenter, 2010; Rosenstock, 1960). The model was developed at a time when there were public health concerns about the widespread reluctance to accept screening for tuberculosis, screening for detection of cervical cancer, immunizations, and other preventive measures that were often free or provided at a nominal charge. The model was viewed as potentially useful to predict individuals who would or would not use preventive measures and to suggest interventions that might increase the willingness of resistant individuals to engage in preventive behaviors.

The HBM is derived from social psychology and Lewin's classic value-expectancy theory. Lewin, a cognitive theorist, conceptualized the life space in which an individual exists as composed of regions, some regions having negative valence, some having positive valence, and others being relatively neutral. Illnesses are conceived to be regions of negative valence exerting a force that moves the person away from the regions of positive valence. Preventive behaviors are strategies for avoiding the negatively valenced regions of illness. An example of how the revised HBM can be applied to a risk behavior such as smoking is presented in Figure 2–1.

Evidence has shown that individuals will take action if two conditions are present: (1) There is a perceived threat (illness susceptibility and severity) to personal health, and (2) the individual is convinced that the benefits of taking action to protect health outweigh the barriers that will be encountered. Beliefs about personal susceptibility and the seriousness of a specific illness (for example, lung disease) combine to produce the degree of threat or negative valence of that illness. Perceived susceptibility reflects feelings of personal vulnerability or risk (pack years smoked) for a specific health problem. Perceived seriousness may be judged either by the degree of emotional arousal created by the thought of having the disease, or by the medical, clinical, or social difficulties (family and work life) that individuals believe a given health condition would create for them. Perceived benefits are beliefs about the effectiveness of recommended actions (more energy, save money) in preventing the health threat. Perceived barriers are perceptions about the potential negative aspects of taking action such as unpleasantness (craving cigarettes, perceived possible weight gain), inconvenience, and time required. Cues to action are events, internal (shortness of breath) or external (anti-smoking campaigns, provider advice), that trigger action. Modifying factors such as demographic, social, psychological, and structural variables, as well as cues to action, indirectly affect an individual's tendency to take action.

The HBM continues to be used to explain preventive and health promotion behaviors as well as sick role behaviors, including breast self-examination and breast cancer early diagnosis behaviors (Ahmadian, Samah, Redzuan, & Emby, 2012; Ersin & Bahar, 2011), condom use (Asare, Sharma, Bernard, Rohas-Guyler, & Wang, 2013), contraceptive behavior (Hall, 2012), and physical activity in children (Ar-yuwat, Clark, Hunter, & James, 2013).

The individual constructs of the HBM model have varied in their predictive ability. Perceived barriers and benefits are considered to be the most powerful HBM dimensions for explaining various preventive behaviors, followed by perceived susceptibility (Carpenter, 2010). In general, these constructs predict behavior when the goal is prevention of a negative outcome. This is consistent with Rosenstock's original purpose of the model to predict the adoption of preventable behaviors. The weak predictability of perceived susceptibility and severity may due to indirect effects that are mediated by perceived threat instead of direct effects as proposed in the model. These relationships should be explored as indirect effects in future research.

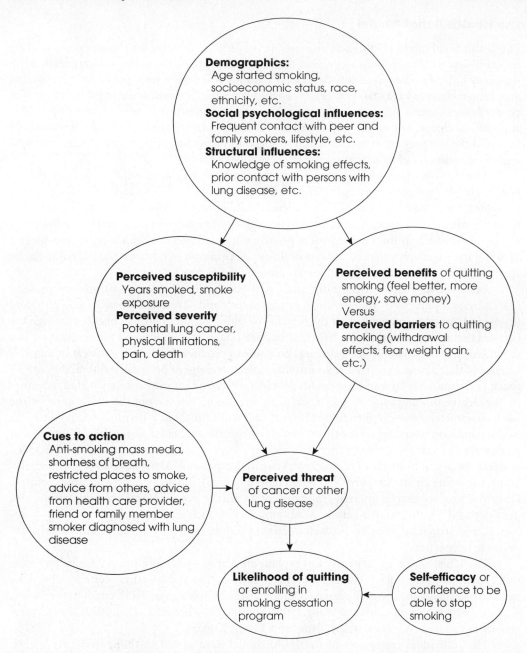

FIGURE 2–1   The Revised Health Belief Model Applied to Smoking as a Health Behavior Risk

Thirty years after the model was introduced, Rosenstock and his colleagues expanded the model components to consider feelings of confidence in one's ability to perform a behavior (self-efficacy) as an explanatory variable and suggested that it be incorporated in interventions using the model. When the HBM was first developed, it was intended for application to one-time behaviors such as immunization. However, application of the model to more complex behavioral risks such as smoking and unsafe sexual practices necessitates attending to individual perceptions of competence, or self-efficacy, to repeatedly engage in preventive behaviors over a long period of time. The extended HBM has been tested in multiple studies. For example, the extended model has been used to predict breast self-examination and mammography in women (Ahmadian, Samah, Redzuan, & Emby, 2012; Ersin & Bahar, 2011). In these studies self-efficacy predicted the health behavior under investigation. The extended HBM has also been used to develop culturally appropriate weight management materials for African American women (James, Pobee, Oxidine, Brown, & Joshi, 2012). Women were interviewed about their susceptibility to obesity as well as their perceived barriers and benefits to losing weight, cues to taking action for initiating weight loss, and their perceived self-efficacy in enacting behaviors to lose weight. The generated themes were used to develop weight management materials for the women to use in a weight management program. Results of research with the extended model substantiate the addition of self-efficacy.

Theory of Reasoned Action and Theory of Planned Behavior

In the theory of reasoned action (TRA), a person's intention to perform a behavior is considered the most immediate determinant and best predictor of that behavior. Attitudes and subjective norms, and intrapersonal factors, constitute the fundamental building blocks of the theory (Fishbein & Ajzen, 1975). Attitudes and subjective norms determine behavioral intention. Attitude toward a behavior is an overall positive or negative evaluation of the consequences (outcomes) of performing the behavior. When the evaluation of the behavior outcome is primarily desirable, the result is a positive attitude; a negative attitude results when the evaluation is primarily undesirable. Subjective norms are individual beliefs about whether significant others expect them to engage in the behavior—that is, whether important others would approve or disapprove—and the motivation of the individual to comply with others' expectations. The relative importance of attitudes and subjective norms in predicting any given behavior varies, depending on the target behavior, the context, and the population being studied.

The TRA is based on the assumption that both attitudes and subjective norms are amenable to change. Interventions by health care professionals may target attitudes by addressing beliefs about outcomes and subjective norms, which influence individuals' values related to the outcomes, by focusing on their perceptions about normative expectations of others and their motivation to comply with what others expect. Research has shown that components of the TRA influence a range of health behaviors.

The TRA assumes that behavior is under an individual's volitional control, in other words, individuals can make choices related to their behaviors. Ajzen, one of the original authors of the TRA, believed that behavior is not completely under the control of the individual. He added a third variable, perceived behavioral control, and labeled the extended theory the *theory of planned behavior* (*TPB*; Ajzen, 1991, 2011). Perceived behavioral control is an individual's expectancy that performance of the behavior is within his or her control and is measured by beliefs about the opportunities to engage in the behavior as well as the power of various factors to inhibit or facilitate the behavior. Perceived behavioral control is similar to Bandura's self-efficacy concept (Sutton, 2010).

The TPB has been widely applied in research to explain many health behaviors, including physical activity (Plotnikoff, Costigan, Karumamuni, & Lubans, 2013), healthy eating (Kothe, Mullan, & Butow, 2012), beverage consumption (Zoellner, Estabrooks, Davy, Chen, & You, 2012), and cardiovascular risk prevention (Krones, Keller, Becker, Sonnichsen, Baum, & Donner-Banzhoff, 2010). However, most studies have been observational or descriptive. In a meta-analysis of the predictive ability of the TPB for physical activity and diet behaviors in adolescents, behaviors assessed in the shorter term were better predicted. Behaviors assessed with self-report measures were better predictors than objective measures (McEachan, Conner, Taylor, & Lawton, 2011). The type of behavior predicted, age, and type of measures (subjective versus objective) moderated the relationships among model components, indicating the need to take these variables into account when using the model. Despite the popularity of the TPB, there have been suggestions to include additional variables to further increase understanding of behavior. The TPB has been extended to include habit strength, which relates to behavioral factors, such as unawareness in performing the behavior (automatic), difficulty in controlling the behavior, and mental efficiency in performing the behavior. This addition acknowledges the influence of past behavior on current and future behavior (Manstead, 2011). Although the interaction of habits with intention has been in the literature for many years, the role of habit has received little attention due to measurement issues. Now, however, reliable and valid measures are available, and the relationship has been tested in several studies in which both habit strength and TPB concepts have been measured. Findings indicate that habit strength interacts with intentions in explaining behavior (Manstead, 2011). When habit strength is strong, intentions are weakly correlated with behavior. When habit strength is weak, intention is a stronger predictor of behavior. These findings provide a beginning explanation for the limited success in breaking strong unhealthy habits.

The TBM model has been criticized for assuming that the predictor variables are linearly related to the outcomes (Manstead, 2011). This criticism has led to a better understanding of the interaction effects of the model concepts. For example, intention has now been shown to predict behavior to the extent that intentions are stable over time (intention stability). Further study and expansion of the model are needed to contribute to the science of behavior change.

Self-Efficacy and Social Cognitive Theory

In social cognitive theory (SCT), personal factors, the environment in which behavior is performed, and behaviors interact with each other. This is called *reciprocal determinism*. The core components include knowledge of health risks and benefits of reducing risks; perceived self-efficacy, or the belief that one has the ability to change one's health habits; both positive and negative outcome expectations about changing behavior; personal health goals and strategies for achieving them; and perceived facilitators and structural impediments to achieving them (Bandura, 1985, 1986, 2004). Although SCT is the only social cognition model that includes the environment, the concept has been operationalized narrowly as the social environment, and in general, it has been overlooked in most research with the model (Burke, Joseph, Pasick, & Barker, 2009).

Self-efficacy plays a central role in personal change and is the foundation of human motivation and action. Knowledge is a precondition for change. However, individuals must believe they have control to change the behavior in order to take action. Health behaviors are also influenced by outcome expectancies and goals set by the individual, as they serve as incentives for change. Both facilitators and impediments are determinants of behavior and must be taken into account when assessing self-efficacy. Bandura also recognizes the role of impediments outside one's personal control. An application of the model to physical activity behavior is presented in Figure 2–2.

According to social cognitive theory, self-beliefs formed through self-observation and self-reflective thought greatly influence human functioning. Self-efficacy expectations develop through mastery experiences (personal accomplishments), vicarious learning (role models), verbal persuasion, and somatic responses to particular situations to build competencies and confidence. The greater one's perceived efficacy, the more vigorously and persistently an individual

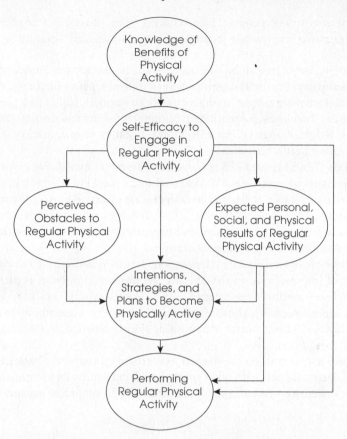

FIGURE 2–2   The Social Cognitive Theory Applied to Physical Activity Behavior

will engage in a behavior, even in the face of obstacles and aversive experiences. Individuals with high levels of self-efficacy expectations are more likely to set higher goal challenges, expect that their efforts will produce favorable change, and believe that obstacles are surmountable.

Self-efficacy beliefs are behavior specific and are measured in terms of three parameters: magnitude, strength, and generality. *Magnitude* refers to the level of difficulty of the behavior and is an assessment of individuals' perceived capability of their level of performance. Individuals with low self-efficacy expectations feel capable of performing only very simple behaviors. *Strength* refers to the individual's confidence in performing the behavior. *Generality* refers to the extent of expectations across situations. The self-efficacy concept is one of the most widely measured in behavior change research; therefore, measures for almost all health behaviors are available in the literature.

Four main sources of self-efficacy beliefs have been described. Mastery or performance expectations are evidence of whether or not one can accomplish the tasks necessary for perform-ing the behavior. Vicarious experiences or modeling refers to seeing others perform a behavior and observing the consequences of their actions. Vicarious experiences supply the strategies and techniques needed to accomplish the behavior. Verbal persuasion, the most widely used tech-nique, is used to convince individuals to perform a positive behavior or stop a negative behavior. Somatic or affective states refer to the emotional or physiological arousal or tensions created by performing an activity. For example, pain resulting from exercise is a negative somatic state that may decrease self-efficacy, while feeling energetic as a result of exercising increases one's self-efficacy.

Self-efficacy is considered to be one of the most important predictors of behavior, and research continues to support social cognitive theory in health behavior change. The theory has been used to predict smoking relapse in adolescents (Van Zundert, Nijhof, & Engels, 2009), physical activity (Ashford, Edmunds, & French, 2010), dental brushing and flossing (Buglar, White, & Robinson, 2010), weight change (Wingo, Desmond, Brantley, Appel, Svetkey, Stevens, & Ard, 2013), and many other health behaviors.

Interventions to increase self-efficacy also have been conducted. For example, the "Smart Bodies" school wellness program was a clinical trial to increase knowledge and preference for a diet rich in fruits and vegetables in fourth and fifth graders (Tuuri, Zanovec, Silverman, Geaghan, Solmon, Holston, Guarino, Roy, & Murphy, 2009). Children who participated in the 12-week program had greater nutrition knowledge and expressed confidence (self-efficacy) that they could choose fruits instead of less healthy alternatives.

Meta-analysis of physical activity interventions targeting self-efficacy showed a small, but significant effect of interventions on self-efficacy (Ashford, Edmunds, & French, 2010). Interventions that included feedback techniques and vicarious experiences were associated with higher levels of self-efficacy. Vicarious experiences have also been found to be a source of perceived self-efficacy as a determinant of physical activity in older adults (Warner, Shulz, Knittle, Ziegelmann, & Wurm, 2011).

Further intervention studies are needed to increase efficacy expectations and to understand how the concept interacts with other motivational determinants to improve health behaviors. In addition, the environmental component of the model should be expanded and included in studies using SCT.

The Health Promotion Model

In 1990 Pender published the first test of the initial version of Pender's health promotion model (HPM; Pender, Walker, Sechrist, & Frank-Stromborg, 1990). The HPM proposes a framework for integrating nursing and behavioral science perspectives with factors influencing health behaviors. The model offers a guide to explore the complex biopsychosocial processes that motivate individuals to engage in behaviors directed toward enhancing health.

The original HPM stimulated studies to describe the potential of seven cognitive-perceptual factors and five modifying factors to predict health behaviors. The cognitive-perceptual factors are importance of health, perceived control of health, definition of health, perceived health status, perceived self-efficacy, perceived benefits, and perceived barriers. The modifying factors are demographic and biologic characteristics, interpersonal influences, situational influences, and behavioral factors. Assumptions and theoretical propositions, a summary of empirical support for constructs in the HPM, and studies using the HPM can be reviewed in earlier editions of this text as well as on Pender's website at the University of Michigan (Pender, Murdaugh, & Parsons, 2002).

The HPM is a competence- or approach-oriented model. Unlike prevention models, such as the HBM, the HPM does not include "fear" or "threat" as a source of motivation for health behavior. Although immediate threats to health have been shown to motivate action, threats in the distant future lack the same motivational strength. The HPM is applicable to any health behavior in which threat is not proposed as a major source of motivation for the behavior. The initial model has since been replaced by the HPM (revised).

THEORETICAL BASIS FOR THE HEALTH PROMOTION MODEL

The HPM is an attempt to depict the multidimensional nature of persons interacting with their interpersonal and physical environments as they pursue health. The HPM integrates constructs from expectancy-value theory and social cognitive theory, within a nursing perspective of holistic human functioning.

THE HEALTH PROMOTION MODEL (REVISED)

The revised HPM that first appeared in the third edition of *Health Promotion in Nursing Practice* (Pender, 1996) is shown in Figure 2–3. Three new variables added to the revised model are activity-related affect, commitment to a plan of action, and immediate competing demands and preferences.

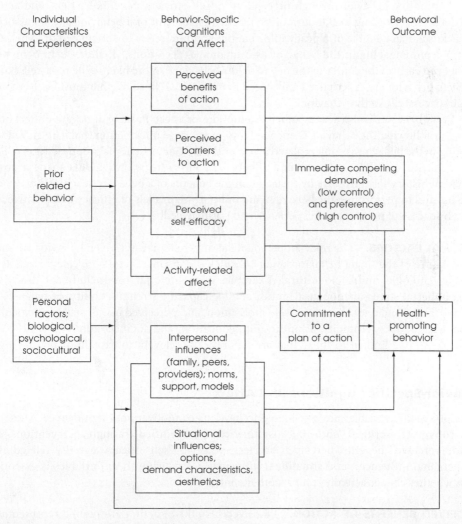

FIGURE 2–3   Health Promotion Model (Revised)

Individual Characteristics and Experiences

Each person has unique personal characteristics and experiences that affect subsequent actions. The importance of their effect depends on the target behavior being considered. Individual characteristics and experiences include prior related behavior and personal factors.

PRIOR RELATED BEHAVIOR.   Research indicates that often the best predictor of behavior is the frequency of the same or a similar behavior in the past. Prior behavior is proposed to have both direct and indirect effects on the likelihood of engaging in health-promoting behaviors. The direct effect of past behavior on current health-promoting behavior may be due to habit formation, predisposing one to engage in the behavior automatically with little attention to the specific details of its execution. Habit strength accrues each time the behavior occurs and is augmented by concentrated, repetitive practice of the behavior.

Consistent with social cognitive theory, prior behavior is proposed to indirectly influence health-promoting behavior through perceptions of self-efficacy, benefits barriers, and activity-related affect. According to Bandura (1985), actual enactment of a behavior and its associated feedback is a major source of efficacy information. Bandura refers to anticipated or experienced benefits from engaging in the behavior as "outcome expectations." If short-term benefits are experienced early in the course of the behavior, the behavior is more likely to be repeated. Barriers to a given behavior are experienced and stored in memory as "hurdles" that must be overcome to engage successfully in the behavior.

Every behavior is also accompanied by emotions or affect. Positive or negative affect before, during, or following the behavior is encoded into memory as information that is retrieved when engaging in the behavior is contemplated at a later time. Prior behavior is proposed to shape all of these behavior-specific cognitions and affects. The nurse helps individuals shape a positive behavioral history for the future by focusing on the benefits of a behavior, teaching how to overcome hurdles to performing the behavior, and building high levels of efficacy and positive affect through successful performance experience and positive feedback.

PERSONAL FACTORS.   The relevant personal factors predictive of a given behavior are shaped by the nature of the target behavior being considered. Personal factors are categorized as biologic, psychologic, and sociocultural. Examples of biologic factors include age, body mass index, pubertal status, menopausal status, aerobic capacity, strength, agility, or balance. Psychologic factors include self-esteem, self-motivation, and perceived health status. Sociocultural factors include race, ethnicity, acculturation, education, and socioeconomic status. Personal factors should be limited to those that are theoretically relevant to explain or predict a given target behavior.

Behavior-Specific Cognitions and Affect

Behavior-specific variables are considered to have major motivational significance. These variables constitute a critical "core" because they can be modified through interventions. They include perceived benefits, perceived barriers, perceived self-efficacy, activity-related affect, interpersonal influences, and situational influences. Measuring these variables is essential to assess whether change actually results from the intervention.

PERCEIVED BENEFITS OF ACTION.   Perceived benefits of action are mental representations of the positive or reinforcing consequences of a behavior. An individual's expectations to engage in a particular behavior hinge on the anticipated benefits. In the HPM, perceived benefits are proposed to directly and indirectly motivate behavior through determining the extent of commitment to a plan of action to engage in the behaviors. According to expectancy-value theory, the motivational importance of anticipated benefits is based on personal outcomes from prior direct experience with the behavior or vicarious experience through observing others engaging in the behavior. Individuals tend to invest time and resources in activities that have a high likelihood of positive outcomes. Benefits may be intrinsic or extrinsic. Intrinsic benefits include increased alertness and energy and increased perceived attractiveness. Extrinsic benefits include monetary rewards or social interactions possible as a result of engaging in the behavior. Initially, extrinsic benefits of health behaviors may be highly significant, whereas intrinsic benefits may be more powerful in motivating sustainability of health behaviors. Beliefs in positive outcome expectations have generally been shown to be a necessary although not sufficient condition to engage in a specific health behavior.

PERCEIVED BARRIERS TO ACTION.   Barriers consist of perceptions about the unavailability, inconvenience, expense, difficulty, or time-consuming nature of a particular action. Barriers are often viewed as mental blocks, hurdles, and personal costs of undertaking a given behavior. Barriers usually arouse motives of avoidance in relation to a given behavior. Anticipated barriers have been repeatedly found to affect intentions to engage in a particular behavior. Loss of satisfaction from giving up health-damaging behaviors such as smoking or eating high-fat foods to adopt a healthier lifestyle may also constitute a barrier.

When readiness to act is low and barriers are high, action is unlikely to occur. Perceived barriers to action in the revised HPM affect health-promoting behavior directly by serving as blocks to action as well as indirectly through decreasing commitment to a plan of action.

PERCEIVED SELF-EFFICACY.   Self-efficacy is the judgment of personal capability to organize and carry out a particular course of action. Self-efficacy involves judgments of what one can do with whatever skills one possesses. Judgments of personal efficacy are distinguished from outcome expectations. Perceived self-efficacy is a judgment of one's abilities to accomplish a certain level of performance, whereas an outcome expectation is a judgment of the likely consequences (benefits, costs) the behavior will produce. Perceptions of skill and competence in a particular domain motivate individuals to engage in behaviors in which they excel. Feeling efficacious and skilled is more likely to encourage one to engage in the targeted behavior more frequently than is feeling inept and unskilled.

The HPM proposes that perceived self-efficacy is influenced by activity-related affect. The more positive the affect, the greater are the perceptions of efficacy. In reality, however, this relationship is reciprocal. Greater perceptions of efficacy, in turn, increase positive affect. Self-efficacy influences perceived barriers to action, with higher efficacy resulting in lowered perception of barriers. Self-efficacy motivates health-promoting behavior directly by efficacy expectations and indirectly by affecting perceived barriers and level of commitment or persistence in pursuing a plan of action.

ACTIVITY-RELATED AFFECT.   Activity-related affect consists of three components: emotional arousal to the act itself (act related), the self-acting (self-related), and the environment in which the action takes place (context related). The resultant feeling state is likely to affect whether an individual will repeat the behavior again or maintain the behavior long term. Subjective feeling states occur prior to, during, and following an activity, based on the stimulus properties associated with the behavioral event. These affective responses may be mild, moderate, or strong and are cognitively labeled, stored in memory, and associated with subsequent thoughts of the behavior. The affect associated with the behavior reflects a direct emotional reaction or gut-level response to the behavior, which can be positive or negative—is it fun, delightful, enjoyable, disgusting, or unpleasant? Behaviors associated with positive affect are likely to be repeated, whereas those associated with negative affect are likely to be avoided. Both positive and negative feeling states are induced for some behaviors. Thus, the relative balance between positive and negative affect prior to, during, and following the behavior is important to ascertain. Activity-related affect is different from the evaluative dimension of attitude proposed by Fishbein and Ajzen (1975). The evaluative dimension of attitude reflects affective evaluation of the specific outcomes of a behavior rather than the response to the stimulus properties of the behavioral event itself.

For any given behavior, the full range of negative and positive feeling states in relation to the act, self as actor, and context for action should be measured. In many measures of affect, negative feelings are elaborated more extensively than positive feelings. This is not surprising because anxiety, fear, and depression are studied much more than are joy, elation, and calm. Emotional responses and their induced physiologic states during a behavior serve as sources of efficacy information (Bandura, 1985). Thus, activity-related affect is proposed to influence health behavior directly as well as indirectly through self-efficacy and commitment to a plan of action.

INTERPERSONAL INFLUENCES.   Interpersonal influences are cognitions involving the behaviors, beliefs, or attitudes of others. These cognitions may or may not correspond with reality. Primary sources of interpersonal influence on health-promoting behaviors are family, peers, and health care providers. Interpersonal influences include social norms (expectations of significant others), social support (instrumental and emotional encouragement), and modeling (vicarious learning through observing others). These three interpersonal influences determine individuals' predisposition to engage in health-promoting behaviors.

Social norms set standards for performance that individuals may adopt or reject. Social support for a behavior taps the sustaining resources offered by others. Modeling portrays the sequential components of a health behavior and is an important strategy for behavior change. The HPM proposes that interpersonal influences affect health-promoting behavior directly as well as indirectly through social pressures or encouragement to commit to a plan of action. Individuals vary in the extent to which they are sensitive to the wishes, examples, and praise of others. Given sufficient motivation, however, individuals are likely to undertake behaviors that will be socially reinforced. Susceptibility to the influence of others may vary developmentally and be particularly evident in adolescence. Some cultures place more emphasis on interpersonal influences than do others. For example, *familismo* among Hispanic populations may encourage individuals to engage in a particular behavior for the good of the family rather than for personal gain.

SITUATIONAL INFLUENCES.   Personal perceptions and cognitions of any situation or context facilitate or impede behavior. Situational influences on health-promoting behavior include perceptions of options available, demand characteristics, and characteristics of the environment in which a given behavior is proposed to take place. Individuals are drawn to and perform more competently in situations or environmental contexts in which they feel compatible, related, and safe and reassured.

In the revised HPM, situational influences have been reconceptualized to directly and indirectly influence health behavior. Situations may directly affect behaviors by presenting an environment "loaded" with cues that trigger action. For example, a "no smoking" environment creates demand characteristics for nonsmoking behavior. Company regulations for hearing protection to be worn create demand characteristics for employees to comply with regulations. Both situations enforce commitment to health actions.

Situational influences have received moderate support as determinants of health behavior and are now considered an important key to develop new and more effective strategies to facilitate the acquisition and maintenance of health-promoting behaviors in diverse populations.

Commitment to a Plan of Action

Commitment to a plan of action initiates a behavioral event. Commitment propels the individual into action unless there is a competing demand that cannot be avoided or a competing preference that is not resisted. Individuals generally engage in organized rather than disorganized behavior. In the revised HPM, commitment to a plan of action implies the following underlying cognitive processes: (1) commitment to carry out a specific action at a given time and place and with specified persons or alone, irrespective of competing preferences (implementation intention), and (2) identification of definitive strategies for eliciting, carrying out, and reinforcing the behavior. Identification of specific strategies to be used at different points in the behavioral sequence goes beyond intentionality to further the likelihood that the plan of action will be successfully implemented. For example, the strategy of contracting consists of a mutually agreed-upon set of actions to which one party commits with the understanding that the other party will provide some tangible reward or reinforcement if the commitment is sustained. Strategies are selected to energize and reinforce health behaviors according to individual preferences. Commitment alone without associated strategies often results in "good intentions" but failure to perform the health behavior. Commitment to a plan is similar to the concept of implementation intentions in which strong commitment is supplemented with when, where, and how the commitment will be realized.

Immediate Competing Demands and Preferences

Immediate competing demands or preferences refer to alternative behaviors that intrude into consciousness immediately prior to the intended occurrence of a planned health-promoting behavior. Competing demands are alternative behaviors over which individuals have a relatively low level of control because of environmental contingencies such as work or family care responsibilities. Failure to respond to a competing demand may have untoward effects for the self or for significant others. Competing preferences have powerful reinforcing properties over which individuals exert a relatively high level of control. The extent to which an individual resists competing preferences depends on the ability to be self-regulating. Examples of "giving in" to competing preferences are selecting a food high in fat rather than low in fat because of taste or flavor preferences, or driving past the recreation center where one usually exercises to stop at the mall based on a preference for shopping rather than physical activity. Both competing demands and preferences can derail a plan of action. Competing preferences are differentiated from barriers such as lack of time, because competing preferences are last-minute urges based on one's preference hierarchy that derail a plan for positive health action.

Individuals vary in their ability to sustain attention and avoid disruption of health behaviors. Some individuals may be predisposed developmentally or biologically to be more easily swayed from a course of action. Inhibiting competing preferences requires the exercise of self-regulation and control capabilities. Strong commitment to a plan of action may sustain dedication to complete a behavior in light of competing demands or preferences. In the HPM, immediate competing demands and preferences are proposed to directly affect the probability of occurrence of health behavior as well as to moderate the effects of commitment.

Behavioral Outcome

HEALTH-PROMOTING BEHAVIOR.   Health-promoting behavior is the end point or action outcome in the HPM. However, health-promoting behavior is ultimately directed toward attaining positive health outcomes for the client. Health-promoting behaviors, particularly when integrated into a healthy lifestyle, result in improved health, enhanced functional ability, and better quality of life at all stages of development.

Studies continue to be conducted to support the HPM model constructs. Most studies have focused on testing the predictability of the model rather than serve as a theoretical basis for developing and testing interventions to study the mechanisms of change proposed in the model. The model has been used to predict physical activity, nutrition, oral health, and hearing protection. An ongoing issue is that only partial testing of the HPM model is conducted in many studies, rather than measuring all of the model concepts. A possible reason may be the complexity of the model and the large number of concepts that need to be measured to test the full model. In spite of its limitations, the HPM model continues to make significant contributions in the prediction of health behavior in nursing and public health. In the 2012–2013 time period, over 150 papers using the HPM were documented in Google Scholar. In addition, studies are beginning to document the effectiveness of the model for guiding health behavior interventions (Dehdari, Rahimi, Aryaeian, & Gohari, 2013). Research has substantiated that it is a motivational model for understanding the major determinants of health behaviors. Pender has developed clinical assessment plans that can be used by nurses and other health care professionals to assess the eight model belief concepts. The concepts assessed are prior behavior, personal factors, behavioral specific cognitions, personal affect, interpersonal influences, situational influences, competing demands and preferences, and commitment to an action plan. The assessment can provide valuable information for developing counseling strategies to help clients change negative behavior or adopt a new healthy behavior. These plans are available at the University of Michigan website.

STAGE MODELS OF BEHAVIOR CHANGE

The fundamental assumption underlying a stage model of change is that differences exist in people in their likelihood of action, and different explanations are necessary for different stages of change. Stage models differ from continuum models in that the latter assume a linear relationship between predictors and behaviors, while stage models propose that individuals go through qualitatively different stages during behavior change and that predictors of behaviors change across stages (Parschau, Richert, Koring, Ernsting, Lippke, & Schwarzer, 2012). Interventions can be tailored to the individual's stage of change.

The best known health behavior stage model is the transtheoretical model of change. Another stage model is the precaution adoption process model, a seven-stage model that focuses on risk and changing behavior to reduce risks (prevention). Further information on this model is available in the literature.

Transtheoretical Model

The transtheoretical model, derived from psychotherapy and theories of behavior change, is an integrative framework to describe how individuals progress toward adopting and maintaining behavior change (Proschaska, Johnson, & Lee, 2009). The premise of the model is that health-related behavior change progresses through five stages, regardless of whether the client is trying to quit a health-threating behavior or adopt a healthy behavior (Prochaska & DiClemente, 1983). These stages are as follows:

- *Precontemplation:* An individual is not thinking about quitting or adopting a particular behavior, at least not *within the next six months* (no intention to take action).
- *Contemplation:* An individual is seriously thinking about quitting or adopting a particular behavior *in the next six months* (aware of the problem and intends to change).
- *Planning or Preparation:* An individual is seriously thinking about engaging in the behavior change *within the next month* (making small or sporadic changes).
- *Action:* The individual has made the behavior change and it has persisted *for less than six months* (actively engaged in behavior change).
- *Maintenance:* The change has been in place for at least six months and is continuing (sustaining the change over time).

The model contains three concepts in addition to the stages of change: decisional balance, situational self-efficacy, and processes of change (Di Noia & Prochaska, 2010). The concept of *decisional balance* from Janis and Mann's decision-making model (Janis & Mann, 1977) is integral to the model. The Janis and Mann conflict model assumes that sound decision making involves comparison of all potential pros and cons. Behavior should occur when the potential gains of engaging in the behavior outweigh the losses. Similar to previously described social cognition models, the benefits outweigh the barriers to change.

Situational self-efficacy also is considered a core concept in the model. Self-efficacy shifts in a predictable way across the stages of behavior change, with clients progressively becoming more self-confident. The concept is also a component in the social cognition models described earlier in the chapter.

Change processes refer to interventions used to facilitate change. Different strategies or techniques need to be used at different stages to facilitate movement through the stages of behavior change. The eight processes of change are presented in Table 2–2. They are categorized as either cognitive or behavioral processes or strategies for change.

In the early stages of change, cognitive processes are more important than behavioral processes for understanding and predicting progress. These processes are to a large extent internally focused on behavior-linked emotions, values, and cognitions. Behavioral processes are more important for understanding and predicting the transition from preparation to action, and from action to maintenance. Behavioral processes focus directly on behavioral change. After an individual's stage has been assessed, appropriate processes are implemented to help the client progress from stage to stage.

Many studies have been conducted using the transtheoretical model. Most of them have focused on smoking, followed by physical activity. Other topics have included stress management, bullying prevention, condom use, and obesity. Behavior change is most successful when all of the core concepts are integrated, not just the stages of change. However, the stages are more commonly used without attention to the other model concepts. Evidence also supports that those who are ready to change respond more to stage-based interventions than those who are not ready

TABLE 2–2	Cognitive and Behavioral Processes Involved in Behavior Change
Process	**Definition**
Cognitive	
Information Seeking	Exploring, reading, and learning about the desired health behavior.
Evaluating Barriers and Benefits	Assessing the pros and cons of the behavior change.
Acknowledging Contextual Influences	Recognizing the pressure of work, peer, and family attitudes on promoting healthy behaviors.
Behavioral	
Substituting Behaviors	Choosing positive behaviors to replace old, unhealthy ones.
Accepting Support	Obtaining help from family and friends to change the behavior.
Setting Realistic Goals	Creating obtainable steps to reach long-term health behavior goals.
Practicing Self-Discipline	Believing in one's ability to change, and actively prioritizing, committing, and performing the new behavior.
Managing Environment	Rearranging one's activities and social contacts to avoid old behaviors and promote the new health behavior.

(Horwath, Schembre, Motl, Dishman, & Nigg, 2013). In a dietary intervention program for youth using transtheoretical model concepts, stages of changes and processes were consistent mediators of program effects, providing some evidence for mechanisms producing the intervention effects (Di Noia & Prochaska, 2010).

Despite the success of the model in helping explain health behavior, additional concepts have been recommended. Rather than solely focusing on stages of change, studies are needed on the processes of change needed to promote behavior change (Armitage, 2009). Finally, using stage-specific interventions is theoretically appealing; however, whether the stage interventions produce more effective and sustained behavior changes than nonstage interventions is not known.

STRATEGIES FOR HEALTH BEHAVIOR CHANGE

Increasing healthy behaviors and decreasing risky or health-damaging behaviors are the major challenges facing health professionals. Thus, a core question is: What are the critical strategies or interventions, based on health promotion and prevention models and theories, which will enable nurses to assist clients to make desired changes in health-related behaviors? Behavior-change strategies based on the theories presented here are used to illustrate evidence-based counseling and behavioral interventions.

Raising Consciousness

The transtheoretical model emphasizes the importance of raising consciousness when the client either is not considering making a behavior change or is just beginning to consider changing a behavior. Awareness of the benefits of adopting a healthy behavior or discontinuing a risky behavior is enhanced by providing clients information and interpreting information in light of their personal situation. The nurse's role is to raise awareness of the problem behavior and any health concerns related to the problem behavior. Information should be provided about health-related issues relevant to the target behavior, including the short- and long-term consequences for the individual. It is important to assess possible reasons for not wanting to commit to a change, such as lack of knowledge, lack of skills, lack of resources and supports, and lack of time. The client should be given information needed to make the decision to change using literacy and culturally appropriate audiovisual aids as well as the client's personal assessment profile. Eliciting client feedback and response to the information should be done in a nonjudgmental manner. Consciousness raising is vital to assist the client in becoming aware of the health problem or behavior that that needs to be addressed.

The way in which the message is framed, rather than the actual content, is more effective in motivating behavior change (Grady, Entin, Entin, & Brunye, 2011). Message framing involves manipulation of information to promote health behaviors (Myers, 2010). Gain-framed messages, or those that focus on the positive consequences (benefits) of behavior change, have consistently been shown to be more effective than loss-framed messages that emphasize the negative consequences (costs). Gain-framed messages are more effective than loss-framed ones in prevention and changing behavior long term. These findings provide support for raising consciousness using positive health messages to increase clients' awareness and to promote behavior change.

Reevaluating the Self

Self-reevaluation, a process identified in social cognitive theory, is based on the premise that change results from the arousal of an affective state of dissatisfaction within oneself. This dissatisfaction leads to an appraisal of one's values related to the problem behavior. The client may ask questions such as: Will I like myself better if I quit smoking or become more physically active? If the client has a contradiction between personal values and current behavior, the issue is resolved by engaging in behavior change. Strong intentions to meet personal standards likely will increase performance of the behavior and eventually lead to sustained behavior change.

Self-reevaluation may involve mental contrasting, in which clients are asked to name the most important health behavior they wish to change (physical inactivity), state the most positive outcome of successfully changing the behavior (feeling better, losing weight), and describe the most critical obstacle standing in the way of accomplishing the wish (family responsibilities). When clients believe they can overcome the obstacles, they are more likely to change the behavior. When they do not believe they can change, the nurse's role is to assess the client's reasons for not engaging in change, including the value or perceived importance of making the change as well as perceived barriers to making the change.

Setting Goals for Change

Once clients are prepared to change, they must make a commitment to change by developing a plan of action (Delahanty & Heins, 2013). Making a commitment is an effective strategy to initiate the change process. Goals enable clients to implement the proposed action plan or initiate a new behavior. Goals are action plans implemented by the client. Well-planned goals focus the client's attention on the activities necessary to change the behavior (Pearson, 2012). Goals should be set by the client, with input as requested and needed from the nurse, and shared with the nurse and supportive others. Effective goals are specific and short term, action oriented, and can be realistically attained (Medynskiy, Yarosh, & Mynatt, 2011). The goals should be quantifiable and realistically attainable within a one- to two-week time frame so that progress can be seen to build self-efficacy in the ability to initiate a new behavior. For example, the client may set a goal to walk 10 minutes every other day for one week. If the goal is reached, a new goal is set. It is important for the goal to be tied to an action over which the client has control. Last, the client must be confident that the goal is attainable, as this builds self-confidence and self-efficacy. If clients have difficulty setting goals initially, the nurse should provide a menu of potential options for addressing the proposed behavior. Providing options enables the client to choose, enhancing personal control over the proposed behavior. As goals are met they should become more challenging, while remaining realistic and achievable.

Goals that include specific actions or intentions to implement the behavior are more likely to be achieved than those without an implementation plan. Implementation intentions are behavioral plans that detail the where, when, and how of what one will do to achieve the goal (Sniehotta, 2009). Implementation intentions have been called "goal primes," as they specify how the goal intention will be carried out (Van Koningsbruggen, Stroebe, Papies, & Aarts, 2011). For example, one may set a short-term goal of walking 15 minutes a day for five days to reach the long-term goal of becoming more physically active. The implementation intention may state that the individual will use the first 15 minutes of the lunch hour to walk on the path around the building at work with a fellow worker each day. Specifying implementation intentions has been shown to facilitate goal attainment (Rodgers, Selzler, Haennel, Holm, Wong, & Strickland, 2013).

Promoting Self-Efficacy

The most powerful input to self-efficacy is successful performance of the behavior. Whenever possible, the client should be facilitated to perform the target behavior and receive ongoing positive feedback about successful performance. For example, when the client selects low-fat foods from a display of food models, providing immediate feedback on the healthy choices increases self-efficacy. Immediate positive feedback builds self-efficacy relevant to the particular behavior. It is also important to provide the client with realistic strategies to overcome the barriers to performing the behavior, as this also increases the client's confidence in overcoming barriers to change. Learning from the experiences of others as well as observing the behaviors of others is one of the most effective social cognitive strategies for enhancing self-efficacy.

Observation of others engaging in the desired behavior is critically important for clients initiating a new behavior to help refine their performance capabilities and enhance self-efficacy. Modeling behavior by others is especially helpful when clients have articulated specific health goals but are uncertain about the exact behaviors that should be developed to move toward the goals. The following considerations are important to effectively use modeling to facilitate self-efficacy and resultant behavior change:

- Clients should share characteristics with the model, such as gender, age, ethnicity, race, and language.
- Clients should have an opportunity to observe the desired behavior.
- Clients should have the requisite knowledge and skills to engage in the behavior.
- Clients need to perceive benefits from engaging in the target behavior.
- Clients need to have the opportunity to practice the target behavior.

Enhancing the Benefits of Change

Behavioral beliefs in the TPB as well as outcome expectations in social cognitive theory are considered necessary conditions for behavior change. Planning for reward or reinforcement is a unique way to expand the benefits or positive outcomes derived from behavior change. The importance of reinforcement is based on the premise that all behaviors are determined by their consequences. If positive consequences result, the probability is high that the behavior will occur again. If negative consequences occur, the probability is low that the behavior will be repeated. Positive reinforcement (reward) rather than negative reinforcement (removal of an aversive condition) or punishment (aversive experience) provides the most effective motivation for behavioral change. When self-modification is the focus of an intervention, clients select the behavior they will change and the rewards they desire to receive for change. Behaviors that are to be reinforced must be clearly identified and a plan or contract for change negotiated between the client and the health care provider.

If a client wishes to increase performance of a specific health-promoting behavior or decrease a health-damaging behavior, one strategy is to obtain an initial frequency count of the behavior (baseline data), so that extent of progress toward the desired change can be accurately assessed.

This type of behavior promotes self-monitoring, a technique to promote awareness of personal risk change behavior (Van Achterberg, Huisman-de Wall, Ketelaar, Oostendorp, Jacobs, & Wollersheim, 2010). Self-monitoring has consistently been shown to contribute to successful behavior change. An example of a daily record of smoking behavior is presented in Figure 2–4.

Behavior to Be Observed:	Smoking		
Observation Categories:	Morning Afternoon Evening		
Method of Coding Behavior:		E = Smoking after or during eating and drinking S = Smoking while nervous in a social situation D = Smoking while driving the car O = Smoking at other times	
Smoking Record			
Date: Tuesday, August 26			
Morning		Afternoon	Evening
E E D O S S S E		O S S D S E E E	E O
Date: Wednesday, August 27			
Morning		Afternoon	Evening
E E E D D S S E E		S S S S D D E E E E	S E O

FIGURE 2–4   Self Observation Sheet   *Source:* Adapted from Watson D. L. & Tharp, R. G. (2003). *Self-directed behavior: Self-modification for personal adjustment.* (8th ed.). Monterey, CA: Brooks/Cole Publishing Co.

Benefits are classified as tangible, social, or self-generated and serve to reinforce desired behavior. Tangible benefits include visible objects or activities, such as making a purchase of a desired article such a piece of jewelry, or participating in a favorite activity. Tangible benefits also include weight loss or lower blood pressure or blood lipids. Social benefits include spending time with friends or family. Self-generated benefits include self-praise and self-compliments. Immediate and continuous reinforcement is important, particularly in the early phases of change, as it promotes rapid learning of the desired behaviors. Intermittent reinforcement applied later stabilizes the behavior and makes it resistant to extinction.

Many behaviors are too complex or require conditioning or adaptation to be acquired all at once, such as beginning a walking program after a long period of inactivity, or reducing the sodium content in one's diet. Gradually shaping desired behaviors is an effective approach to make permanent changes in lifestyle. An example of shaping is the following:

- Brisk walk for 15 minutes 2 days the first week
- Brisk walk for 20 minutes 3 days the second and third weeks
- Brisk walk for 30 minutes 3 days the fourth and fifth weeks
- Brisk walk for 45 minutes 4 days the sixth and seventh weeks
- Brisk walk for 60 minutes 5 days the eighth and ninth weeks

Each step toward the final behavior should be mastered before the next step is attempted.

After the client starts engaging in a desired behavior, the intrinsic rewards, such as losing weight, feeling more relaxed, or feeling more energetic, have reinforcing properties. When the behavior begins to offer its own reward, the nurse counsels the client that extrinsic rewards to enhance the benefits of the behavior may no longer be necessary.

Using Cues to Promote Change

Internal prompts coupled with external prompts encourage action; for example, "feeling good after brisk walking" coupled with "the invitation from spouse to take a walk." Synergistically, this provides powerful stimuli for behavior change. Table 2–3 presents an overview of possible cues that prompt health-promoting behaviors.

TABLE 2–3   Possible Cues for Health-Promoting Actions

Internal Cues

- Bodily states; e.g., feeling good, feeling energetic, recognizing aging, fatigue, cyclical discomfort
- Affective states; e.g., enthusiasm, motivation for self-preservation, high level of self-esteem, happiness, concern

External Cues

- Interactions with significant others; e.g., family, friends, colleagues, nurse, and physician
- Impact of communication media; e.g., motivational messages from television, radio, newspapers, advertisements, and special mailings
- Visual stimuli from the environment; e.g., passing a diabetic screening clinic, billboards, attendance at a health fair, passing a gym or exercise center, or viewing others participating in target activity

Three types of cues may be used to promote healthy behaviors and eliminate problem behaviors: cue elimination, cue restriction, and cue expansion. In *cue elimination,* cues for undesired behaviors are decreased to zero, for example, eating meals only with nonsmokers if cessation of smoking is the goal. In successful cue elimination, extinction of the behavior results.

Frequently, cues cannot be totally eliminated but can be reduced or restricted. In *cue restriction,* for example, the cues to eating may be reduced to one room in the house, the kitchen or dining room. By localizing the cues that activate behavior, arrangements for limited encounter with these cues are possible. In *cue expansion*, the number of prompts to desired behaviors is increased. For example, whereas personal preparation of food at home in one's own kitchen may prompt small servings of meats, fruits, and vegetables, the environment of a restaurant may prompt selection of rich entrées and desserts. In *cue expansion*, a menu at a restaurant provides cues for looking only at salad and vegetable options rather than scanning the dessert section. By expanding the range of cues that elicit specific responses, desirable behaviors may occur more frequently and with greater regularity. Using environmental cues conducive to the behavior through the elimination, restriction, or expansion of cues assists clients in creating internal and external conditions to support positive health practices.

Managing Barriers to Change

Barriers to change are central constructs in the health belief model, the social cognitive model, and the health promotion model. Behavior change is facilitated by working with the client to minimize or eliminate barriers to action. It is futile to encourage clients to take actions that are highly likely to be blocked or cause frustration or are unrealistic. Internal barriers may include the following:

- Unclear short-term and long-term goals
- Lack of knowledge and/or skills needed to make change
- Lack of resources
- Perceptions of lack of control
- Lack of motivation
- Lack of support

Barriers such as these often need to be addressed early in the change process using consciousness raising and self-reevaluations prior to initiating the change.

The interaction of level of readiness and barriers to action is depicted in Table 2–4. Consequences and appropriate interventions also are presented. When clients have a high level of readiness to engage in health-promoting or preventive behaviors and barriers are low, a low-intensity cue, such as a telephone or e-mail reminder, is sufficient to activate behavior. A high-intensity cue under these conditions may actually be a negative force. When readiness is high and barriers to action are formidable, barriers must be reduced or eliminated. When both readiness and barriers are low, the initial focus should be to promote readiness through raising self-awareness, clarifying misconceptions or concerns, and providing information and access to resources. When readiness is low and barriers are high, both factors should be addressed, or behavior change is unlikely to occur.

Significant others may be a barrier to health actions. As noted in the TPB and the HPM, social norms play a role in behavior change. When family members or other persons disagree or

TABLE 2–4   Interrelationships among Level of Readiness to Take Health Actions, Barriers, Consequences for Clients, and Nursing Interventions

Level of Readiness	Barriers to Action	Consequences for Client	Nursing Interventions
High	Low	Action	Support and encouragement; provide low-intensity cue
High	High	Conflict	Assist client in lowering barriers to action
Low	Low	Conflict	Provide high-intensity cue
Low	High	No action	Assist client in lowering barriers to action and then provide high-intensity cue

are neutral or apathetic toward health behaviors, the constraints created for the client depend on the following factors:

- Importance of disagreeing persons to the client: Is this person influential in the client's life?
- Extent of disagreement of important persons: Is this person voicing a large disagreement or is it a minor concern?
- Number of persons important to the client who disagree with the behavior: How many important persons are against the action?
- Extent to which the client is self-directed rather than other dependent: Is it a significant concern to the client if important others are not on board with the change?

Membership in support groups may be beneficial at this point to provide needed support not provided by family or friends, to identify barriers likely to be encountered in making changes, and to suggest strategies to overcome the identified constraints.

TAILORING BEHAVIOR CHANGE INTERVENTIONS

Tailoring is a process for creating individualized communication to meet the unique needs of an individual (Wanyonyi, Themessl-Huber, Humphris, & Freeman, 2011). Tailored health materials are personalized, based on characteristics unique to that person, related to the outcome of interest, and derived from an individual assessment. Tailored materials are considered more effective than generic or targeted communication in terms of engaging individuals, building self-efficacy, and improving health behaviors, and they are more likely to be read, remembered, and viewed more positively, as they are personally relevant. Generic communication is not personalized in any way, and targeted communication messages are developed for a certain segment of the population. Computer-tailoring is a form of tailored communication that involves a combination of strategies to reach a specific person based on that person's unique characteristics related to the health behavior and the results of an individual assessment (Krebs, Prochaska, & Rossi, 2010).

Tailoring print and interactive computer communications in health promotion and prevention offers exciting opportunities for nurses to engage in individualized behavior-change strategies. The computer provides the nurse–client team with more power to collect and process information, collaboratively set goals, and tailor strategies to assist individuals and families in achieving health goals. "One-size-fits-all" health education materials are rapidly becoming outdated as information technology expands the range of possibilities for using complex, interactive behavior change strategies that are relevant to clients, practical for providers, and cost effective for health care systems. The one-size-fits-all approach cannot address the range of details that vary from person to person and effectively guide individuals' health-related decisions and health behaviors.

Tailored health messages, defined as the delivery of health education based on an assessment of the client's health profile and behavior change models, are becoming more common in primary health care. These interventions combine behavior change models with health communication to provide education to address specific concerns or behaviors that are personally relevant to clients. Behavior change models guide the development of the health messages to maximize readiness for change or to motivate sustainability of the changed behavior. For example, if the transtheoretical model with its stages of change is the basis for the intervention, interventions are tailored to the stages most likely to promote change. Tailored interventions with the HBM involve tailoring information based on clients' perceived threats as well as perceived benefits and barriers to changing behavior. A tailored intervention using the TPB targets the individual's attitudes, subjective norms, and perceived behavioral control. Social cognitive theory–tailored interventions focus on changing efficacy expectations to meet the individual's desired outcomes (outcome expectations), such as helping clients identify behaviors that are under their control and easy to change initially, to increase self-efficacy. The selected theory provides the conceptual structure for designing the communication message to match client characteristics. Tailored health messages may be delivered through many channels: print, interactive computer programs, telephone, audio, video, the Internet, or face-to-face. A meta-analysis of face-to-face tailored health messages found that these messages have a positive effect on clients' health behaviors (Wanyonyi, Themessl-Huber, Humphris, & Freeman, 2011). Findings reinforce the importance of a readiness and needs assessment prior to initiating health education for effectively delivering health messages.

The advantage of computer-tailored interventions has been documented (Lustria, Cortese, Noar, & Glueckauf, 2009). Web-based tailored programs offer many advantages, including the ability to be delivered to wider audiences and to overcome geographical and temporal barriers. Computer-tailored health interventions delivered over the Web have a large diversity of formats and features. Interventions vary in level of sophistication, ranging from computer-assisted health risk assessments with immediate feedback to customized, longer-term, complex health programs with multiple opportunities for program access. Most programs are self-guided with minimal contact with the experts and consistently focus on four areas—health behavior, stage of change, risk factors, and information needs—and are delivered by print, CD-ROM–based applications, computer kiosks, or the Internet. Clearer guidance is needed for tailoring, and health outcomes must be evaluated.

Mobile telephones also have been effective for tailoring behavior change interventions. Mobile telephone interventions allow for instantaneous delivery of short messages at any time, place, or setting; can be tailored to individuals; allow for quantifiable interaction between the participant and the interventionist; and are more cost-effective than other telephone or print-based interventions (Fjeldsoe, Marshall, & Miller, 2009). The potential use of the mobile telephone is significant, as the higher-frequency user groups are adolescents, young people, socioeconomically disadvantaged populations, less educated, and people who rent and change addresses frequently. Of 33 mobile telephone studies identified, 14 met inclusion criteria for review (Fjeldsoe et al., 2009). Significant positive behavior changes were noted in eight studies, and positive changes occurred in 13 of the 14 studies. Important features of the interventions included how the intervention was initiated, how the short messages were initiated, origin of the content, and interactivity. The mobile telephone intervention has positive short-term behavioral outcomes. As the quality of the studies improves, the full potential of this technology will be realized.

MAINTAINING BEHAVIOR CHANGE

Maintenance of health behavior raises special challenges for the client. Changes in behavior that are transient accomplish little in enhancing one's health status. The behavior must be sustained in the environment in which it is learned, and the behavior must also be generalized to other situations. Factors important for continuation of positive health behaviors are similar to those necessary for initiating behavior change and include the following:

- Extent of personal skill to carry out the behavior
- Number of personal beliefs and attitudes that support the target behavior including beliefs about self-efficacy
- Extent of positive emotional response (positive affect) and cognitive commitment (intention) to perform the behavior
- Ease of incorporating behavior into lifestyle
- Absence of environmental constraints (barriers) to performing the behavior
- Extent to which the new behavior is intrinsically rewarding
- Extent to which there is social support for the behavior
- Consistency of behavior with self-image

The maintenance phase of health behavior extends from beginning stabilization of the new behavior throughout the client's life span. Habit formation facilitates maintenance of behaviors. Habits are behaviors that become automatic with little conscious effort. (See the discussion of habits in the Theory of Reasoned Action and Theory of Planned Behavior and Health Promotion Model sections.) Habit formation results in stable patterns of behavior. For example, a client who has incorporated exercise into the daily routine, such as walking at noon in the company fitness center, three to five days a week, is likely to continue to exercise as routinely as brushing teeth or showering.

ETHICS AND BEHAVIOR CHANGE

Although the Ottawa Charter is considered the ethical cornerstone for world health promotion, the charter is considered abstract and does not address the ethical issues facing individual health promotion. Ethical issues in health promotion are broad and found in all aspects of behavior change, beginning with defining the health problems, setting goals, intervention approaches used for change, and assessment of outcomes (Puhl & Heuer, 2010). As health care professionals work with individuals in health promotion, the goal is to help individuals to change their lifestyles to promote healthy behaviors. Concepts in the behavior change models are used to influence individuals to change, raising ethical concerns (Tengland, 2012).

Common ethical issues include personal responsibility versus government obligation, persuasion tactics, cultural sensitivity, and labeling and stigmatization (Puhl & Heuer, 2010; Carter et al., 2011).

Personal responsibility is an underlying assumption in the social cognition and stage theories of change reviewed in this chapter. It is based on the premise that individuals are free to make choices about their health behavior practices and therefore should take responsibility for changing behaviors. Although targeting individuals can be empowering for many, it is also seen by some as blaming the victim. Victim blaming, or locating the source of the problem within individuals or shaming individuals for not adopting change, de-emphasizes the role of social and environmental factors in behavior change.

Ethical issues in individual behavior change strategies include communication tactics, cultural insensitivity, and stigmatization. Often, clients do not have the desire to change, so they need be persuaded to do so. Persuasion, a communication strategy, becomes an ethical issue when information is emotionally manipulating, exaggerated, omitted, or misrepresented. Cultural beliefs and customs must be taken into consideration when designing change strategies for individuals (Unger & Schwartz, 2012). However, culture becomes an ethical concern when change strategies ignore or contradict cultural values or are viewed as offensive by the cultural group. Last, stigmatization, which links individuals to negative stereotypes and results in prejudice and discrimination, labels individuals in ways that promote shame. Obesity stigma is an ongoing example. Negative attitudes toward obese people are common in the United States and are considered an important social problem (Puhl & Heuer, 2010). Obesity stigma is similar to other examples throughout history when individuals and groups have been blamed for their disease and considered immoral, unclean, or lazy. Now, however, it is well known that obesity must be framed within the social and environmental conditions that have played a major role in creating the problem.

Additional ethical issues exist in health promotion that may infringe on an individual's autonomy and privacy. These are discussed in detail in nursing and public health ethics textbooks. Nurses must recognize these and other potential ethical issues that may arise in health promotion. Steps must be taken to ensure that ethical principles are applied in practice, as ethically sensitive interventions gain the respect and trust of individuals. Individual models of health behavior have much strength, and their authors now recognize the mandate to address the social, environmental, and political context as well as individual factors. Expansion of the models will enable many of the ethical issues to be addressed.

CONSIDERATIONS FOR PRACTICE IN HEALTH BEHAVIOR CHANGE

Knowledge of individual theories and models of health behavior enables the nurse to select the most appropriate model to guide the development of health promotion strategies and interventions. One's choice of theory takes into account the needs of the individual. For example, barriers such as travel or cost may be significant for a woman who needs to obtain mammography. The Health Belief Model is appropriate to identify perceived barriers and benefits, as well as the perceived threat of breast cancer for this woman in order to design effective strategies to enable her to participate in health screenings. In contrast, self-efficacy may be important to address for individuals who desire to develop new patterns of food shopping and preparation for changing eating patterns. Interactive information technology is available to extend the efforts of the nurse, especially for youth and adolescents.

Intervention strategies vary for different stages of change. For example, raising consciousness has been shown to be an effective strategy in making clients aware of the benefits of behavior change. This strategy is more effective in the early stages when individuals are either beginning to think about change or have not considered making a change. Restructuring the environment is effective when individuals are ready to implement the new behavior to provide cues to trigger the behavior. Having healthy foods, such as fruits and vegetables, available in the house serves as a trigger for healthy family eating. Smoke-free environments are triggers for tobacco avoidance. Community walking paths or bike lanes are visible cues for individuals and families to develop regular physical activity habits.

Existing theories, models, and related strategies enable the nurse to engage in evidence-based counseling and implement tailored interventions for health promotion and prevention. Tailoring interventions enhances the effectiveness of health promotion, as such factors as knowledge level, perceived needs, and health literacy are taken into account in designing health information. Additional information on evidence-based counseling strategies can be found at the Agency for Health Care Research and Quality (AHRQ) website.

OPPORTUNITIES FOR RESEARCH WITH HEALTH BEHAVIOR THEORIES AND MODELS

All of the behavior change models described in this chapter need further testing and expansion to continue to increase our understanding of the mechanisms that promote behavior change. The following are suggested avenues of research:

1. Continue to perform meta-analysis and reviews of research that has been conducted with the models to identify concepts that have consistently predicted health behaviors across social and cultural contexts. Design and test interventions using these robust concepts.
2. Identify the major sociocultural-environmental concepts that can be integrated into social cognition models and develop hypotheses to test these concepts in diverse groups and geographic settings.
3. Develop protocols to evaluate both short-term and long-term effectiveness of computer-tailored interventions.
4. Identify and test biologic concepts that can be incorporated as long-term outcomes of behavior change in the social cognition models.
5. Develop reliable and valid objective measures of concepts identified to expand the social cognition models.

Research requires collaboration of scientists from multiple disciplines to design and test the expanded models and to develop and test the effectiveness of new behavior-change interventions.

Summary

This chapter presents an overview of models and theories relevant to individual health behaviors. Development of theories that incorporate a wider range of powerful explanatory and predictive variables for effective health promotion and prevention interventions continues to be a priority. Although progress is being made in addressing the social context, as noted in Bandura's concept of environment, and interpersonal factors in Pender's Health Promotion Model, these concepts are defined narrowly and are static in their approach. The social context is constantly changing, as it is determined by social, cultural, economic, political, legal, and historical factors. All of these factors influence how individuals approach health.

Examples of theory-based behavior-change strategies also are described. These strategies can be implemented to help individuals make desired changes. Health promotion interventions empower clients to engage in a wide array of behavior changes. Effective strategies are tailored to individuals and their context to improve their health and well-being.

Learning Activities

1. Choose one social cognition theory described in the chapter and use it as a guide to develop an intervention to address a selected behavior change for you. Identify the stage of change you are in currently as it relates to the selected behavior.
2. Describe potential barriers that you will face in maintaining your behavior change and identify strategies to overcome them.

3. Write two short-term realistic, measurable goals and implementation strategies to attain the behavior and one long-term measurable goal. State the time frame for achieving the goals.
4. Use the eight beliefs described in Pender's Health Promotion Model to assess an individual and develop an intervention to change one behavior based on the assessment.

References

Ahmadian, M., Samah, A. A., Redzuan, M., & Emby, Z. (2012). Predictors of mammography screening among Iranian women attending outpatient clinics in Tehran, Iran. *Asian Pacific Journal of Cancer Prevention, 13*, 969–974.

Ajzen, I. (1991). The theory of planned behavior. *Organizational Behavior and Human Decision Processes, 50*, 179–211.

Ajzen, I. (2011). The theory of planned behavior: Reactions and reflections. *Psychology and Health, 29*(9), 1113–1127.

Armitage, C. J. (2009). Is there utility in the transtheoretical model? *British Journal of Health Psychology, 14*, 195–210.

Ar-yuwat, S., Clark, M. J., Hunter, A., & James, K. S. (2013). Determinants of physical activity in primary school students using the health belief model. *Journal of Multidisciplinary Healthcare, 6*, 119–126.

Asare, M., Sharma, M., Bernard A. L., Rojas-Guyler, L., & Wang, L. L. (2013). Using the health belief model to determine safer sexual behavior among African immigrants. *Journal of Health Care for the Poor and Underserved, 24*(1), 120–134. doi:10.1353/hpu.2013.0020.

Ashford, S., Edmunds, J., & French, D. (2010). What is the best way to change self-efficacy to promote lifestyle and recreational physical activity? A systemic review with meta-analysis. *British Journal of Health Psychology, 15*, 265–288.

Bandura, A. (1985). Model of causality in social learning theory. In M. J. Mahoney & A. Freeman (Eds.),

Cognition and psychotherapy (pp. 81–99). New York: Plenum Publishing Corporation.

Bandura, A. (1986). *Social foundations of thought and action: A social cognitive theory.* Englewood Cliffs, NJ: Prentice Hall.

Bandura, A. (2004). Health promotion by social cognitive means. *Health Education & Behavior, 31*(2), 143–164.

Buglar, M. E., White, K. M., & Robinson, N. G. (2010). The role of self-efficacy in dental patients' brushing and flossing: Testing an extended health belief model. *Patient Education and Counseling, 78*, 269–272.

Burke, N. J., Joseph, G., Pasick, R. J., & Barker, J. C. (2009). Theorizing social context: Rethinking behavioral theory. *Health Education & Behavior, 36*(suppl 1), 55s–70s.

Carpenter, C. J. (2010). A meta-analysis of the effectiveness of health belief model variables in predicting behavior. *Health Communication, 25*, 661–669.

Carter, S. M., Rychetnik, L., Lloyd, B., Kerridge, I. A., Baur, L., Bauman, A., Hooker, C., & Zask, A. (2011). Evidence, ethics, and values: A framework for health promotion. *American Journal of Public Health, 101*(3), 465–472.

Dehdari, T., Rahimi, T., Aryaeian, N., & Gohari, M. R. (2013). Effect of nutrition education intervention based on Pender's health promotion model in improving the frequency and nutrient intake of breakfast consumption among female Iranian students. *Public Health Nutrition, 1–10.*

Delahanty, L. M., & Heins, J. (2013). Tools and techniques to facilitate nutrition intervention. In A. Coulston,

C. Brouchey, & M. Ferruzzi (Eds.). *Nutrition in the prevention and treatment of disease* (3rd ed., pp. 169–189). Waltham, MA: Academic Press-Elsevier.

Di Noia, J., & Prochaska, J. O. (2010). Mediating variables in a transtheoretical model dietary intervention program. *Health Education & Behavior, 27*(5), 753–757.

Ersin, F., & Bahar, Z. (2011). Effect of health belief model and health promotion model on breast cancer early diagnosis behavior: A systematic review. *Asian Pacific Journal of Cancer Prevention, 12*, 2555–2562.

Fishbein, M., & Ajzen, I. (1975). *Belief, attitude, intention and behavior: An introduction to theory and research.* Boston, MA: Addison-Wesley.

Fjeldsoe, B. S., Marshall, A. L., & Miller, Y. D. (2009). Behavior change interventions delivered by mobile telephone short-message service. *American Journal of Preventive Medicine, 36*(2), 165–173.

Grady, J., Entin, E. B., Entin, E. E., & Brunye, T. T. (2011). Using message framing to achieve long-term behavioral changes in persons with diabetes. *Applied Nursing Research, 24*, 22–28.

Hall, K. S. (2012). The health belief model can guide modern contraceptive behavior research and practice. *Journal of Midwifery and Women's Health, 57*, 74–81.

Horwath, G. C., Schembre, S. M., Motl, R. W., Dishman, R. K., & Nigg, C. R. (2013). Does the transtheoretical model of behavior change provide a useful basis for interventions to promote fruit and vegetable consumption? *American Journal of Health Promotion, 27*(6): 351–357.

James, D. C., Pobee, J. W., Oxidine, D., Brown, L., & Joshi, G. (2012). Using the health belief model to develop culturally appropriate weight-management materials for African American women. *Journal of the Academy of Nutrition and Dietetics, 112*, 664–670.

Janis, I. L., & Mann, L. (1977). *Decision making: A psychological analysis of conflict, choice and commitment.* New York, NY: Free Press.

Kothe, E. J., Mullan, B. A., & Butow. P. (2012). Promoting fruit and vegetable consumption: Testing an intervention based on the theory of planned behavior. *Appetite, 58*, 997–1004.

Krebs, P., Prochaska, J. O., & Rossi, J. S. (2010). A meta-analysis of computer tailored interventions for health behavior change. *Preventive Medicine, 51*, 214–221.

Krones, T., Keller, H., Becker, A., Sonnichsen, A., Baum, E., & Donner-Banzhoff, N. (2010). The theory of planned behavior in a randomized trial of a decision aid on cardiovascular risk prevention. *Patient Education and Counseling, 78*, 169–176.

Lustria, M. L., Cortese, J., Noar, S. M., & Glueckauf, R. L. (2009). Computer-assisted health interventions delivered over the web: Review and analysis of key components. *Patient Education and Counseling, 74*, 156–173.

Manstead, A. S. R. (2011). The benefits of a critical stance: A reflection on past papers on the theories of reasoned action and planned behavior. *British Journal of Social Psychology, 50*, 366–373.

McEachan, R., Conner, M., Taylor, N., & Lawton, R. (2011). Perspective prediction of health-related behaviors with the theory of planned behavior: A meta-analysis. *Health Psychology Review, 5*(2), 97–144.

Medynskiy, Y., Yarosh, S., & Mynatt, E. (2011). Five strategies for supporting healthy behavior change. Work in Progress, CHI, May 7–12, 2011, Vancouver, BBC, Canada, ACM978-1-4503-0268-5/11/05.

Myers, R. E. (2010). Promoting healthy behaviors: How do we get the message across? *International Journal of Nursing Studies, 47*, 500–512.

Parschau, L., Richert, J., Koring, M., Ernsting, A., Lippke, S., & Schwarzer, R. (2012). Changes in social-cognitive variables are associated with stage transitions in physical activity. *Health Education Research, 27*(1), 129–140.

Pearson, E. S. (2012). Goal setting as a health behavior change strategy in overweight and obese adults: A systematic literature review examining intervention components. *Patient Education and Counseling, 87*, 32–42.

Pender, N. J. (1996). *Health promotion in nursing practice* (3rd ed.). Stamford, CT: Appleton & Lange.

Pender, N. J., Murdaugh, C. L., & Parsons, M. A. (2002). *Health promotion in nursing practice* (4th ed.). Upper Saddle River, NJ: Prentice Hall.

Pender, N. J., Walker, S. N., Sechrist, K. R., & Frank-Stromborg, M. (1990). Predicting health-promoting lifestyles in the workplace. *Nursing Research, 38*, 326–332.

Plotnikoff, R. C., Costigan, S. A., Karunamuni, N., & Lubans, D. R. (2013). Social cognitive theory used to explain physical activity behavior in adolescents: A systematic review and met-analysis. *Preventive Medicine, 56*(5): 245–253.

Prochaska, J. O., & DiClemente, C. C. (1983). Stages and processes of self-change of smoking: Toward an integrative model of change. *Journal of Consulting and Clinical Psychology, 51*, 390–395.

Prochaska, J. O., Johnson, S., & Lee, P. (2009). The transtheoretical model of change. In S. Shumaker, J. Ockene, & K. Riekert, (Eds.), *The handbook of behavior change* (3rd ed., pp. 59–84). New York, NY: Springer Publishing Co.

Puhl, R. M., & Heuer, C. A. (2010). Obesity stigma: Important consideration for public health. *American Journal of Public Health, 100*(6), 1019–1028.

Rodgers, W. M., Selzler, A. M., Haennel, R. G., Holm, S., Wong, E. Y., & Strickland, M. K. (2013). An experimental assessment of the influence of exercise versus social implementation intentions on physical activity during and following pulmonary rehabilitation. *Journal of Behavioral Medicine.* doi:10.1007/s 10865-013-9503-z

Rosenstock, I. M. (1960). What research in maturation suggests for public health. *American Journal of Public Health, 50*, 295–301.

Sniehotta, F. F. (2009). Towards a theory of intentional behavioral change: Plans, planning and self-regulation. *British Journal of Health Psychology, 14,* 261–273.

Sutton, S. (2010). Using social cognition models to develop health behavior interventions: The theory of planned behavior as an example. *Health Psychology,* 122–134.

Tengland, P. (2012). Behavior change or empowerment: On the ethics of health promotion strategies. *Public Health Ethics, 5*(2), 140–153.

Tuuri, G., Zanovec, M., Silverman, L., Geaghan, J., Solmon, M., Holston, D., Guarino, A., Roy, H., & Murphy, E. (2009). Smart Bodies school wellness program increased children's knowledge of healthy nutrition practices and self-efficacy to consume fruit and vegetables. *Appetite, 52,* 445–451.

Unger, J. B., & Schwartz, S. J. (2012). Conceptual considerations in studies of cultural influences on health behaviors. *Preventive Medicine, 55,* 353–355.

Van Achterberg, T., Huisman-de Wall, G. G., Ketelaar, N. A., Oostendorp, R. A., Jacobs, J. E., & Wollersheim, H. C. (2010). How to promote health behaviors in patients? An overview of evidence for behavior change techniques. *Health Promotion International, 26*(2), 148–162.

Van Koningsbruggen, G. M., Stroebe, W., Papies, E. K., & Aarts, H. (2011). Implementation intention as goal primes: Boosting self-control in tempting environments. *European Journal of Social Psychology, 41,* 551–557.

Van Zundert, R. M, Nijhof, L. M., & Engels, R. C. (2009). Testing social cognitive theory as a theoretical framework to predict smoking relapse among daily smoking adolescents. *Addiction Behavior, 34*(3), 281–286. doi:10.1016/j.addbeh.2008.11.004. Epub 2008 Nov 21.

Wanyonyi, K. L., Themessl-Huber, M., Humphris, G., & Freeman, R. (2011). A systematic review and meta-analysis of face to face communication of tailored health messages: Implications for practice. *Patient Education and Counseling, 85,* 348–355.

Warner, L. M., Schulz, B., Knittle, K., Ziegelmann, J. P., & Wurm, S. (2011). Sources of perceived self-efficacy as predictors of physical activity in older adults. *Applied Psychology: Health and Well-Being, 3*(2), 172–192.

Wingo, B. C., Desmond, R. A., Brantley, P., Appel, L., Svetkey, L., Stevens, V., & Ard, J. (2013). Self-efficacy as a predictor of weight change and behavior change in the PREMIER trial. *Journal of Nutrition Education and Behavior, 45*(4): 314–321.

Zoellner, J., Estabrooks, P. A., Davy, B., Chen, Y., & You, W. (2012). Exploring the theory of planned behavior to explain sugar-sweetened beverage consumption. *Journal of Nutrition Education and Behavior, 44*(2), 172–177.

CHAPTER 3

Community Models to Promote Health

OBJECTIVES

This chapter will enable the reader to:

1. Describe commonalities and differences in the various definitions of communities.
2. Discuss the key concepts and features of social-ecological models of health promotion.
3. Describe the characteristics of social capital and the role of social support in this approach.
4. Define the steps in the PRECEDE-PROCEED model in planning health promotion programs.
5. Compare and contrast the diffusion of innovation and social marketing models as effective models for health communication.

Health professionals' attention to community-based approaches to promote health and prevent disease has dramatically increased in recent years. The increased emphasis is due to many factors, including a greater understanding of the complex etiologies of health problems, an appreciation of the relationship of individuals with their environment, and recognition of the limitations of focusing only on individual behaviors to promote health. A greater understanding of the role of the sociocultural, physical, and political environments in achieving health has resulted in multiple approaches to promoting wellness. Individual approaches to health promotion identify a finite number of lifestyle areas that can be quantified and targeted for intervention. Community-based models move beyond individual lifestyles to distal factors that influence health, such as working and living conditions. In a community-based view, the social, political, institutional, legislative, and physical environments in which behavior occurs can be targeted to promote health. Community approaches emphasize populations and communities as clients and acknowledge that the greater environment influences individual health behaviors.

Although health care professionals recognize that attention to the social, physical, and political environment is necessary for health promotion, community-based models are not intended to neglect the individual. Individuals make up communities, so although the community may be targeted, individuals play a critical role in providing leadership. Community-based strategies for health promotion are community-led strategies, as control is placed with individuals who reside in the community. This chapter introduces the concepts in community models and provides an overview of the major community models and theories in the literature.

THE CONCEPT OF COMMUNITY

Community has been defined in multiple ways. The World Health Organization (WHO) was a pioneer in defining the community as a collective body of individuals identified by geography, common interests, concerns, characteristics, or values (WHO, 1974). A community can be considered a self-generated gathering of common people or citizens who have the creativity and capacity to solve problems. The definition of community has evolved from a structural focus on geographic boundaries, to a functional focus of people interacting in social units and sharing common interests. Whatever the definition of *community,* residents have a sense of community or identity, shared values, social norms, communication modes, and helping patterns, and identify themselves as being of the same community.

The community in which individuals live, work, and play is critical to health promotion and prevention. The community context refers to the interdependence that exists between selected aspects of a given environment or setting. The context includes personal, physical, cultural, and social aspects of environments and the relationship between them that may influence an individual's mental and physical health, opportunities, achievement, and developmental outcomes (Kegler, Rigler, & Honeycutt, 2011). The relationship between individuals and the context or social system in which they interact is reciprocal, as individuals may work to change their neighborhood context, just as the context influences the individual. For example, lack of street lighting may prevent persons from walking later in the evening. However, individuals can work together to get appropriate lighting installed in their community to facilitate safe walking.

The context encompasses social institutions and resources within a community, surroundings, and social relationships. Social institutions include cultural and religious organizations, economic systems, and political structures. Surroundings include neighborhoods, workplaces, towns, and cities; and social relationships include position in the social hierarchy, social group, and social networks. Health care professionals need to take all of these aspects into consideration to understand the relationship between the context and health (Miller, Pollack, & Williams 2011).

A risk environment is an example of a context in which factors interact to increase the chances of dangerous behaviors and harm. Risk environments have two key dimensions: the type of environmental influence (i.e., physical, social, economic, or policy), and the level of environmental influence (i.e., micro or macro; Caspi, Kawachi, Subramanian, Tucker-seeley, & Sorensen, 2013). Examples of the physical environment that may increase risks include lack of safe running water, inadequate public transportation, and heavy street traffic with noise and air pollution. Micro level influences that may increase risk include social networks, social norms, values and rules, peer and social influences, and the setting where one works and lives. Macro level influences take into account one's economics, gender, ethnicity, and culture, as well as the legal and policy environment, including state and federal laws. Micro and macro level influences intersect with the environment to either increase risks or enable individuals to promote health. Knowledge of the environmental context is necessary to create an enabling environmental context in which potential risks are reduced to maximize healthy behavior.

The client becomes the community when the focus is on the collective or the common good of the population instead of the individual (Shuster & Goeppinger, 2009). In the community models discussed in this chapter, the nurse works with individuals and groups. However, the outcomes of health promotion programs are expected to affect the entire community. For example, the nurse may work with parents to get safe walking tracks for adults and recreational parks for children. These changes improve the health of the community. In community health promotion, change occurs at multiple levels, beginning with the individuals and moving to the community as a whole. In other words, healthy individuals result in healthier communities. Policy changes may be necessary at the societal level for community-wide change to occur. When the community is the client, the nurse and the community work together to achieve mutual goals, as community members are at the heart of the process.

COMMUNITY INTERVENTIONS AND HEALTH PROMOTION

Community interventions differ from interventions within a community. Community interventions target either the majority of the population in a community or the community as a whole, as the goal is to change the entire setting. Community interventions have multiple advantages. First, they have the potential to make large-scale changes. Interventions based on community models focus on both high-risk persons and the larger community to promote health. The interventions are relevant for the population in the community. Other benefits include a high level of exposure to the intervention and increased generalizability of the intervention to other communities. Second, the interventions are likely to be valuable in the development of public health policies. Community changes are integrated into existing structures within the community, thereby changing the system that influences health behaviors.

Community models are based on four underlying assumptions (Minkler & Wallerstein, 2012). First, communities shape individual behaviors through community values and norms. Second, communities can be mobilized to change individual behaviors by legitimizing the desirable behaviors and changing environments to facilitate the new behaviors. The third assumption is that participation of community leaders is crucial for community ownership; and last, members of the community must have a sense of responsibility and control over the planned change. In other words, they must own the planned change for it to be successful. People are more likely to commit to and sustain change if they participate in identifying the problem, as well as in developing and implementing the program to address the problem (Torjman & Makhoul, 2012). Community interventions must engage participants to guide the change. Members are engaged early in the planning process to identify needs, develop priorities, and plan programs to promote health. Community-based models take into consideration individuals in interaction with their families, cultures, and social structures, as well as the actual physical environment. Community empowerment and community participation were identified decades ago as the twin pillars of community-based programs, and they are still considered the cornerstone for effective community change today.

Community empowerment is a social action process by which people and communities are enabled to participate and act to transform their lives and their environments (Minkler, 2000). The concept of empowerment refers to a process by which people and communities work together to gain mastery over factors that shape their lives and health. Empowerment principles are essential components in health promotion. Empowered communities are visible when people within the community participate in equal partnership with health professionals in defining their health problems and developing solutions. In addition, community members receive the benefits of the interventions and are partners in evaluating the effectiveness of the intervention. Community empowerment is not new in public health; public health nurses have long recognized the need for members to take control of the health of their community.

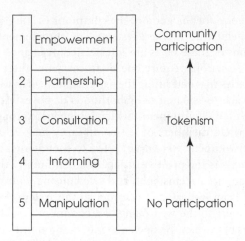

1	Empowerment	Community Participation
2	Partnership	
3	Consultation	Tokenism
4	Informing	
5	Manipulation	No Participation

FIGURE 3–1   Continuum of Community Involvement (Control) in Decisions

Community participation is the process of taking part in activities, programs, or discussions to promote planned change to improve the community. Community participation is a basic principle in health education and has been the major focus of chronic disease prevention. Community participation is expected to empower individuals and communities through group decision making and knowledge of resources, as well as creating new networks and opportunities. Participation of community members results in greater buy-in, higher participation, and greater sustainability. Empowerment and community participation go hand in hand, as empowered members participate in the health agenda for the community.

Community participation varies from little or no participation and control to high participation or engagement with leadership and control over the proposed action (Dooris & Heritage, 2011). The amount of community participation can be viewed on a continuum, which describes participation ranging from manipulation (no control) to empowerment (complete control over the project; Davidson, Johnson, Lizarralde, Dikmen, & Sliwinski, 2007; Dooris & Heritage, 2011). As Figure 3–1 depicts, empowering people enables the community to fully participate and have control of the project or program, including identifying the problem and making all key decisions for the program. Community empowerment involves shifts in power relations among individuals, groups, and institutions within a community. These shifts occur as people and institutions come together for social action. The nurse's role is to create opportunities to enable community members to become empowered to gain control over the factors that determine their health.

COMMUNITY ECOLOGICAL MODELS AND THEORIES

An overview of systems theory is helpful to understand ecological models. Systems theory was originally described by von Bertalanffy (1975) in the biological sciences as a complex of elements mutually interacting. These elements include multiple aspects of the physical environment and the social environment as well as personal attributes of the individual. Some of the major terms used in systems theory include *boundary, adaptation, entropy, negentropy, equifinality,* and *feedback.* In social-ecological models, communities are open systems in which there are interactions within a community among its members, as well as between community members and their environment. A community is made of many interrelated and independent parts that are organized to function for the good of the community. These parts include school systems, healthcare systems, churches, welfare systems, law enforcement, economics, and recreational areas. The functions of these parts are interrelated: A change in one part affects other parts of the community. Functions require energy to carry out their activities. Communities have geographical boundaries that determine the external borders as well as internal boundaries within the community, such as isolated neighborhoods of poverty or wealth. Communities experience change within their environments, which is managed through the process of adaptation. Adaptation occurs when members of the community make changes, or changes occur within the community environment. *Negentropy* refers to energy used by the system for maintenance or growth. *Negentropy* is the positive aspect of a community that promotes well-being, such as adequate social support systems, jobs, and safe housing. *Entropy* is the tendency of the system to break down. It is an indicator of disorder in the system. Entropy refers to negative aspects that do not contribute to the well-being of a community, such as deteriorating conditions seen in communities of poverty. As open systems, communities have inputs, throughputs, and outputs. *Inputs* take energy into the system. Inputs come from sources outside the system as well as members within the community. *Throughput* refers to the process of using inputs, such as community activities, and *outputs* are the results of these activities. Feedback occurs through communication of the subparts of the community as they interact to facilitate effective functioning of the whole community.

The term *ecology* has its roots in biology and refers to the interrelations between organisms and their environments. The concept has evolved to provide an understanding of the interactions of people with their physical and sociocultural environments (see Richard, Gauvin, & Raine, 2011 for a historical review). Ecological models emphasize the social, institutional, and cultural contexts of people in interaction with their environment.

Social-Ecological Model

Stokols (2000, 2004) expanded the concept of an ecology model to a social-ecological approach to health promotion. He described certain core assumptions about human health and the development of strategies to promote personal and collective well-being. First, the healthfulness of an environment and the well-being of its individuals are assumed to be influenced by both physical and social environmental components as well as the personal attributes of the individual. Second, environments are multidimensional and complex and can be described in physical and social terms; as objective or subjective (perceived), proximal or distal, and other attributes, such as noise, group size, and so on; or as constructs, such as social climate. Third, individuals within an environment can be described at multiple levels, such as individuals; families; groups or organizations, including schools; and populations. Finally, system theory concepts—including interdependence, homeostasis, and feedback—facilitate understanding of the interrelationships between people and their environments. Environments are viewed as complex systems, and efforts to promote well-being must take into account the interdependence among all components and levels of the environment. Figure 3–2 is an example of an ecological model developed by Sallis and colleagues (2006) to describe the environmental and political influences on four domains of active living: recreation, transport, occupation, and household.

In an ecological perspective, health promotion interventions target multiple levels: intrapersonal, interpersonal, organizational, community, and public policy (Golden & Earp, 2012). Intrapersonal factors include knowledge, beliefs, and related concepts in the individual

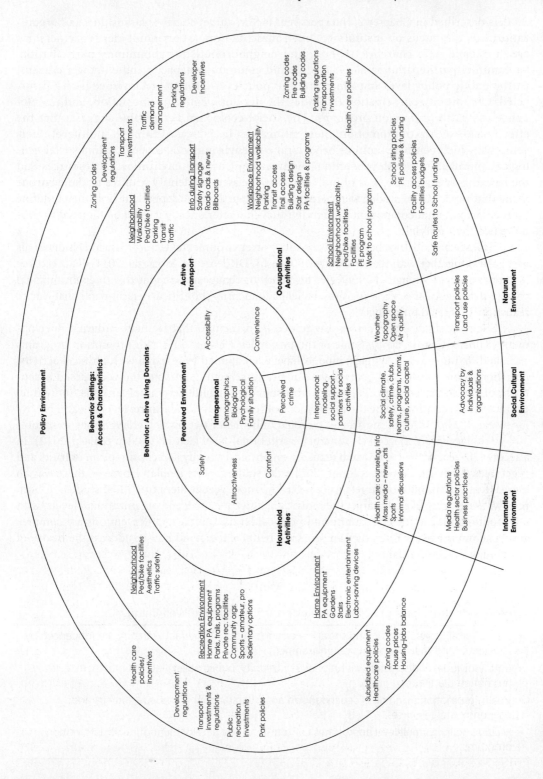

FIGURE 3-2 Ecological Model of Four Domains of Active Living   *Source:* Sallis, J., Cervero, R., Ascher, W., et al. (2006). An ecological approach to creating active living communities. *Annual Review of Public Health, 27*, 297–322.

models described in Chapter 2. Interpersonal factors target social relationships, and organizational factors focus on institutional environments. At the community level partnerships are developed with churches, schools, and neighborhoods for community participation. Community participation is necessary to build community capacity and empower citizens. At the public policy level, implementation of policies to promote or improve health is targeted. Community participation facilitates the development, implementation, and maintenance of health promotion programs. The social-ecological perspective suggests that the effectiveness of health promotion interventions can be increased through multilevel interventions, which combine multiple behavioral and environmental strategies. In a social-ecological approach to health promotion, the interplay between environmental resources and the health habits and lifestyles of individuals is assessed to identify features of the environment that promote or hinder well-being. Identifying the interdependent links helps define both environmental components and individual characteristics that must be targeted to promote healthy lifestyles.

Ecological models go beyond a focus solely on environmental factors to include individuals and groups together with the environment (Crosby, DiClemente, & Salazar, 2011). This is a key feature and major strength, as strategies for behavior change are integrated with environmental change strategies. However, it is also a challenge to identify the critical determinants that can be realistically targeted for change.

Social-ecological approaches are guided by principles that facilitate program development (Sallis & Owens, 2008). Some of the principles relevant for health promotion programs are listed in Table 3–1. Ecological models have been applied to research with physical activity, nutrition, tobacco use, and sexual behavior health screening. Despite the widespread acceptance of the social-ecological approach and support for multilevel interventions, individual characteristics continue to be the major focus of research. In a 20-year review of health behavior research, two thirds of the articles targeted only one or two levels. Interventions in schools and workplaces were more likely to target institutional-level factors (Golden & Earp, 2012). In a second 20-year review of research focusing on physical activity and consumption of fruits and vegetables (Richard, Gauvin, & Raine, 2011), the findings were similar. However, there was an increase in the number of targets to three in the more recent literature. Most studies in both reviews were more likely to target the individual, interpersonal, and organizational levels, with few studies aimed at the community and political levels. Multilevel interventions are complex and time intensive; however, they enable us to better understand how to address the health of individuals and communities.

TABLE 3–1 Principles of Ecological Models for Health and Well-Being

- The physical, psychological, and social dimensions of health interact with and are influenced by individuals and their socio-physical environment.
- Both individual and societal (institutional, community, public policy) factors influence health promotion planning.
- Health promotion planning is dependent on an understanding of individual needs and environmental resources.
- Multidisciplinary, multilevel approaches contribute to the development of health promotion programs.

Social Capital Theory

The theory of social capital focuses on how individuals and groups interact and how these interactions result in benefits for individuals as well as their communities (Brunie, 2009). The theory focuses on actions taken to either maintain or gain resources or valued goods in a society.

Although a definition of social capital lacks consensus, in most definitions, trust and reciprocity are central components. There is agreement on the conceptual meaning of social capital; however, it has been measured at many levels, leading some to question the usefulness of the concept. In his classic research, Putnam (2000) suggested that the core elements of social capital—trust and cooperation—are learned behaviors, indicating that social capital can be created. Putnam defined five characteristics of social capital: (1) measures of community organizational life or human interactions, such as clubs, churches, and other group organizations; (2) measures of engagement in civic affairs, such as participation in local and national elections or other types of political involvement; (3) measures of community voluntarism; (4) measures of reciprocity or mutual help among members of a community; and (5) measures of social trust. Social capital has also been conceptualized into five types of assets needed for communities to thrive (Manzi, Lucas, Lloyd-Jones, & Allen, 2010). These five capital assets are human capital (skills and education), social capital (social networks), built capital (access to amenities), natural capital (access to green space), and economic capital (income, resources).

Differences have also been described between bonding (within groups) social capital and bridging (across groups) social capital. Bonding social capital refers to the reinforcement of links between similar people. It builds strong ties but can also build higher walls to exclude those who are different. Bonding social capital is assumed to be a critical factor in creating and nurturing the group solidarity seen in close neighborhoods and ethnic groups. Bridging social capital refers to building connections between heterogeneous groups. Bridging social capital facilitates linkages among different agencies and organizations in a community around a common purpose. Linking social capital is how communities are vertically networked with institutions and political structures. However, the concept has been defined in multiple ways, so conceptual clarity has not been achieved. In studies of the link between the social capital dimensions of bonding and bridging neighborliness, both were associated with better self-related health (Beaudoin, 2009; Nogueira, 2009). Bonding and bridging social capital have also been found to be associated with neighborhood deprivation and self-rated health (Poortinga, 2012). In an intervention to increase social networking in young adult cancer survivors, those identified with weak bonding social capital used the network as a way to fulfill needs that were not being met (McLaughlin, Nam, Gould, Pade, Meeske, Ruccione, & Fulk, 2012). This study is an example of interventions that can be implemented to increase social capital. Although bonding and bridging were measured with different questions in the studies, they substantiate the value of both dimensions of social capital. Table 3–2 provides examples of components that have been used to assess bonding, bridging, and linking social capital.

A key ingredient of social capital is social support, as this is the initial informal link among individuals. It is important to note the difference between *social support,* a component of social capital, and *social capital,* as some authors believe they are the same. Social capital is a property of communities, and social support is a property of individuals. Debate continues over the extent to which social capital represents a new concept, because social support and social competence have been in the literature for many years. In addition, the similarities and differences between social capital and community capacity and their relationship to health have been investigated (Jung & Viswanath, 2013).

The social support component of social capital draws attention to the significant role of one's family and social connections as a builder and source of social capital through nurturance, caregiving, socialization, values, attitudes, expectations, and habitual patterns of behavior.

TABLE 3–2   Social Capital: Characteristics and Examples

Characteristics	Example
Bonding	
Neighborhood cohesion	The extent to which individuals in a neighborhood pull together to improve the neighborhood
Neighborhood trust and belonging	The extent to which individuals trust others in the neighborhood; the extent of feeling a sense of belonging to the neighborhood
Civic participation	The extent to which individuals in a neighborhood are involved in groups, clubs, or organizations on an ongoing basis
Bridging	
Social cohesion	Extent to which people from multiple backgrounds in a community get along together
Mutual respect	Extent to which ethnic differences in a community are recognized and valued
Heterogeneity	The extent to which an individual's friends are of the same ethnic group and have similar income and educational backgrounds
Linking	
Political participation and activism	The amount of contact community members have with people in their local organization; the extent to which individuals currently attend public meetings or have signed a petition
Political influence	Extent to which citizens believe they can influence decisions affecting their community
Political trust	The amount of trust members of a community have in their local government, the police, and the federal government

This component has also been referred to as *network social capital,* or the resources accessed through one's social connections (Legh-Jones & Moore, 2012). Participation in networks has been linked to health, the enhancement of social relationships, and social capital. Building trust, a component of social capital, begins with the attachment process in infancy and continues throughout early life. Family relationships and behavior also help establish the principle of reciprocity, the idea of receiving and giving in return, which is another major component of social capital.

Research to test the relationship between social capital and community health promotion has expanded dramatically in the past 25 years. Descriptive studies provide evidence for a link between social capital and physical activity, adolescent risk taking, and physical health (Thorlindsson, Valdimarsdottir, & Jonsson, 2012). An ongoing issue is the lack of consistency in defining and measuring social capital. Some authors focus on the individual, and others focus on community social capital. Multiple definitions may be required; however, they need to be generalizable across populations and measured consistently. Social capital is a complex concept that continues to be clarified and refined, providing evidence of its significance for understanding its influence on health.

COMMUNITY PLANNING MODELS FOR HEALTH PROMOTION

The PRECEDE-PROCEED Model

The PRECEDE-PROCEED model was designed to guide the planning and development of health education programs (Green & Kreuter, 2005). The model (Figure 3–3) provides a structure to identify and implement the most appropriate intervention strategies. It can be considered a road map that provides all possible routes; in contrast, theories suggest which avenues to follow. Two fundamental propositions of the model are as follows: (1) Health and health risks have multiple determinants, and (2) efforts to change the behavioral, physical, and social environments must be multidimensional and participatory.

The PROCEED framework can be considered an ecological planning model as it takes into consideration individuals as well as the physical and social environments. The model consists of two separate components, PRECEDE and PROCEED. *PRECEDE* stands for Predisposing, Reinforcing, and Enabling Constructs in Educational/Ecological Diagnosis and Evaluation. *PROCEED* stands for Policy, Regulatory, and Organizational Constructs in Educational and Environmental Development.

The PRECEDE planning and assessment process consists of three phases in sequential order. Planning begins with a social assessment to learn people's perceptions of their own needs and life quality. This step involves a community assessment, including problem-solving capacity, strengths, and readiness for change. In step 2, an epidemiologic assessment

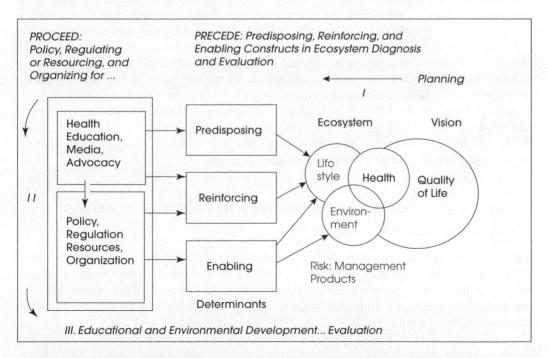

FIGURE 3–3 The PRECEDE-PROCEED Model for Health Promotion Planning and Evaluation
Source: Green, L. W., & Kreuter, M. W. (2005). The PRECEDE-PROCEED model of health program planning and evaluation. In *Health Promotion Planning: An Educational and Ecological Approach* (4th ed.). New York: McGraw-Hill. Reprinted by permission.

is performed to identify the health problems that are most important. Secondary sources of data (e.g., state and national surveys) can be used to identify major health problems in the community. Step 3 consists of an educational and ecological assessment to identify the predisposing, reinforcing, and enabling factors that must be in place to initiate and sustain the proposed change. Predisposing and reinforcing factors target individual-level factors, whereas enabling factors focus on community-level factors such as programs, services, and resources needed. Individual- and community-level theories are relevant to guide appropriate interventions. In step 4, administration and policy assessment and intervention alignment, development of intervention strategies, and planning for implementation occur. Policies and resources are identified that may facilitate or hinder program implementation. Resources needed, barriers to implementation, and organization policies that may affect implementation are assessed. In step 5, implementation of the planned intervention takes place, and both impact and outcome evaluations are performed in steps 6–8. Objectives, which are written at each step, are the basis for evaluating accomplishments.

The PRECEDE-PROCEED model has been widely used to plan health promotion programs (Glasgow, 2011). Despite its success, several weaknesses have been identified. Application of the model requires significant human and financial resources, as the model is data driven. The planning process is time intensive, which may dampen enthusiasm of community members who want to implement change strategies quickly. Cole and Horacek (2009) have developed a consolidated version to shorten the time frame needed to implement the assessment. Demographic, behavioral, organizational, and administrative data are obtained with a single survey instead of in distinct steps. Focus groups, made up of planning and steering committee members, are conducted to obtain environmental, organizational, and policy assessment data. The consolidated PRECEDE-PROCEED model overcomes the time needed to conduct the assessment while remaining a participatory planning model. The strength of the model is its comprehensiveness, as it incorporates both individual and community perspectives and can be used in a variety of settings. Application of the model by nurses includes development of a faith-based healthy eating program for African Americans (Buta, Brewer, Hamlin, Palmer, Bowie, & Gielen, 2011), health program planning in breast cancer (Tramm, McCarthy, & Yates, 2011), and changing cardiovascular risk behaviors in women (Peterson, 2012). In addition, a bibliography of more than 1000 published papers reporting application of the model as well as adaptations of the model is available.

COMMUNITY DISSEMINATION MODELS TO PROMOTE HEALTH

Diffusion of Innovations Model

The diffusion of innovations model was developed to help disseminate health behavior interventions that have been successfully tested into the mainstream for practical use (Rogers, 2003). The framework enables one to understand the process of innovation diffusion and the various stages involved in adopting a new idea, thereby narrowing the gap between what is known and what is put to use.

Diffusion has been defined as the process through which an innovation is communicated through certain channels, over time, among members of a social system (Rogers, 2003). It is a special kind of communication to spread messages about new ideas that might represent a certain degree of uncertainty to the individual or organization. Diffusion is a type of social change, as social changes may occur when new ideas are adopted. The terms *dissemination* and *diffusion* are used interchangeably in the diffusion of innovations model.

The four main elements of diffusion of new ideas are (1) innovation, (2) communication channels, (3) time, and (4) social system. These elements are found in every diffusion program. An *innovation* is an idea that is thought to be new. An innovation is broad and can be almost any new idea or novel approach to an old way of doing things. An example of an innovation is electronic books instead of traditional hard copies of books. It does not matter if the idea is not new, as it is perceived newness that decides how individuals will react. Individuals progress through five stages, known as the innovation-decision process, as they are evaluating an innovation for adoption (Weigel, Rainer, Hazen, Cegielski, & Ford, 2012). These stages are knowledge, persuasion, decision, implementation, and confirmation. In the persuasion stage potential adopters form either a positive or a negative attitude toward the innovation. According to Rogers (2003), the perceived characteristics of the innovation influence the adopter's attitudes.

The characteristics that also help explain the relative speed of adoption of an innovation include relative advantage, compatibility, complexity, trialability, and observability. *Relative advantage* is the degree to which the innovation is perceived to be better than the current, older idea. It does not matter if the innovation has no true advantage. What matters is whether an individual thinks the innovation will be better. Relative advantage may be perceived in economic terms or as social prestige, convenience, or satisfaction. *Compatibility* is the degree to which an innovation is perceived to fit with existing values and past experiences. Innovations that are consistent with the existing values and norms of the social system are more likely to be adopted. For example, an incompatible innovation might be the use of contraceptives in a traditionally Catholic community, as it is unlikely that the majority would adopt it. *Complexity* is the degree to which the innovation is thought to be difficult to understand or use. In general, new ideas that are simple to understand are more easily adopted than complex ones. *Trialability* is the extent to which the innovation may be considered tentative for a limited time period. Ideas that can be tried in installments are usually adopted more quickly than those that cannot be divided. Last, *observability* is the degree to which the results of the innovation are visible to others. The easier it is to see results, the more likely the idea will be adopted. Relative advantage and compatibility have been found to be most important in the rate of adoption of an innovation. Additional characteristics include the influence of the innovation on social relationships, the ability to reverse the innovation, the ability to easily communicate the innovation, the time and commitment needed to adopt the innovation, and the ability to modify the innovation over time. Communication must take place for an innovation to spread. Mass media channels are used to reach large audiences to provide initial information about the innovation. Because diffusion is a process of people talking to people, interpersonal or face-to-face communication channels are effective in forming and changing attitudes toward a new idea. Social media, the "participative Internet," is a new, cost-effective communication strategy for reaching large numbers of people (Korda & Itani, 2013). Social media include Internet-based social network services (Facebook, MySpace) Twitter, blogs, and mobile messaging platforms. As with other types of communication, social media require careful application to achieve the desired outcomes.

Innovativeness refers to the degree to which individuals, organizations, or systems adopt new ideas or practices. Five adopter categories have been described: innovators, early adopters, early majority, late majority, and laggards (see Figure 3–4). These patterns of adoption have been

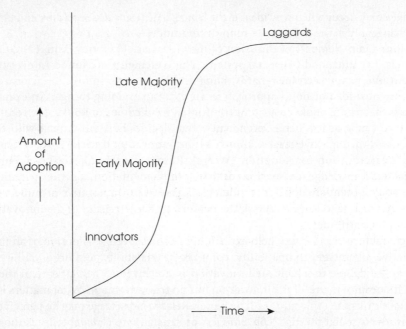

FIGURE 3–4   The Diffusion Process for Adoption of an Innovation

shown to be predictable in a variety of populations and settings. *Innovators* are active information seekers and can cope with high levels of uncertainty about a new idea. They are open to
taking risks and the first to adopt a new idea. Innovators are role models for others in the social
system. *Early adopters* have the greatest degree of opinion leadership in most social systems and
are considered to be the persons to check with before adopting the innovation. The *early majority* may deliberate before adopting, so they seldom lead in adoption of an idea. The *late majority*
view innovations with skepticism and may adopt only because of increasing pressure from peers,
or because they feel it is safe to adopt. The laggards tend to be suspicious of innovations and
change. They want to be sure that the innovation will not fail before they adopt and often slow
down the innovation diffusion process. Identification of adopter categories facilitates implementing new health behavior programs or behaviors, as it is important to know that not everyone will accept the change in the same time frame. Laggards, for example, will need more time
and evidence that the innovation is effective and safe. Early adopters, the opinion leaders in a
social system who can influence others, should be identified early in the process, as they will
help facilitate change.

Preventive innovations are defined as new ideas that require action at one point in time
in order to avoid unwanted consequences at a future point in time (Rogers, 2002). The rewards
of adopting a preventive innovation are delayed and intangible, and unwanted consequences
may never occur, resulting in a low relative advantage of the innovation. Because relative
advantage is one of the important predictors of the rate of adoption of an innovation, it is
understandable why preventive innovations may be slow or fail to be adopted. To increase the
rate of adoption of a preventive innovation, perceived relative advantages should be identified
and made as visible as possible. For example, the relative advantage of dietary changes for those
at risk for hypertension is low, as hypertension does not have immediate or obvious symptoms.

Perceived relative advantages, such as weight loss, should be identified and communicated. Strategies to speed up the adoption of preventive innovations include increasing the relative advantage, using role models to devote personal influence to promote the innovation, changing the system norms through peer support, placing educational ideas in entertainment messages, and activating peer and social media communication networks.

The innovation diffusion model has been applied with varying success. One possible reason for unsuccessful outcomes is that the nature of the innovation receives priority without attending to resource constraints. Additional reasons for unsuccessful innovations have been identified (Dearing, 2009). For example, authority may be confused with influence. Persons with formal authority may not be the influential leaders. The solution is to find the informal authority leaders and seek their advice on diffusing the intervention. Another potential reason for unsuccessful innovations is failure to distinguish between change agents, authority figures, opinion leaders, and innovation champions. An evaluation or assessment process will enable these role functions to be evident.

Diffusion of an innovation is a complex, multilevel change process, as change must occur at multiple levels across different settings, using multiple strategies to promote widespread behavior change. Understanding the diffusion process enables health care practitioners to implement behavior changes at multiple levels. The theory is based on many years of research in diffusion of innovations to change behaviors, programs, and policies to promote health. The theory incorporates strategies to promote widespread, long-term change and takes into account social structures and communication systems, as well as characteristics of the innovation, to promote successful change.

The innovation diffusion model needs more research to capture current Internet communication trends, as mentioned earlier. The diffusion innovations model presents communication channels as either mass media or interpersonal. However, communication channels that capture current communication trends, such as YouTube, will lead to new forms of health interventions. The benefits of technology for promoting health have been seen with mobile telephone- and computer-based messages. However, the increasing importance of new Internet communication channels points to the need for applying hybrid communication channels to models of health promotion communication.

Social Marketing Model

Compared to traditional models of behavior change, social marketing promotes voluntary behavior change by offering potential benefits, reducing barriers, and using persuasion to convince the target audience that the product (intervention) is the solution to the problem being addressed. In a social marketing model, commercial marketing technologies are applied to plan, implement, and evaluate programs to change the behavior of target audiences to improve health (Morris & Clarkson, 2009). Marketing practices that have traditionally been used in business advertising are applied to social purposes to adopt an idea, product, or behavior. Core principles are adhered to in social marketing. These include (1) a consumer orientation, (2) knowledge of competition, (3) mutual exchange of tangible or intangible goods, (4) segmentation of populations and careful selection of target audiences, and (5) marketing and intervention mix. A marketing approach goes beyond education to change behavior, as social marketers attempt to increase the attractiveness of the desired behavior so that consumers will desire the new behavior. Efforts are made to provide immediate effects, as immediate reinforcement has a greater potential to shape behavior.

The social marketing model is a set of principles rather than a theory. The framework considers the "Four Ps": product, price, place, and promotion. The *product* is the desired health behavior change, such as eating five fruits and vegetables daily. *Price* refers to the social, emotional, and monetary costs associated with adoption of the program or behavior. Higher-priced products are more difficult to implement than less expensive ones. *Place* is the distribution point or location of the intervention program. The more convenient the place, such as exercise facilities, the more likely the adoption will occur. *Promotion* refers to the behavior being promoted and strategies used to persuade adoption of the desired behavior. Both mass media and interpersonal communication channels are used to promote the change. An additional concept is the product's competition, or the existing behavior that must be changed.

The interrelated components and basic principles serve as guides to design implementation strategies for target populations. The product must provide a solution to problems that consumers believe are important to them. Consumers are confronted with choosing between the new behavior and the current risk behavior, so the benefits of the new behavior (product) must outweigh those of the current risk behavior. Price, from the consumer's perspective, is the cost, such as the cost of a joining a health club to exercise. Costs may also be time, effort, and emotional discomfort in changing behaviors such as smoking cessation. Place is also an important component for consumers, and social marketers must assess when and where the target audience will be most receptive to messages, or where and when they are ready to purchase products. Promotion to motivate change includes communication objectives for the target audience; strategies for designing attention-getting, effective messages; and credible, trustworthy spokespersons. Strategies may include mass communication, public information, consumer education, direct mail, public relations, and printed materials. Additional promotion strategies that may be implemented include service delivery enhancements, policy changes, and use of coupons to attract consumers. Two additional approaches are "edutainment," the use of traditional entertainment media for educational purposes, and media advocacy, the strategic use of mass media to increase public support to address the change.

The consumer orientation in social marketing distinguishes it from other approaches in health promotion. In a consumer orientation, one must understand the consumer's perception of product benefits, price, the competition's benefits and costs, and other factors that may influence consumer behavior. Research findings are used to identify recommendations for health promotion programs. Recommendations, based on research defining what works best, assist in planning marketing strategies.

Social marketing uses audience segmentation to select target audiences, a process of dividing the population into distinct segments based on characteristics that might influence their response to the marketing program. Segments identify smaller groups that may require different marketing strategies. Group profiles help health care providers decide which groups to target and the best way to reach the targeted segments.

In social marketing, programs should be monitored continuously to evaluate their effectiveness in promoting change. Continuous monitoring also enables identification of activities that need to be revised as well as activities that are most effective. The target audience is constantly checked for their responsiveness to the intervention. The evaluation of social marketing is multidimensional and consists of multiple measures. Criteria include impact, reach, sustainability, cost effectiveness, acceptability, and equity (Langford &

Panter-Brick, 2013). Qualitative and quantitative strategies are used for both formative and outcome evaluations.

The social marketing model can be applied as one component in program development. Social marketing concepts are used to guide qualitative studies to gain insight into individual behaviors prior to implementing change. For example, focus groups were used to conduct a formative assessment to identify health and nutrition perspectives of Native American women (Parker, Hunter, Briley, Miracle, Hermann, Van Delinder, & Standridge, 2011). The four principles of social marketing were applied to gain an understanding of the program components for a diabetes prevention program. Risky driving behaviors of taxi drivers were also identified in a qualitative study using a social marketing approach (Shams, Shojaeizadeh, Majdzadeh, Rashidian, & Montazeri, 2011). In focus groups using the four Ps, insights into what would be involved in an acceptable driving program were elicited. Focus groups were also used with African American adults to inform a social marketing campaign for walking (Wilson et al., 2013). The adults identified an additional "P," the promotion of physical and mental health.

The social marketing model is considered to be one component of multiple actions and theories to produce successful change. In research to reduce barriers to sun protection, social marketing interventions were combined with concepts from individual behavior change models (perceived barriers, attitudes, and knowledge of sun protection and skin cancer) (McLeod, Insch, & Henry, 2011). Marketing models are also recommended to achieve change (Mah, Deshpande, & Rothschild, 2006).

The four Ps in social marketing have been criticized as being outdated (Gordon, 2012). Other weaknesses that have been identified include focusing on short-term rather than long-term change, the static nature of the concepts, and the simplistic approach for contemporary marketing. It has been suggested that the "Ps" should be extended to include place, promotion, process, physical evidence, and people to promote a more consumer-oriented model. Although the debate continues, a common theme is to engage the stakeholder and the community. Focusing on upstream concepts, instead of the current downstream approach, also is recommended [see Gordon (2012) for a review]. Last, due to its simplicity, the addition of theories of behavior change to social marketing has the potential to increase its effectiveness in changing behaviors.

The social marketing strategy also has been criticized for having a negative impact on health equity, as the interventions have differential effects between socioeconomic groups (Langford & Panter-Brick, 2013). This is due to the social marketing focus on proximal downstream effects that target individual behaviors, rather than confronting upstream, environmental issues. Health equity in social marketing can be achieved by extending social marketing strategies to an in-depth understanding of the individual as well as the social environment in which the individual lives and works.

CONSIDERATIONS FOR PRACTICE USING COMMUNITY MODELS OF HEALTH

The concepts and principles of community models of health promotion are relevant for practice in assessing, planning, designing, and evaluating interventions and programs. Communities must be assessed prior to implementing health promotion programs. Assessment of an individual's physical and social environments, including social capital, will provide helpful information about facilitators and barriers to healthy lifestyle practices in the community. Knowledge of the physical environment will shed light on the resources (or lack thereof) in a neighborhood—such as safe walking areas and access to grocery stores or transportation—that influence one's ability to practice healthy behaviors. Focus groups incorporating concepts and principles of social capital are appropriate to gain an understanding of essential factors to consider in planning interventions. The diffusion of innovations model, as well as the social marketing approach, are useful in facilitating change within a community. Learning to identify individual characteristics of adopters will enable the nurse to choose specific strategies that must be stressed for successful change, depending on, for example, whether one is an innovator or laggard. Social marketing strategies that target specific populations as well as their environment offer opportunities for large-scale health promotion. As the nurse gains a broader understanding of the role of the community and greater social system in promoting health, small-scale interventions can be piloted to develop evidence to gain support for larger-scale, more complex programs.

OPPORTUNITIES FOR RESEARCH WITH COMMUNITY-BASED MODELS

The limited success of individual-level theories and models in achieving long-term changes in health behavior has led to an increase in the use of community theories and models in health promotion. Community-level theories and models are complex, as multiple dimensions of both the individual and the environment are addressed. The costs and complexity of designing and testing multilevel interventions have resulted in their limited use. Research is needed to develop consistent measures of the concepts and to test and refine the concepts and theories. Additional research in the following areas is recommended:

1. Perform state-of-the-science reviews and meta-analyses to identify the consistently significant concepts in the social-ecological model as well as missing concepts to target for interventions.
2. Develop and test reliable and valid measures of social capital.
3. Identify culturally sensitive and measurable community outcomes of health promotion.
4. Design and test multilevel community models of behavior change.
5. Expand and test the effectiveness of the diffusion innovation model to produce community-level changes in health behaviors.

Summary

The ongoing interest in community-based models to promote healthy behaviors has occurred because of a greater need to understand the complex etiologies of health problems, an appreciation of the interrelationship between individuals and their social and physical environments, and recognition of the limited effectiveness of individual models in promoting health. Community-based models focus on contextual factors that influence health, such as social conditions, and the political, institutional, legislative, and physical environments in which behaviors occur. Tests of community-level interventions show promising results.

Additional research is needed to identify the most effective models to guide health promotion interventions. Diffusion of innovations and social marketing models have the potential to promote widespread change.

Learning Activities

1. Describe three ways in which people in communities can be empowered to participate in their health.
2. What elements in a community would you assess using a social-ecological model for health behavior?
3. Apply the eight steps in the PRECEDE-PROCEED model to design a program to improve a specific health behavior such as physical activity for adolescents. Which individual and community theories would you choose to implement the program?
4. Using principles described in the social marketing framework, interview four individuals prior to designing a behavior change intervention. Interview minority women between the ages of 50 and 65 years, or minority men from ages 25–40 years. What additional factors in the environment need to be assessed in the interviews to be able to design an effective intervention?

References

Beaudoin, C. E. (2009). Bonding and bridging neighborliness: An individual-level study in the context of health. *Social Science & Medicine, 68*(12), 1–8.

Brunie, A. (2009). Meaningful distinctions within a concept: Relational, collective, and generalized social capital. *Social Science Research; 38*, 251–265.

Buta, B., Brewer, L., Hamlin, D. L., Palmer, M. W., Bowie, J., & Gielen, A. (2011.) An innovative faith-based health eating program: From class assignment to real-world application of PRECEDE-PROCEED. *Health Promotion Practice, 12*(6), 867–875.

Caspi, C. E., Kawachi, I., Subramanian, S. V., Tucker-Seeley, R., & Sorensen, G. (2013.) The social environment and walking behavior among low-income housing residents. *Social Science & Medicine, 80*, 76–85.

Cole, R. E., & Horacek, T. (2009.) Applying PRECEDE PROCEED to an intuitive eating nondieting approach to weight management pilot program. *Journal of Nutrition Education and Behavior, 41*, 120–126.

Crosby, R. A., DiClemente, R. J., & Salazar, L. F. (2011). Ecological approaches in the new public health. In R. J. DiClemente, L. F. Salazar, & R. A. Crosby (Eds.), *Emerging theories in health promotion practice and research* (pp. 231–249). San Francisco, CA: Jossey Bass.

Davidson, C. H., Johnson, C., Lizarralde, G., Dikmen, N., & Sliwinski, A. (2007). Truths and myths about community participation in post-disaster housing projects. *Habitat International, 31*, 100–115.

Dearing, J. W. (2009). Applying diffusion of innovation theory to intervention development. *Research on Social Work Practice, 19*(5), 503–518.

Dooris, M., & Heritage, Z. (2011). Healthy cities: Facilitating the active participation and empowerment of local people. *Journal of Urban Health,* doi:10.1007/s11524-011-9623-0

Glasgow, R. E. (2011.) Planning models and theories integrating components for addressing complex challenges. *Journal of Public Health Dentistry, 71*, S17.

Golden, S. D., & Earp, J. A. (2012). Social ecological approaches to individuals and their contexts: Twenty years of *Health Education & Behavior* health promotion. *Health Education & Behavior, 39*(3), 364–372.

Gordon, R. (2012). Re-thinking and re-tooling the social marketing mix. *Australasian Marketing Journal, 20*, 122–126.

Green, L. W., & Kreuter, M. W. (2005). *Health promotion program planning: An educational and ecological approach* (4th ed.). Boston, MA: McGraw-Hill.

Jung, M., & Viswanath, K. (2013). Does community capacity influence self-rated health? Multilevel contextual effects in Seoul, Korea. *Social Science & Medicine, 77*, 60–69.

Kegler, M. C., Rigler, J., & Honeycutt, S. (2011). The role of community context in planning and implementing community-based health promotion projects. *Evaluation and Program Planning, 34*, 246–253.

Korda, H., & Itani, Z. (2013). Harnessing social media for health promotion and behavior change. *Health Promotion Practice, 14*(1), 15–23.

Langford, R., & Panter-Brick, C. (2013). A health equity critique of social marketing: Where interventions have impact but insufficient reach. *Social Science & Medicine, 83*, 133–141.

Legh-Jones, H., & Moore, S. (2012). Network social capital, social participation, and physical inactivity in an urban adult population. *Social Science & Medicine, 74,* 1362–1367.

Mah, M. W., Deshpande, S., & Rothschild, M. I. (2006). Social marketing: A behavioral change technology for infection control. *American Journal of Infection Control, 34,* 452–457.

Manzi, T., Lucas, K., Lloyd-Jones, T., & Allen, J. (Eds.). (2010). *Social sustainability in urban areas: Communities, connectivity, and the urban fabric.* London: Earthscan.

McLaughlin, M., Nam, Y., Gould, J., Pade, C., Meeske, K. A., Ruccione, K. S., & Fulk, J. (2012). A video sharing social networking intervention for young adult cancer survivors. *Computers in Human Health, 38,* 631–641.

McLeod, G., Insch, A., & Henry, J. (2011). Reducing barriers to sun protection—Application of a holistic model. *Australasian Marketing Journal, 19,* 212–222.

Miller, W. D., Pollack, C. E., & Williams, D. R. (2011). Healthy homes and communities: Putting the pieces together. *American Journal of Preventive Medicine, 40*(1S1), S48–S57.

Minkler, M. (2000). Health promotion at the dawn of the 21st century: Challenges and dilemma. In M. S. Jamner & D. Stokols (Eds.), *Promoting human wellness* (pp. 349–377). Berkeley: University of California Press.

Minkler, M., & Wallerstein, N. (2012). Improving health through community organization and community building. In M. Minkler (Ed.), *Community organizing and community building for health and welfare* (3rd ed., pp. 37–58). New Brunswick, NJ: Rutgers University Press.

Minkler, M., Wallerstein, N. B., & Wilson, N. (2008). Improving health through community organization and community building. In K. Glanz, B. K. Rimer, & K. Viswanath (Eds.), *Health behavior and health education theory, research and practice* (4th ed., pp. 279–311). San Francisco, CA: Jossey-Bass.

Morris, Z. S., & Clarkson, P. J. (2009). Does social marketing provide a framework for changing healthcare practice? *Health Policy, 91*(2), 135–141.

Nogueira, H. (2009). Healthy communities: The challenge of social capital in the Lisbon metropolitan area. *Health & Place, 15*(1), 133–139.

Parker, S., Hunter, T., Briley, C., Miracle, S., Hermann, J., Van Delinder, J., & Standridge, J. (2011). Formative assessment using social marketing principles to identify health and nutrition perspective of Native American women living within the Chickasaw Nation boundaries in Oklahoma. *Journal of Nutrition Education and Behavior; 43*(1), 55–62.

Peterson, J. A. (2012). One theoretical framework for cardiovascular disease prevention in women. *Journal of Cardiovascular Nursing, 27*(4), 295–302.

Poortinga, W. (2012). Community resilience and health: The role of bonding, bridging, and linking aspects of social capital. *Health & Place, 18,* 286–95.

Putnam, R. (2000). *Bowling Alone: The collapse and revival of American community.* New York, NY: Simon & Schuster.

Richard, L., Gauvin, L., & Raine, K. (2011). Ecological models revisited: Their uses in health promotion over two decades. *Annual Review of Public Health, 32,* 307–326.

Rogers, E. M. (2002). Diffusion of preventive innovations. *Addictive Behaviors. 27,* 989–993.

Rogers, E. M. (2003). *Diffusions of innovations* (5th ed., pp. 5–34). New York, NY: Free Press.

Sallis, J. F., Cervero, R. B., Ascher, W., Henderson, K. A., Kraft, M. K., & Kerr, J. (2006.) An ecological approach to creating active living communities. *Annual Review of Public Health, 27,* 297–332.

Sallis, J. F., & Owens, N. (2008). Ecological models of health behavior. In K. Glanz, B. K. Rimer, & F. M. Lewis (Eds.), *Health behavior and health education theory, research and practice* (4th ed., pp. 464–484). San Francisco, CA: Jossey-Bass.

Shams, M., Shojaeizadeh, D., Majdzadeh, R., Rashidian, A., & Montazeri, A. (2011). Taxi drivers' views on risky driving behaviors in Tehran: A qualitative study using a social marketing approach. *Accident Analysis and Prevention, 43,* 646–651.

Shuster, G. F., & Goeppinger, J. (2009). Community assessment and evaluations. In M. Stanhope & J. Lancaster (Eds.), *Foundation of public health nursing in the community* (3rd ed., pp. 216–235). St. Louis, MO: Mosby Elsevier.

Stokols, D. (2000). The social ecological paradigm of wellness promotion. In M. S. Jamner & D. Stokols (Eds.), *Promoting human wellness* (pp. 21–37). Berkeley: University of California Press.

Stokols, D. (2004). Ecology and health. In N. J. Smelzer & P. B. Bolten (Eds.), *International encyclopedia of the social and behavioral sciences* (pp. 21–37). Berkeley: University of California Press.

Thorlindsson, T., Valdimarsdottir, M., & Jonsson, S. H. (2012). Community social structure, social capital and adolescent smoking: A multilevel analysis. *Health & Place, 18,* 796–804.

Torjman, S., & Makhoul, A. (2012). *Community-led development.* Ottawa, ON: Caledon Institute of Social Policy.

Tramm, R., McCarthy, A., & Yates, P. (2011). Using the PRECEDE-PROCEED model of health program planning in breast cancer nursing research. *Journal of Advanced Nursing, 68*(8), 1870–1880.

von Bertalanffy, L. (1975). General systems theory. In B. D. Ruben & J. Y. Kim (Eds.), *General systems theory and human communication.* Rochelle Park, NJ: Hayden Book Co.

Weigel, F. K., Rainer, R. K., Hazen, B. T., Cegielski, C. G., & Ford, F. N. (2012). Use of diffusion of innovations theory in medical informatics research. *Journal of Healthcare Information Systems and Informatics, 7*(3), 44–56.

Wilson, D. K., St. George, S. M., Trumpeter, N. N., Coulon, S. M., Griffin, S. F., Wandersman, A., . . . Brown, P. V. (2013). Qualitative developmental research among low income African American adults to inform a social marketing campaign for walking. *International Journal of Behavioral Nutrition and Physical Activity, 10,* 33.

World Health Organization. (1974). *Community health nursing: Report of a WHO expert committee.* Report No.559, Geneva.

CHAPTER 4

Assessing Health and Health Behaviors

OBJECTIVES

This chapter will enable the reader to:

1. Describe the expected outcomes of a nursing health assessment.

2. Identify the components of a nursing health assessment conducted for an individual client.

3. Examine life span, language, and culturally appropriate nursing health assessment tools for children, adults, and older adults.

4. Compare the similarities and differences among the various approaches to assessing the family, mindful of cultural influences.

5. Evaluate the criteria for conducting a screening in the community.

6. Compare the similarities and differences among the various approaches to assessing the community.

A thorough assessment of health and health behaviors is the foundation for tailoring a health promotion-prevention plan. Assessment provides the database for making clinical judgments about the client's health strengths, health problems, nursing diagnoses, desired health or behavioral outcomes, as well as the interventions likely to be effective. This information also forms the nature of the client–nurse partnership such as the frequency of contact and the need for coordination with other health professionals. The portfolio of assessment measures depends on the characteristics of the client, including developmental stage and cultural orientation. The nurse assesses age, language, and cultural appropriateness of the various measures selected.

Cultural competence is the ability to communicate effectively with people of different cultures. Providing culturally competent care is the cornerstone of the nursing assessment. The nurse's awareness of her own attitude toward cultural differences and her cultural worldview and characteristics are critical to her understanding and knowledge of various cultures. Recognizing that diversity exists in all cultures based on educational level, socioeconomic status, religion, rural/urban residence, and individual and family characteristics will ensure a more successful encounter (The Office of Minority Health, 2013). An online cultural educational program, designed specifically for nurses and featuring videotaped case studies and interactive tools, is available.

The Enhanced National Standards for Culturally and Linguistically Appropriate Services, based on a definition of culture expanded to include geography, spirituality, language, race and ethnicity, and biology, provides a practical guide to culturally and linguistically sensitive care (The Office of Minority Health, 2013).

Technology is having a significant impact on health care. The Electronic Health Record (EHR) promotes involvement of the client in developing a dynamic, tailored database. The EHR offers great promise to improve health and increase the client's satisfaction with his care. Data aggregation, cross-continuum coordination, and clinical care plan management are critical components of the EHR. It allows storage and almost instantaneous access to data while improving quality and efficiency in health care and improving communication among providers, insurers, and consumers (Figure 4–1).

Promising developments in EHRs are facilitating widespread usage. Among these are cooperation between health care providers and technology companies to create standards for seamless communication, regardless of vendor; cost subsidization of implementing EHRs to encourage physician usage; and incentives offered by Centers for Medicare and Medicaid Services (CMS).

The Health Information Technology for Economic and Clinical Health (HITECH) Act of 2009 provides incentives to physicians and hospitals to make "meaningful use" of EHRs by meeting objectives that positively affect the care of their patients. For example, one objective states that more than 50% of patients who request an electronic copy of their health information should have it within three business days. Clients should be encouraged to request their electronic health information so that they know what is in their record and can participate more fully in their care (CMS.gov, 2009).

Data Aggregation

- Data acquisition and exchange platforms for ADT feeds, claims and clinical data
- Ability to import provider directory files
- Algorithms and analytics for inclusion/exclusion criteria by population
- Processes, algorithms for patient-provider attribution

Cross-Continuum Coordination

- Shared care plans
- Activity tracking and real-time notification of encounters (ED, admission, discharge)
- Disease registries
- Health information exchanges
- Enhanced communication aides for care team connectivity
- Patient outreach and messaging

Clinical Care Plan Management

- EMR, case and utilization management systems
- Workflow automation and rules engines
- Assessment tools, clinical care protocols, and work lists
- Analytics for high-risk patient identification
- Telehealth and home monitoring capabilities

FIGURE 4–1 IT Support for Care Management Progresses Beyond EHR Functionality *Source:* Comstock, J. Asthmapolis, now Propeller, moves beyond asthma. *Mobilhealthnews.* September 10, 2013; Propeller Health, available at http://propellerhealth.com/, accessed September 25, 2013. The Advisory Board Company interviews and analysis.

While there are many benefits of the EMR, there are also questions to answer about best practices for the successful implementation of *patient-accessible* EMRs. These questions include cost, security, privacy, consumer and provider education, and user-friendly systems. To overcome some of the current issues, researchers are investigating tamper-resistant and portable health folders and evidence-based designs to evaluate consumer health informatics (Chen, Lu, & Jan, 2012; Li, Lee, Jian, & Kuo, 2009). In addition, access to web-based portal links (electronic patient portals) for patients to view and modify their record encourages adoption by patients.

Doctors who are more willing to open their doctors' notes via secure Internet portals, and patients who take advantage of the opportunity to access them, create transparency between providers and patients. This ensures more open communications and shared responsibility for the patient's health. Most patients are willing to accept some compromises to privacy in order to have more access to their health records and to make records more transparent (Robert Wood Johnson Foundation, 2009).

With the implementation of EMRs, computers are showing up in more and more health care settings. The introduction of computers into the examination room potentially is a barrier to meaningful provider/patient relationships. Health care providers should face the client while they are entering data, being careful to maintain eye contact and engagement with the client. To do otherwise is to focus on the technology, and not the client.

The Personal Health Record (PHR) is a another application to help consumers take charge of their health and has the potential to improve care, lower costs, and help clients obtain and manage the care they need. The PHR belongs to the user and is distinct from physician records (Figure 4–2).

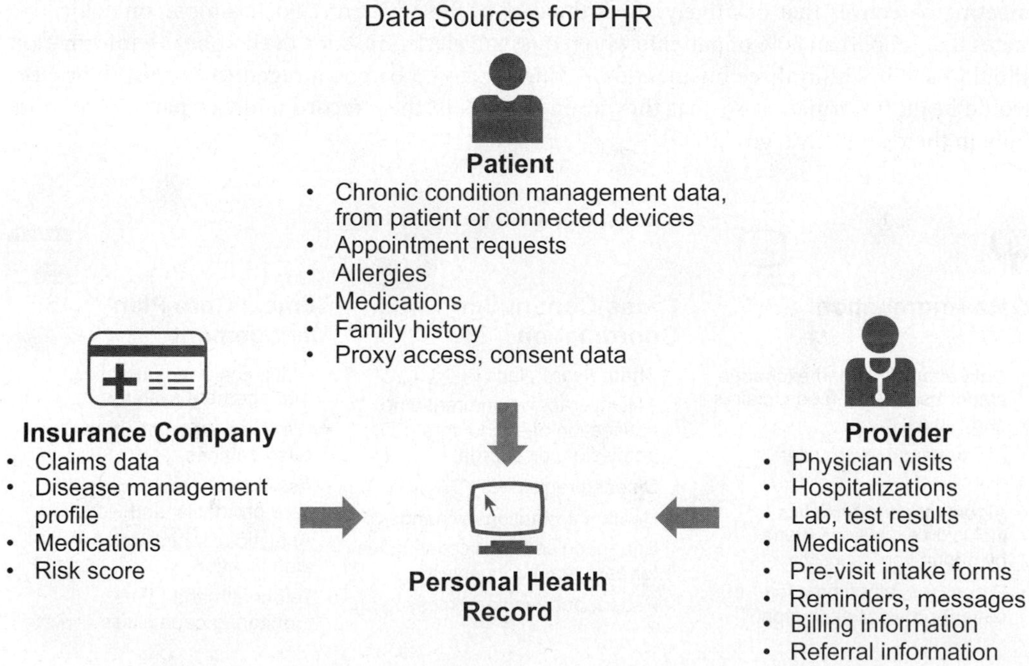

Data Sources for PHR

Patient
- Chronic condition management data, from patient or connected devices
- Appointment requests
- Allergies
- Medications
- Family history
- Proxy access, consent data

Insurance Company
- Claims data
- Disease management profile
- Medications
- Risk score

Personal Health Record

Provider
- Physician visits
- Hospitalizations
- Lab, test results
- Medications
- Pre-visit intake forms
- Reminders, messages
- Billing information
- Referral information

FIGURE 4–2 PHRs: Allowing Patients to Actively Manage Their Data   *Source:* The Advisory Board Company Interviews and Analysis, 2013.

GPS Device on Inhaler Provides Accurate Information on Asthma Complications

Inhaler usage automatically tracked, shared with physician

Physician reviews patterns and trends with patient during next scheduled visit

Physician able to proactively reach out to patient between visits if usage increases

Passive Tracking Improves Outcomes

80% Increase in medication adherence among users

>66% Proportion of app users who were well-controlled

Case in Brief: Propeller Health

- Health care technology firm based in Madison, Wisconsin
- Attachable GPS device for asthma and COPD inhalers sends real-time breathing and medication adherence data to provider

FIGURE 4–3 New Technologies Fostering Self-Care *Source:* The Advisory Board Company Interviews and Analysis, 2013.

CMS initiated a pilot PHR program in 2009 for clients to add supplemental information to their health record, authorize access to third parties such as family members, and track and view claims. The evaluation of this pilot showed the preferences of consumers to include download-able data, direct on-line communication between client and provider, simplified log-ins, and strong technical support.

Nursing clinics, community health centers, and primary care centers are using EHRs, PHRs, and/or cell phone technology to offer comprehensive resources, including easily cus-tomized and self-managed online portfolios (see Figure 4–3). The smartphone, named one of the top medical trends for 2013, increases greatly the option of clients' involvement in their health care. Governmental approval of mobile software applications such as ones that help clients monitor potential skin cancers, or that provide doctors with a mobile electrocar-diogram, are being promoted as ways to fight disease and get health care costs under control (ANA, SmartBrief, 2012).

Social media such as Facebook and Twitter optimize communications with clients. Tai-lored health information, delivered through these new informatics interventions, has the poten-tial for enhancing self-efficacy, improving decision making, increasing healthy behaviors, and fostering self-care. The potential for consumers to be involved in the ownership and mainte-nance of their health record with "cradle-to-grave" information is especially relevant for com-puter users and technology-savvy consumers who interface with providers and health systems. Age, race, and culture are significant discriminators of computer/Internet home usage, with 65 and older people's usage at 29.8% and all other age groups' usage ranging from 55.2% to 62.6%. Whites (56.1%) are more likely to use a home computer to connect to the Internet than Blacks (41.7%) and Hispanics (35.4%) are. Age is the greatest influence on the focus of Internet searches; for example, persons 45 years and older conduct Internet searches about health care more

TABLE 4–1   Reported Activity of People Using the Internet, by Selected Individual Characteristics: 2010 Population age 15 and over Number in thousands

Selected characteristics	Total connected to the Internet	Percent of those connected to the Internet who engage in each type of Internet activity			
		Take a course online	Search about healthcare	Search for government services	Search for a job
Total	145,286	11.4	35.5	33.2	24.8
Age					
15–24 years	30,687	13.4	17.6	19.8	31.5
25–34 years	27,963	13.5	35.3	34.1	34.3
35–44 years	26,471	12.2	38.1	36.4	27.0
45–64 years	47,917	10.2	42.8	39.1	19.1
65 years and over	12,248	4.3	46.2	34.6	4.0
Race and Hispanic Origin					
White	119,892	11.2	36.0	33.2	23.6
Non-Hispanic	106,947	11.4	37.0	33.8	23.1
Black	14,953	12.0	30.1	30.9	32.3
Hispanic (of any race)	14,309	9.7	27.5	27.8	27.9
Gender					
Male	70,229	10.9	29.6	32.0	25.1
Female	75,057	11.8	41.0	34.3	24.5
Language spoken at home					
Speaks English only at home	126,776	11.6	36.1	33.4	24.5
Speaks Spanish at home	11,141	8.8	27.1	27.6	26.3
Speaks other language at home	7,368	11.5	37.9	37.7	28.6

Source: U.S. Department of Commerce. 2010 Census Report

frequently than do those under 45 (Table 4–1; U.S. Department of Commerce Census, 2012). Non-computer users and vulnerable populations are at greater risk, which may exacerbate health disparities unless a safeguard system protects these groups. Safeguards include developing the concept of health care partners, opportunities for clients to access a computer, and staff available to enter information at the client's request.

Another technology making a significant impact on health care is telehealth, the use of electronics and telecommunications to support long-distance care. Health assessment occurs in a variety of settings including hospitals, clinics, offices, community centers, schools, and

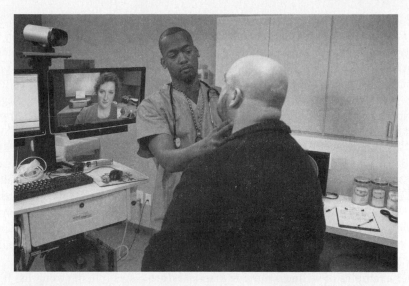

FIGURE 4–4 Telehealth Improves Access to Care   *Source:* http://www.telehealth.va.gov

homes; and the home is becoming a primary setting for assessing and delivering health services due in large measure to telehealth. The Veterans Administration is a major player in funding, developing, and using telehealth. As technology improves and cost decreases, telehealth is likely to have an even greater impact on health care (Figure 4–4). Three points are spurring adoption of telehealth:

- Governmental support and integration into accountable care organizations
- Consumer demand
- Technological innovation

NURSING FRAMEWORKS FOR HEALTH ASSESSMENT

Health assessment performed by the nurse is a collaborative partnership with the client that promotes mutual input into decision making and planning to improve the client's health and well-being. The initial assessment provides a valuable baseline to compare subsequent assessments.

The desired outcomes describe the following:

1. Health assets
2. Health problems
3. Health-related lifestyle strengths
4. Key health-related beliefs
5. Health behaviors that put the client at risk
6. Changes that improve the quality of life

Nursing frameworks are available for nurses to assess and diagnose health and health behaviors. *Nursing assessment* is the systematic collection of data about a client's health status, beliefs, and behaviors relevant to developing a health promotion-prevention plan, whereas nursing diagnosis is the identification and enhancement of assessment to maximize health status.

Nursing diagnostic classification systems (taxonomies) primarily focus on the individual and aspects of illness. Hence, positive health states (or strengths) of the individual, family, or community are not always adequately addressed in these taxonomies. As health promotion and prevention knowledge expands, taxonomies continue to include new definitions supportive of a health promotion/wellness perspective.

The North American Nursing Diagnosis International (NANDA-I) nursing diagnosis taxonomy responds to the nine human response patterns: exchanging, communicating, relating, valuing, choosing, moving, perceiving, knowing, and feeling (National Association of Nursing Diagnosis-International, 2013). The defining characteristics of each diagnosis, as well as related factors and risk factors, provide guidance about the critical assessment areas for the diagnosis. The NANDA-I classification provides a way to diagnose and intervene in selected health promotion and wellness processes and problems across the span of nursing practice (Popkess-Vawter, 2008). For example, stress overload occurs when the client presents feelings of tension and pressure that interfere with effective decision making, resulting in physical or psychological distress. Potential interventions, including active listening and decision-making support, address the stress overload diagnosis (Lunney, 2008).

Other examples of wellness nursing diagnoses/processes (client strengths) include the following:

1. Nutrition adequate to meet or maintain body requirements
2. Exercise level appropriate to maintain wellness state
3. Strength derived from one's spirituality

Case studies and sample care plans are available to illustrate how diagnostic statements provide direction for health promotion-prevention care planning.

Gordon (2009) grouped the NANDA-I diagnoses into 11 functional health patterns to assist in classifying nursing diagnoses:

1. Health perception–health management
2. Nutritional–metabolic
3. Elimination
4. Activity–exercise
5. Sleep–rest
6. Cognitive–perceptual
7. Self-perception–self-concept
8. Role–relationship
9. Sexuality–reproductive
10. Coping–stress tolerance
11. Value–belief

Gordon provides guidelines to conduct a nursing history and examination to assess clients' functional health patterns. As assessment proceeds, diagnostic hypotheses generate targeted or more detailed data collection. Refer to Gordon's *Manual of Nursing Diagnosis* for recommended formats to assess functional health patterns in infants and young children, adults, families, and communities (Gordon, 2009).

The Omaha Visiting Nurse Association System is a useful guide for community health nursing practice, a method of documentation, and a framework for community management. The Omaha System incorporates the needs of individuals and families in the categories of environment, psychosocial, physiological, and health behavior needs. These categories use key words such as *individual*, *family*, or *health promotion* in the individual and family categories. Nurse researchers have shown the usefulness of the Omaha System in quantifying nursing practice in community health, rural nursing practice, primary care, and wellness centers. A difficulty in developing nursing classification systems for communities is that nursing diagnoses/problem classifications focus on nursing practice, whereas community problems focus more on interdisciplinary practice.

Nursing Interventions Classification (NIC), a system that generates standardized nursing actions and interventions for providing care, is relevant for community health because nursing services are categorized and linked to direct reimbursement (Bulechek, Butcher, Dochterman, & Wagner, 2013). However, NIC does not have categories for the health behaviors of communities. The Nursing Outcomes Classification (NOC) system measures the responses of an individual, family, and community behavior/perception to a nursing intervention and is useful in all settings with individuals, families, and communities (Moorhead, Johnson, Maas, & Swanson, 2013).

The next phase of knowledge generation in nursing is the integration of terminologies into EHR information systems to support standards of care across settings worldwide. Integration will make it easier to describe and share interventions that work or do not work to help people be healthy and reduce costs. Research using data from information systems embedded with nursing standards and terminology builds nursing knowledge and documents the contribution of nursing to health care.

GUIDELINES FOR PREVENTIVE SERVICES AND SCREENINGS

An increasing emphasis on the prevention of disease has resulted in the development of varying sets of guidelines for the delivery of preventive services to individuals, families, and communities across the life span. These guidelines focus on clinical care directed toward prevention of specific diseases such as HIV disease and behavioral morbidity such as substance abuse.

The Guide to Clinical Preventive Services (U.S. Preventive Services Task Force, 2012) is an authoritative source for making decisions about preventive services. In 2009, the U.S. Preventive Services Task Force (USPSTF) recommended limiting the use of screening mammography. The recommendation garnered the media's attention and, according to one study, the percentage of women screened the year following the recommendation declined by 4.3%, suggesting that the recommendation had a chilling effect on the willingness of women to get mammograms. However, Block and colleagues examined data from the Behavioral Risk Factor Surveillance Study and observed no change in rates among women who had mammograms the previous year, but did observe lower rates of mammogram use among women who reported no mammogram in the previous year (Block, 2013).

Other experts report 1.3 million overdiagnosed breast cancers over 30 years, meaning that their screening detected tumors that would never lead to clinical symptoms (Bleyer & Welsh, 2012). However, the American Cancer Society and the American Radiology Association continue to recommend that women undergo a yearly mammogram beginning at age 40.

Screening is not right for everyone or every health problem. Screenings to detect particular, unrecognized health problems in individuals who are members of at-risk groups reduce false alarms. However, data are not sufficient to address all the uncertainties of general screenings.

Screenings uncover health problems in an efficient and economically feasible manner when the following factors are present:

1. The specific population has a high prevalence of the disease or health problem.
2. Treatment is available if the condition is identified.
3. Screening instruments are valid and reliable.

The cost of conducting screenings bears on the decision to offer large-scale screenings. For example, conducting a screening to detect osteoporosis requires special equipment, and the cost may be high due to the number of machines needed to screen in a timely, efficient manner. In addition to cost, targeted screenings should consider race/ethnicity, age, and low income and how these factors relate to increased or decreased willingness to participate in screenings, along with the risks and benefits (Kressin, Manze, Russell, Katz, Claudio, Green, & Wang, 2010).

Elective Preventive Services Selector (ePSS) is a quick, hands-on tool available to primary care providers to identify screening services that are appropriate for particular clients based on the recommendations of the U.S. Preventive Services Task Force, and can be searched by client characteristics, such as age, sex, and behavioral risk factors. ePSS is available as Web and Mobile applications for the iPhone, iPad, and other mobile devices. Through these application nurses and other clinicians have preventive information—recommendations, clinical considerations, and selected practice tools—available at the point of care (U.S. Preventive Services Task Force, 2012). *Guide to Clinical Preventive Services* (U.S. Department of Commerce Census, 2012) and *Bright Futures: Guidelines for Health Supervision of Infants, Children, and Adolescents* (Hagan, Shaw, & Duncan, 2008) also are important guidelines for nurses to be familiar with and use to ensure that clients across the life span benefit from state-of-the-art preventive services.

ASSESSMENT OF THE INDIVIDUAL CLIENT

Assessment of the individual client in the context of health promotion extends beyond physical assessment to include a comprehensive examination of other health parameters and health behaviors. The purpose of the assessment, setting, culture, and age determine the components of health assessment. The components are as follows:

- Functional health patterns
- Physical fitness
- Nutrition
- Life stress
- Spiritual health
- Social support systems
- Health beliefs and lifestyle

Functional assessment of health patterns comprises a health history, including hereditary and family characteristics, and physical assessment. Assessment components focus on individuals and have particular relevance for health promotion and prevention.

Physical Fitness

Physical activity is an important part of personal health status (see Chapter 6). Determining one's level of physical fitness is a critical part of the nursing assessment. A sedentary lifestyle, for many individuals, begins early in childhood and continues into adulthood. The assessment is applicable to clients of all ages, with restrictions on some components for physically compromised individuals. Skill-related physical fitness and health-related physical fitness focus on different qualities.

Skill-related fitness focuses on qualities that contribute to successful athletic performance: agility, speed, power, and reaction time. Health-related fitness focuses on qualities that contribute to general health and include **cardio-respiratory endurance** (aerobic capacity); **muscular endurance, strength,** and **flexibility;** and **body composition.**

CARDIO-RESPIRATORY (CR) ENDURANCE (AEROBIC CAPACITY). Aerobic capacity is the *most important component* of fitness. Fitness reflects the ability of the CR system to efficiently adjust to and recover from exercise. Research shows that individuals with an acceptable aerobic capacity have a reduced risk of obesity, diabetes, high blood pressure, and other health problems.

MUSCULAR ENDURANCE, STRENGTH, AND FLEXIBILITY. The goal of muscular endurance, strength, and flexibility tests is to determine the functional health status of the musculoskeletal system. It is important to have strong muscles that maintain body structure and endurance. The strength and endurance of the upper body muscles are good indicators of overall fitness. Flexibility, the ability to move muscles and joints through their maximum range of motion, also is an important component of physical fitness. Flexibility decreases with age and chronic illness. The lack of ability to flex or extend muscles or joints often reflects poor health habits, such as sedentary lifestyle, poor posture, or faulty body mechanics. Loss of flexibility greatly decreases one's ability to move about with ease and comfort.

BODY COMPOSITION. The increased prevalence of overweight and obesity in children and adults in the United States is a concern for both the public and private sectors. The availability of high-fat and low-cost fast foods and the decline in levels of physical activity contribute to these trends. Increased levels of body fat are associated with cardiovascular disease, diabetes, and stroke in adults; and diabetes, hypertension, and increased cholesterol levels occur more frequently in overweight and obese children.

Estimates of body fat include underwater weighing, bioelectrical impedance, skin fold measures, and other anthropometry measures such as the Body Mass Index (BMI). Each method has limitations leading to measurement errors of 2% to 3% for estimates of body fat, with the BMI error rate as great as 6% because body weight includes bone and muscle mass and not just fat composition.

Bioelectrical impedance analysis (BIA) provides a measure of body fat when a small, safe electrical current passes through the body, carried by water and electrolytes of the fluid spaces. Impedance is greatest in fat tissue, which contains only 10 to 20% water, while muscle tissue, which contains 70 to 75% water, allows the signal to pass more easily. Height and weight, body type, gender, age, fitness level, and BIA are measures used to calculate percentage of body fat, muscle mass, and hydration level (American College of Sports Medicine, 2009).

BIA is useful in healthy, young, normally hydrated teens and adults, and for monitoring these groups for changes in body fat composition over time. Body fat scales (similar to bathroom scales) and handheld body fat analyzers, both available at reasonable cost, also provide a measure of BIA. While technology is improving, it is difficult to get an accurate body fat composition from commercially available body fat analyzers.

Anthropometric (measures of body fat) methods are simple, convenient, and inexpensive. Skin fold estimates, conducted while maintaining standards and using high-quality skin fold calipers, provide an accurate measure of body fat and compare favorably with bioelectrical impedance. The combination of weight, anthropometric methods, and BIA is an excellent predictor of total body fat composition.

A physical fitness assessment is an essential component of health assessment. Careful attention to assessment will optimize the fit of the exercise prescription to the physical capabilities of the client. The Presidential Youth Fitness Program adopted *FITNESSGRAM,* a research-based assessment developed by the nonprofit Cooper's Institute, and recommends implementation in all public schools. The *FITNESSGRAM* program assesses cardiovascular fitness, body composition, muscle strength, muscular endurance, and flexibility in children 4 to 17 years of age. *The American College of Sports Medicine (ACSM) Resource Manual for Guidelines for Exercise Testing and Prescription* (American College of Sports Medicine, 2013) is an excellent guide for physical fitness assessment tools for adults.

Nutrition

Good nutrition is one of the primary determinants of good health. *Effective* planning for health promotion requires an assessment of the nutritional status of the client to establish a baseline. Anthropometrical measurements and/or BIA analysis, laboratory values, and dietary history are useful assessment tools.

Anthropometrics assessment measures include height and weight, circumference of various areas of the body, and skin-fold thickness. BMI is the best method to assess healthy weight (American College of Sports Medicine, 2013). BMI does not assess body fat composition or fat distribution, but it is a useful screening tool for overweight or obesity. It has been determined that childhood BMI is associated with adult adiposity. The classification of overweight and obesity by BMI, waist circumference, and associated disease risks standards for adults is available in Table 4–2.

Healthy and unhealthy weight guidelines are in Table 4–3. The *waist-to-hip* ratio assesses the amount of fat distributed in the abdomen versus fat distributed below the waist. The ratio is the waist circumference over the hip circumference. The higher the value of the waist-to-hip ratio, the greater the potential that health problems are present or will occur (American College of Sports Medicine, 2013; WHO Expert Consultation, 2008).

Biochemical analyses of blood and urine help to identify nutritional deficiencies. In addition to laboratory tests for cholesterol, triglycerides, glucose, and high-density lipoproteins, tests for protein (creatinine index, serum protein, serum albumin, total lymphocyte count, blood urea nitrogen, uric acid), serum or plasma vitamin levels (water-soluble, fat-soluble), and minerals (calcium, sodium, potassium, iron, phosphorus, magnesium) are used to assess

TABLE 4–2   Classification of Overweight and Obesity by BMI, Waist Circumference, and Associated Disease Risk*

	BMI (kg/m^2)	Disease Risk* Relative to Normal Weight and Waist Circumference	
		Men ≤ 40 in. Women ≤ 35 in.	Men > 40 in. Women > 35 in.
Normal†	18.5–24.9	—	—
Overweight	25.0–29.9	Increased	High
Obesity	30.0–or above	High	Very High

*Disease risk for type 2 diabetes, hypertension, and CVD.

†Increased waist circumference can also be a marker for increased risk even in persons of normal weight.

Source: Adapted from *Preventing and Managing the Global Epidemic of Obesity.* Report of the World Health Organization Consultation of Obesity. WHO, Geneva, June 1997. http://www.nhlbi.nih.gov/guidelines/obesity/e_txtbk/txgd/411.htm

TABLE 4–3   Healthy and Unhealthy Weight Guidelines

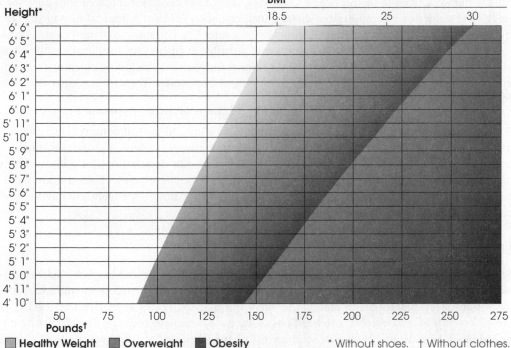

Are you at a healthy weight?

☐ **Healthy Weight**   ☐ **Overweight**   ■ **Obesity**   * Without shoes.   † Without clothes.

The BMI (weight-for-height) ranges shown are for adults. They are not exact ranges of healthy and unhealthy weights. However, they show that health risk increases at higher levels of overweight and obesity. Even within the healthy BMI range, weight gains can carry health risks for adults.

Directions: Find your weight on the bottom of the graph. Go straight up from that point until you come to the line that matches your height. Then look to find your weight group.

BMI of 24.9 defines the upper boundary of healthy weight.

BMI of 25 to 29.9 defines overweight.

BMI of 30 or higher defines obesity.

Source: Report of the Dietary Guidelines Advisory Committee on the Dietary Guidelines for Americans. (2000). http://www.cnpp.usda.gov/Publications/DietaryGuidelines/2000/2000DGCommitteeReport.pdf, p. 11.

nutritional status. Three particularly important values in assessing nutritional status are serum albumin less than 3.5 g/dL, total lymphocyte count less than $1800/mm^3$, and an involuntary loss of body weight greater than 15%. These three indicators correlate significantly with nutritional status (Gupta & Lis, 2010; Nishida & Sakakibara, 2010).

The dietary diary, available as either a paper or Web-based option, is one common measure used to assess nutritional status. SuperTracker, a diet planning and tracker tool is a Web-based dietary assessment that is easy to access and use. It incorporates both the 2010 Dietary Guidelines for Americans and the 2008 Physical Activity Guidelines. After the client, or nurse, enters the requested dietary information, the results are a part of a tailored nutrition plan that empowers the client to make healthier food choices. ChooseMyPlate also has a Spanish-language food icon *MiPlato* to guide Spanish-speaking consumers in making healthy food choices.

With the *paper option* dietary diary, clients keep a record of everything eaten for three days during the week prior to their office or home visit. Daily food choices, compared with published daily food guides or a computerized dietary analysis package, identify unusual or poor dietary patterns (see Nutrition and Health Promotion, Chapter 7). The nurse and nutritionist work together to prepare materials and/or recommend websites to ensure that the client has the latest and most accurate research findings about nutritional supplements, including vitamins and minerals (calcium, iron) as well as proteins and complex carbohydrates. Tools for assessing nutrition in primary care settings are available.

Culture and socioeconomic level influences eating patterns, obesity, and malnutrition. Assessment of nutritional status and dietary habits is a critical part of comprehensive health assessment for individuals, families, and specific target groups, such as high-school students, pregnant women, and the elderly. An analysis of assessment data determines which interventions are most appropriate to improve the nutritional status of the client/family. Understanding cultural influences on nutrition and dietary patterns is essential in both assessment and intervention to affect change.

Life Stress

Stress is a potential threat to mental health and physical well-being and is associated with illnesses such as cardiovascular disease, cancer, and gastrointestinal disorders, as well as depression, poor sleep patterns, and inability to carry out daily activities at an effective level. Life stress is a part of a comprehensive health assessment. Assessment begins with helping the client identify sources of stress. One strategy is to have the client write down the issues, concerns, and challenges that trigger stress responses in his or her life. Some of the stressors will be internal, and others will be external events. External stressors are events and situations that happen *to* individuals.

Examples of external stressors include the following:

1. Some events may be happy ones such as marriage, birth of a child, and a new home, while some may be negative, such as death of a loved one, loss of a job, and an unplanned pregnancy. Stress results from *both positive and negative events.*
2. The interaction between the individual and the environment involves subjective perception and assessment of stressors. Common events—such as a barking dog, a crying baby, and extreme weather conditions—may cause stress.
3. Much of life is unpredictable, and one's personality influences responses to change and unplanned-for events. Unpredictable events include dealing with unexpected house guests, increased rent, or a sick child.
4. Family stressors include conflicts and arguments between children and spouses, issues resulting from the health problems of family members, and multigenerational households.
5. Common stressors in the workplace include long working hours, difficult coworkers, and urgent deadlines.
6. Social stressors include commitments to family, friends, and organizations balanced with the need for downtime for oneself, and pressure from peers.

Internal stressors are self-induced thoughts and feelings that lead to unrest and anxiety.

Examples of internal stressors include the following:

1. Common fears such as flying, heights, and public speaking.
2. The inability to *predict* behaviors such as use of alcohol and not knowing the outcome of medical tests.
3. Attitudes and expectations exhibited toward job loss or unexpected guests.

Despite the high prevalence of stress-related health problems, including substance abuse, primary care providers screen too few clients for these problems. Regular screenings enable earlier identification of problems and earlier treatment. Screening tools include the following:

STRESS SCALES.   Assessing a person's vulnerability to stress and strength to cope provides an essential measure of mental and physical well-being. The Derogatis Stress Profile (Derogatis & Lazarus, 1997) assesses personal and professional stress in adolescents and adults. The Perceived Stress Scale (Cohen, Kessler, & Gordon, 1997) measures moods and feelings about life stressors and is considered a measure of global stress.

HASSLES AND UPLIFTS.   Hassles are the irritating, frustrating, distressing demands such as traffic jams, losing items, and arguments that characterize everyday life. Uplifts, the counterpart of hassles, are the positive experiences or joys of life, such as getting a good night's rest, receiving an email from a friend, or spending time with a pet. The assessment of daily hassles and uplifts is a better predictor of health or illness than the usual assessment of life events. An example of a hassles and uplifts scale is the Adolescent Hassle Scale (AHS; Wright, Creed, & Zimmer-Gembeck, 2010).

ANXIETY INVENTORY.   Anxiety level is a part of the life-stress review. The State-Trait Anxiety Inventory consists of 20 items that assess the extent of anxiety one feels at that moment (state anxiety) and 20 items that assess how one generally feels (trait anxiety; Spielberger, Gorsuch, Lushene, & Vagg, 1983). A State-Trait Anxiety Inventory is available for children ("How I Feel Questionnaire"; Spielberger et al., 1983). Both instruments and administration manuals are available from Mind Garden, Palo Alto, California.

STRESS WARNING SIGNALS INVENTORY.   Clients should understand and be aware of the symptoms of an elevated stress level. When clients are aware of their own stress signals, they can use stress-management techniques (see Chapter 8) more effectively. Symptoms of stress may be physical, behavioral, emotional, or cognitive as shown in Figure 4–5.

COPING MEASURES.   Coping is an individual's ongoing efforts to manage specific internal and external demands that exceed personal resources. A commonly used tool to measure coping is the Ways of Coping Questionnaire developed by Folkman and Lazarus (1988). The scale measures both the emotion- and problem-focused coping strategies an individual uses when responding to a stress situation. The Schoolager's Coping Strategies Inventory is used to measure the type, frequency, and effectiveness of children's stress-coping strategies, and additional instruments to measure stressors in children are available [Ryan-Wenger, Wilson (Sharrer), & Broussard, 2012].

The Patient Health Questionnaire (PHQ-2) is a two item-screening test that consists of the first two questions of the Patient Health Questionnaire (PHQ-9) tool to assist providers with diagnosing depression. The client that answers positively to one or both of the two items (PHQ-2) then answers the remainder of the seven items on the PHQ-9 (Li, Friedman, Conwell, & Fiscella, 2007). The PHQ-2 is effective in screening large groups to detect undiagnosed depression in a variety of populations.

Stress Warning Signals

PHYSICAL SYMPTOMS

- ☐ Headaches
- ☐ Indigestion
- ☐ Stomachaches
- ☐ Sweaty palms
- ☐ Sleep difficulties
- ☐ Dizziness

- ☐ Back pain
- ☐ Tight neck, shoulders
- ☐ Racing heart
- ☐ Restlessness
- ☐ Tiredness
- ☐ Ringing in ears

BEHAVIORAL SYMPTOMS

- ☐ Excess smoking
- ☐ Bossiness
- ☐ Compulsive gum chewing
- ☐ Attitude critical of others

- ☐ Grinding of teeth at night
- ☐ Overuse of alcohol
- ☐ Compulsive eating
- ☐ Inability to get things done

EMOTIONAL SYMPTOMS

- ☐ Crying
- ☐ Nervousness, anxiety
- ☐ Boredom—no meaning to things
- ☐ Edginess—ready to explode
- ☐ Feeling powerless to change things

- ☐ Overwhelming sense of pressure
- ☐ Anger
- ☐ Loneliness
- ☐ Unhappiness for no reason
- ☐ Easily upset

COGNITIVE SYMPTOMS

- ☐ Trouble thinking clearly
- ☐ Forgetfulness
- ☐ Lack of creativity
- ☐ Memory loss

- ☐ Inability to make decisions
- ☐ Thoughts of running away
- ☐ Constant worry
- ☐ Loss of sense of humor

Do any seem familiar to you?

Check the ones you experience when under stress. These are your stress warning signs.

Are there any additional stress warning signals that you experience that are not listed? If so, add them here.

_____

_____

_____

_____

FIGURE 4–5 Stress Warning Signals   *Source:* From Benson, H., & Stuart, E. M. 1992. *The Wellness Book.* New York, NY: Citadel Press/Kensington Publishing Corp. All rights reserved. Reprinted by arrangement with Citadel Press/Kensington Publishing Corp.

See *Instruments for Clinical Healthcare Research* (Frank-Stromborg, 2004) for a review of instruments on stress, coping, and anxiety and the relevance of each measure to nursing.

Spiritual Health

Spiritual health is the ability to develop one's inner being to its fullest potential. Spiritual health includes the ability to discover and articulate one's basic purpose in life; to learn how to experience love, joy, peace, and fulfillment; and to help oneself and others achieve their fullest potential.

The assessment of spiritual health is critical in a holistic approach to health as spiritual beliefs affect a client's interpretations of life events and health. Acquiring a better understanding of clients' spiritual needs will enable health care providers to develop tailored and effective spiritual interventions (Monod, Rochat, Bula, & Spencer, 2010).

Examples of spirituality measures include the following:

- The Spiritual Needs Assessment for Patients (SNAP) is a 23-item multidimensional survey instrument to describe and measure spiritual needs (Galek, Flannelly, Vane, & Galek, 2012).
- The Spiritual Involvement and Beliefs Scale (SIBR) measures actions as well as beliefs across religious traditions (Litwinczuk & Groh, 2007). This instrument and the previous one provide supportive data for understanding the client's spiritual beliefs and their impact on health needs and care.
- The Spiritual Perspective Scale (SPS) is a 10-item instrument that measures one's perceptions of the extent to which one's spiritual beliefs and one's daily interactions are consistent (Chung, Wong, & Chan, 2007).

Additional measures are available in *Instruments in Clinical Healthcare Research* (Frank-Stromborg, 2004).

Social Support Systems

Two approaches for reviewing the social support networks of clients are useful in providing the client and nurse increased insight into existing support resources. When assessing the adequacy of support systems, it is important to be cognizant of factors that may cause the assessments to vary. Such things as the client's culture, age, social context (school, home, work), and role context (parent, student, professional) influence perceived and received support. Using the Internet to expand one's social contacts is increasing in popularity and can be included in assessing the client's social support system. Definitive measures for assessing social support are abundant in the literature. They can also be found on educational websites, such as Stanford University.

SUPPORT SYSTEMS REVIEW.   One straightforward, useful approach to assess support systems is to ask the client to list individuals who provide informational, emotional, appraisal, or instrumental support. Then ask the client to indicate the relationship with the persons listed. Next, identify persons who have been sources of support for five years or more. This list enables the client to become aware of the stability of personal support systems. Last, identify the frequency and types of contacts. These may be face-to-face or telephone and e-mail communication. Examining the social network enables the client and the nurse to assess the adequacy of support. If it is inadequate, generate strategies to enhance existing social networks. Figure 4–6 shows a sample of a completed support system review.

After reviewing the client's social support systems, explore the following questions:

- In what areas do you need more support: informational, emotional, instrumental, appraisal?
- Who within your present support system might provide the needed support?
- Who else do you think needs to become a part of your support system?
- What can you do to add the people you believe you need to your support system?

Answers to these questions suggest actions the client can take to expand sources of personal support.

List individuals who provide support to you. Next indicate the following relationships: Family member (FM); Fellow worker (FM); or Social Acquaintance (A). Frequency of Contact: Daily (D); Weekly (W); Monthly (M); or Rarely (R). Types of Contact: Face-to-Face (F); Telephone (T); or Email (EM). If individual has been supportive for 5 years or more, place the number 5.

Individual	Relationship	Frequency	Type	Time
John	FM (husband)	D	F	5
Peter	FM (son)	D	F	5
Helen	FM (daughter)	D	F	5
Ted	FM (father)	W	T	5
Andrew	FW	D	F	-
Frances	FW	W	F	-
Rose	FW	W	T	5
Elsa	A	M	E	-
Jack	A	M	E	5

Ask the client to identify the type of support provided by individuals in the list. They may provide more than one type of support.

Sources of Emotional Support

FAMILY	WORK	SOCIAL GROUP
John	Frances	Elsa
Peter	Rose	Jack
Helen	Andrew	
Ted		

Sources of Instrument Support

FAMILY	WORK	SOCIAL GROUP
John	Andrew	Jack
Ted		

Sources of Information Support

FAMILY	WORK	SOCIAL GROUP
John	Andrew	Jack
Ted	Rose	

Sources of Appraisal Support

FAMILY	WORK	SOCIAL GROUP
John	Rose	Elsa

FIGURE 4–6 Support System Review: Social Network and Type of Support

EMOTIONAL SUPPORT DIAGRAM. Diagrams are effective ways to assess the strength and sources of support. Figure 4–7 presents a sample emotional support diagram that indicates strong, moderate, and weak sources of support, as well as current conflicts with supportive individuals. The length of each line indicates geographical proximity to the client. This approach is particularly appropriate for clients who need a visual presentation of their emotional support system to take action to sustain or enhance emotionally satisfying relationships.

An integral part of the assessment is a review of sources of social support. A review enables the client to recognize current sources of support and identify barriers in social relationships that may block desirable health actions. The nurse must always be alert to client

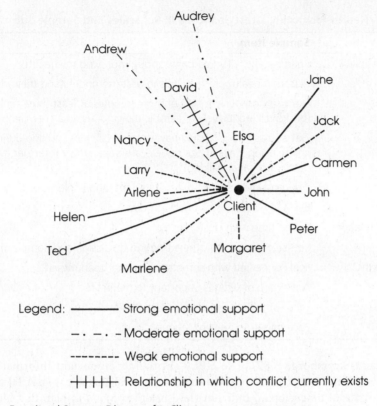

FIGURE 4-7 Emotional Support Diagram for Client

situations in which social support is minimal or nonexistent. Extensive review of support systems may cause anxiety and depression, and in this case, a more informal, nonthreatening approach is useful.

Social support instruments represent the broad spectrum of measures used in clinical settings as well as research. The Social Support Questionnaire is a six-item measure of perceived social support and satisfaction with social support. Each item presents a specific scenario for which respondents list the people who would be available for support in that situation. Respondents are also asked to rate their satisfaction with the support available (Sarason, Shearin, Pierce, & Sarason, 1987).

Lifestyle Assessment

In the context of health, *lifestyle* defines discretionary activities that are a regular part of one's daily pattern of living and significantly influences health status. Health-promoting behavior is an expression of the human actualizing tendency that optimizes well-being, personal fulfillment, and productive living. The 52-item Health-Promoting Lifestyle Profile II (HPLP-II), a revision of the original instrument, consists of six subscales to measure major components of a health promoting lifestyle: health responsibility, physical activity, nutrition, interpersonal relations, spiritual growth, and stress management. Scores are obtained for each subscale, or a total scale score is calculated to measure overall health-promoting lifestyle (Sechrist, Walker,

TABLE 4–4   Health-Promoting Lifestyle Profile II: Subscales and Sample Subscale Items

Subscale	Sample Item
Health responsibility	Read or watch TV programs about improving my health.
	Question health professionals in order to understand their instructions.
Physical activity	Exercise vigorously for 20 or more minutes at least three times a week (brisk walking, bicycling, aerobic dancing, using a stair climber).
	Get exercise during usual day activities (such as walking during lunch, using stairs instead of elevators, parking car farther away from destination and walking).
Nutrition	Choose a diet low in fat, saturated fat, and cholesterol.
	Eat 2 to 4 servings of fruit each day.
Interpersonal relations	Spend time with close friends.
	Settle conflicts with others through discussion and compromise.
Spiritual growth	Feel connected with some force greater than myself.
	Am aware of what is important to me in life.
Stress management	Take some time for relaxation each day.
	Pace myself to prevent fatigue.

Pender, & Frank-Stromborg, 1987). The HPLP-II provides important information about a client's lifestyle. Sample items for each of the subscales appear in Table 4–4. A HPLP-II profile provides information to develop an individualized health promotion plan that identifies lifestyle strengths and resources as well as areas for further growth. A Spanish-language version of the HPLPII is available. The Adolescent Lifestyle Profile (ALP) measures seven domains of health-promoting lifestyle (Hendricks, Murdaugh, & Pender, 2006) and is useful for measuring health-promoting behaviors in adolescents.

Additional lifestyle instruments are available at educational websites, including Stanford University.

STAGE OF CHANGE ASSESSMENT.   Clients may be at one of several stages in relation to any given behavior change. Table 4–5 shows the stages of change for positive health behaviors. Recognizing the different stages of change in relation to various health behaviors allows for more tailored interventions.

TABLE 4–5   True–False Statements for Assessing Stages of Behavior Change

1. I currently do not (specify exact behavior, e.g., exercise 30 minutes three times a week, eat 2 to 4 servings of fruit daily) and do not intend to start in the next 6 months. (Precontemplation)
2. I currently do not (specify behavior), but I am thinking about starting to do so in the next 6 months. (Contemplation)
3. I have tried several times to (specify behavior) but am seriously thinking of trying again in the next month. (Planning)
4. I have (specify behavior) regularly for less than 6 months. (Action)
5. I have (specify behavior) regularly for more than 6 months. (Maintenance)

ASSESSMENT OF THE FAMILY

The contemporary family and the reciprocal influence of family health on individual family members reconfirm the family as the primary social structure for health promotion. Health-promoting as well as health-damaging behaviors and lifestyles learned and reinforced within the context of the family are powerful mediating factors in determining how individual members cope with health concerns and challenges. The family—the logical unit of assessment—has the primary responsibility for the following:

1. Developing self-care and dependent-care competencies of its members
2. Fostering resilience of family members to include shared values and shared goals
3. Providing social and physical resources to the family group
4. Promoting healthy individuals while maintaining family cohesion (Peace & Lutz, 2009)

Although women generally carry the major responsibility for health decision making and health education for the family, the task of fostering health and healthy behaviors should be "mainstreamed" as an integral part of family functioning. The milieu for health promotion is likely to differ significantly across families, depending on their composition, structure, socioeconomic status, living environment, culture and cultural context, and family history. A family history is a window on the individual family members' health and an invaluable insight into the risk of inheriting specific diseases, shared environmental factors, and individual health concerns. My Family Health Portrait is an example of an Internet-based family health tool that takes about 20 minutes to complete online, or the form is available to download. The nurse may need to print a copy for the family if the family does not have access to a computer or the skills to access the form. The program assembles the information and builds a family tree. Families can share the information with other family members and enter it into the PHR. As noted by Peace and Lutz (2009), the limitation of this traditional family history representation is evident when applied to diverse families. Genopro is a free (with some restrictions) commercial application for drawing genograms and is more useful in assessing nontraditional family units.

Healthy family traits and family strengths have many different modes of expression. One-parent families, blended families, unmarried parents with children, and gay and lesbian families are examples of the wide variation among families. Variations produced by transitions in family life influence the family assessment as well. Approaches to family assessment are presented below.

A systems approach to family assessment includes five assessment categories: (1) individual members, (2) subsystems (developmental, biological, psychological, social characteristics), (3) interactional patterns (relationships, communication patterns, roles, and attachment patterns), (4) family processing, and (5) change or adaptive abilities (Kaakinen, Gedaly-Duff, Hanson, & Coehlo, 2009).

Three categories of processes underlie a systems model of family assessment: (1) those that regulate exchanges with the environment, (2) processes designed to prevent an overload of the system, and (3) internal processes that regulate the family's ability to adapt and change (Clark, 2007). Assessment based on systems theory provides insight about the internal processes of the family as well as the relationship of the family to the environment and larger social system.

Family decision-making patterns in relation to health identify power structure and health care function. In a structural-functional approach to family assessment, the family is a system with communication patterns, power structure, role structure, family values, affective function, socialization patterns, health care function, family stress, coping, and adaptation mechanisms. Family functional assessment dichotomizes instrumental functioning and expressive functioning. *Instrumental functioning* refers to the routine activities of everyday living, while *expressive functioning* connotes emotional communication, verbal communication, nonverbal communication, circular communication, problem solving, roles, control, beliefs, alliances, and coalitions (Melesis, 2012; Kaakinen, Gedaly-Duff, Hanson, & Coehlo, 2009).

The Calgary Family Assessment Model is adapted for nurses to assess families (Wright & Leahey, 2009). This model consists of family structural assessment, family developmental assessment, and family functional assessment. In structural assessment, the family's *internal* structure includes family composition, rank order, subsystem, and boundary; components of the *external* structure are culture, religion, socioeconomic level, mobility, environment, and extended family.

To assess *family development*, the Calgary model reviews the current stage of the family in relation to family developmental history. Family development focuses primarily on the traditional family developmental cycle, but it also includes assessment of alterations in the family developmental life cycle brought about by separation, divorce, death, single parenthood, and remarriage.

A significant gap in conducting family assessments is the lack of valid and reliable instruments that measure family dimensions of a health-related lifestyle. Family assessment and individual assessment are interrelated processes and complement each other. Table 4–6 lists suggested assessment areas. To provide further guidance, Chapter 5 presents a format for developing a family health promotion-prevention plan.

TABLE 4–6   Components of Family Assessment

Nutrition

1. Meals prepared in the home are generally consistent with MyPlate.
2. Healthy snacks are consumed in the home.
3. Knowledge about healthy eating habits is shared among family members.
4. Mutual assistance occurs among family members for maintenance of recommended weights and avoidance of overweight and underweight.
5. Family members praise each other for healthy eating.
6. Family members encourage each other to drink 6 to 8 glasses of water per day.
7. Family members base purchase decisions on nutritional labels on food.

Physical Activity

1. Many family outings consist of vigorous or moderate physical activity.
2. Exercise equipment is available within the home.
3. Use of home exercise equipment is part of "family time."
4. Family members expect each other to be physically active.
5. A family membership is held in recreational facilities or programs.
6. Time together is seldom spent watching television or playing video games.
7. Family prefers to spend as much time out of doors as possible.

Stress Control and Management

1. Family manages time well to minimize stressful demands on members.
2. Family often relaxes, shares stories, and laughs together.
3. Emotional expression is encouraged within the family.
4. Family members share stressful experiences with each other.
5. Family members offer each other assistance with difficult tasks.
6. Family members seldom criticize each other.
7. Periods of relaxation and sleep are considered important by the family.

Health Responsibility

1. A schedule for preventive care visits is maintained by the family.
2. Family often discusses news and articles about health topics.
3. Family members are encouraged to seek health care early if a problem develops.
4. Personal responsibility for health is encouraged by the family.
5. Family feels a sense of responsibility for the health of the family and each member.
6. Health professionals are consulted about health promotion as well as care in illness.
7. Appropriate protective behaviors are openly discussed and encouraged (abstinence, use of condoms, hearing protection, eye protection, sunscreen, helmets).

Family Resilience and Resources

1. Worship or spiritual experiences are a regular part of family activities.
2. Family members share a sense of "togetherness" despite difficult life events.
3. Family has a common sense of purpose in life.
4. Family members encourage each other to "keep going" when life is difficult.
5. Growth in positive directions is mutually encouraged within the family.
6. Health is nurtured as a positive family resource.
7. Personal strengths and capabilities are nurtured.

Family Support

1. Family has a number of friends or relatives that they see frequently.
2. Family is involved in community activities and groups.
3. Family members frequently praise each other.
4. In times of distress, the family can call on a number of other families or individuals for help.
5. Disagreements are settled through discussion rather than verbal abuse or physical violence.
6. Family members model healthy habits for each other.
7. Professional support services are sought when needed.

ASSESSMENT OF THE COMMUNITY

A third essential component of assessing the health of individuals is an assessment of the community in which they live, work, and play. Community assessment is a complicated and time-consuming undertaking. However, such assessments are critical to identify community strengths and resources as well as to diagnose community problems and/or deficits. Collaboration is required among many individuals in the community as well as health professionals.

A community analysis performed *with* the community, and not *on* or *for* the community, increases the likelihood of success. A team or coalition of local citizens and organizations involved in the assessment process encourages community "ownership" of the program and commitment to implement the plan.

There are four objectives for conducting a community assessment:

1. Identify community strengths and areas for improvement.
2. Identify and understand the status of community health needs.
3. Define improvement areas to guide the community toward implementing and sustaining policy, systems, and environmental changes around healthy living strategies (e.g., increased physical activity, improved nutrition, reduced tobacco use and exposure, and chronic disease management).
4. Assist with prioritizing community needs and consider appropriate allocation of available resources (Centers for Disease Control and Prevention, 2010).

Assessment involves gathering data and input on what the community needs. Assessing community needs gives voice to citizens' concerns and issues and allows that "voice" to influence significantly the program design. Components of a community assessment include human biology, the environment, community lifestyles, and the health system. Table 4–7 lists these components.

An assessment methodology that combines at least three to four data collection methods is more likely to provide a holistic picture of the community than is an assessment that relies on only one or two approaches. Review the advantages and disadvantages of data collection methods at the CDC Healthy Communities website.

Successful implementation of community health promotion-prevention programs depends in large part on a well-developed community plan. Community-level changes such as policy are more sustainable, impact infrastructure, and support social change. For example, an effort to improve family food choices is sustainable only if healthy, affordable, and assessable food locations are available in the community.

TABLE 4–7   Components of Community Assessment

Human Biology

1. Composition of population by age, gender, and race
2. Population patterns of longevity
3. Genetic inheritance patterns by gender and race
4. Disease incidence and prevalence compared to prior years, and to state and national statistics
5. Health status indicators (immunization levels, nutritional status, mobility)

Environment

1. Physical environment (urban/rural/suburban, housing, water supply, parks and recreation, climate, topography, size, population density, aesthetics, natural or manmade resources, goods and services, health risks)
2. Psychologic environment (productivity level, cohesion, mental health status, communication networks, intergroup harmony, future orientation, prevalence of stressors)
3. Social environment (income and education levels, employment, family composition, religious affiliations, cultural affiliations, language[s] spoken, social services, organization profile, leadership and decision-making structures)

Community Lifestyles

1. Consumption patterns (nutrition, alcohol)
2. Occupational groups
3. Leisure pursuits
4. Community health attitudes and beliefs
5. Patterns of health-related behaviors in aggregates
6. History of participation in community health action

Health System

1. Health care services available (health promotion, prevention, primary care, secondary care, tertiary care, mental health)
2. Accessibility of promotive and preventive care (low income, homeless, varying racial and ethnic groups)
3. Financing plans for health care

Source: Clark, Mary Jo, *Community Health Nursing: Caring for Populations,* 4th Edition, © 2003. Reproduced by permission of Pearson Education, Inc., Upper Saddle River, New Jersey.

A community-based action may improve the overall health of the community, but within the community, certain groups may be disenfranchised based on income level or occupation, exacerbating health disparities. Achieving health equality may be at odds with improving the overall health of the community, and priorities must be determined (Institute of Medicine, 2012). The need for transparency is paramount between the decision makers and the community to ensure that the action plan reflects the values and preferences of the citizens.

PRACTICE CONSIDERATIONS IN ASSESSING HEALTH AND HEALTH BEHAVIOR

Use of assessment measures to document areas for improvement to enhance the health status of individuals, families, and communities is an important responsibility of the nurse. Assessment data about health status and behaviors provide the basis for clinical judgments and help plan appropriate individual, family, and community interventions. Nurses' knowledge and influence can ensure that a portfolio of conceptually congruent assessment instruments is available and used in the work setting. The nurse must know how to administer assessment measures and explain the value of conducting systematic assessments to the client. The busy work environment may discourage the use of detailed assessments because they require time to administer and follow up. One strategy to manage the time issue is to seek innovative ways to communicate with clients through videotapes and brochures that explain assessment procedures. Information technology has made computerized assessment possible. Thus, clients may be able to complete self-assessments at home, as time allows, with transmission of the information by computer prior to health care visits.

Practicing nurses must keep up-to-date about new assessment measures and strategies that can be quickly implemented and yield accurate data. Nurses influence the quality of the health promotion plan of the individual, family, and community through a commitment to thorough assessment of health and health behaviors.

OPPORTUNITIES FOR RESEARCH IN HEALTH ASSESSMENT AND HEALTH BEHAVIOR

Research that develops and tests assessment instruments for health and health behaviors of aggregates from diverse racial, cultural, and socioeconomic backgrounds is a high priority. Reliable and valid instruments based on theory and research are needed to perform meaningful assessments. Community interventions should be developed and tested in subgroups. Accurate knowledge of the client, family, and community will facilitate the development and implementation of successful health promotion interventions.

Summary

Health assessment at the individual, family, and community levels is time intensive and costly, so measures must reflect client characteristics and presenting health issues. The nurse and client must mutually establish a relevant plan to ensure its success.

Learning Activities

1. Go to the My Family Health Portrait website and record a traditional family health portrait. Examine the differences between My Family Health Portrait and the commercial application at Genopro.
2. Develop a list of safeguards to ensure that non-computer users are included in the health care technology environment.
3. Develop an assessment plan based on age-specific instruments for a child, a young adult, and an older adult.
4. Using Table 4–2, determine your percentage of body fat and outline a personal goal based on the results.
5. Investigate one approach to assessing a family and discuss its strengths and weaknesses for use in the clinical setting.
6. Identify the relationship between a family and a community assessment and discuss how they affect the health outcomes of the family and community.
7. Discuss factors to consider in a community assessment including those influencing the extent of assessment conducted.

References

American College of Sports Medicine. (2013). *ACSM's resource manual for guidelines for exercise testing and prescription* (9th ed.). Baltimore, MD: Williams and Wilkins.

ANA SmartBrief. (2012). *Mobile apps seen as one of top medical trends for 2013*. New York, NY: Wall Street Journal (12/31).

Bleyer, A., & Welsh, H. (2012). Effect of three decades of screening mamography on breast-cancer incidence. *New England Journal of Medicine, 367*(21),1998–2005.

Block, L. (2013). *USPSTF mommo recommendations: Tempest in a teapot?* Retrieved May 20, 2013, from HealthImaging: http://www.healthimaging.com /topics/womens-health/breast-imaging/uspstf-mammo-recommendations-tempest-teapot.

Bulechek, G., Butcher, H., Dochterman, J., & Wagner, C. (2013). *Nursing Interventions Classification (NIC)* (6th ed.). St. Louis, MO: Mosby.

Centers for Disease Control and Prevention. (2010). *Community Health Assessment and Group Evaluation (CHANGE) action guide: Building a foundation of knowledge to prioritize community needs*. Atlanta, GA: U.S. Department of Health and Human Services.

Chen, Y. Y., Lu, J. C., & Jan, J. K. (2012). A secure EHR system based on hybrid clouds. *Journal Medical Systems, 3*(5), 3375–3384.

Chung, L., Wong, F., & Chan, M. (2007). Relationship of nurses' spirituality to their understanding and practice of spiritual care. *Journal of Advanced Nursing, 58*(2), 158–170.

Clark, M. (2007). *Community health nursing: Advocacy for population health* (5th ed.). Upper Saddle River, NJ: Prentice Hall.

CMS.gov. (2009). Retrieved February 7, 2013, from Centers for Medicare & Medicaid Services: www.cms.gov/Regulations-and-Guidance/legislation/EHRIncentiveProgram.

Cohen, S., Kessler, R., & Gordon, L. (1997). *Measuring stress.* New York, NY: Oxford Press.

Derogatis, L., & Lazarus, R. (1997). *Evaluating stress. The Derogatis stress profile (DSP): A theory driven aproach to stress measurement.* Lanham, MD: Scarecrow Press.

Folkman, S., &, Lazarus, R. (1988). Coping as a mediator of emotion. *Journal of Personality and Social Psychology, 54*(3), 466–475.

Frank-Stromborg, M. (2004). *Instruments for clinical health-care research* (3rd ed.) Sudbury, MA: Jones & Bartlett.

Galek, K., Flannelly, K., Vane, A., & Galek, M. (2012). The Spiritual Needs Assessment for Patients (SNAP): Development and validation of a comprehensive instrument to assess unmet spiritual needs. *Journal of Pain and Symptom Management, 44*(1), 44–51.

Gordon, M. (2009). *Manual of nursing diagnosis* (12th ed.). Sudbury, MA: Jones and Bartlett, Inc.

Gupta, D., & Lis, C. (2010). Pretreatment serum albumin as a predictor of cancer survival: A systematic review of the epidemiological literature. *Nutrition Journal, 9*, 69.

Hagan, J. F., Jr., Shaw, J. S., & Duncan, P. M. (Eds.). (2008). *Bright futures: Guidelines for health supervision of infants, children, and adolescents* (3rd ed.). Elk Grove Village, IL: American Academy of Pediatrics.

Hendricks, C., Murdaugh, C., & Pender, N. (2006). The adolescent lifestyle profile: Development and psychometric characteristics. *Journal of National Black Nurses Association, 17*(2), 1–5.

Institute of Medicine. (2012). *An integrated framework for assessing the value of community-based prevention.* Washington, DC: The National Academy of Sciences.

Kaakinen, J., Gedaly-Duff, V., Hanson, S., & Coehlo, D. (2009). *Family health care nursing: Theory, practice, and research.* Philadelphia, PA: F. A. Davis Co.

Kressin, N., Manze, M., Russell, S., Katz, R., Claudio, C., Green, B., & Wang, M. (2010). Self-reported willingness to have cancer screening and the effects of sociodemographic factors. *Journal of the National Medical Association, 102*(3), 219–227.

Li, M., Friedman, B., Conwell, Y., & Fiscella, K. (2007). Validity of the Patient Health Questionnaire 2 (PGQ-2) in identifying major depression in older people. *Journal of the American Geriatric Society, 55*, 596–602.

Li, Y., Lee, P., Jian, W., & Kuo, C. (2009). Electronic Health Record goes personal world-wide. *Yearbook of Medical Informatics, 10*(1), 40–43.

Litwinczuk, K., & Groh, C. (2007). The relationship between spirituality, purpose in life, and well-being in HIV-positive persons. *Journal of the Association of Nurses in AIDS Care, 18*(3), 13–22.

Lunney, M. (2008). The need for international nursing diagnosis research and a theoretical framework. *International Journal of Nursing Terminologies and Classifications, 19*(1), 28–29.

Melesis, A. (2012). *Theoretical nursing: Development and progress.* Philadelphia, PA: Lippincott, Williams & Wilkins.

Monod, S., Rochat, E., Bula, C., & Spencer, B. (2010). The spiritual needs model: Spirituality assessment in the geriatric hospital setting. *Journal of Religion, Spirituality & Aging, 22*(4), 271–282.

Moorhead, S., Johnson, M., Maas, M., & Swanson, E. (Eds.). (2013). *Nursing outcomes classification (NOC)* (5th ed.). St. Louis, MO: Elsevier.

National Association of Nursing Diagnosis-International. (2013). Retrieved from: www.nanda.org

Nishida, T., & Sakakibara, H. (2010). Association between underweight and low lymphocyte count as an indicator of malnutrition in Japanese women. *Journal of Womens Health, 19*(7), 1377–1383.

Peace, J., & Lutz, K. (2009). Nursing conceptionization of research and practice. *Nursing Outlook, 57*(5), 42–49.

Popkess-Vawter, S. (2008). Wellness nursing diagnosis: To be or not to be? *Journal of Terminologies and Classifications, 2*(1), 19–25.

Robert Wood Johnson Foundation. (2009). *Personal health records.* Retrieved from http://www.rwjf.org/en/search-results.

Ryan-Wenger, N., Wilson (Sharrer), V., & Broussard, A. (2012). Stress, coping, and health in children. In V. H. Rice, *Stress, coping, and health implications for nursing research, theory, and practice* (pp. 226–253). Los Angeles, CA: Sage.

Sarason, B., Shearin, E., Pierce, X., & Sarason, J. (1987). A brief measure of social support: Practical and theoretical implications. *Journal of Social and Personal Relations, 4*, 497–510.

Sechrist, K., Walker, S., Pender, N., & Frank-Stromborg, M. (1987). Development and psychometric evaluation of the Exercise benefits/Barriers Scale. *Journal of Nursing Research, 10*, 357–365.

Spielberger, C., Gorsuch, R., Lushene, R., & Vagg, P. (1983). *Manual for state-trait anxiety inventory.* Palo Alto, CA: Consulting Psychologists Press Inc.

The Office of Minority Health. (2013). *Cultural competency.* Retrieved January 30, 2013, from Minority

Health, Health & Human Services: http://aspe.hhs
.gov/sp/reports/2010

U.S. Department of Commerce Census. (2012). *Selected
individual characteristics 2010.* Washington, DC: U.S.
Government Printing Office.

U.S. Preventive Services Task Force. (2012). *The Guide to
Clinical Preventive Services.* Washington, DC: Agency
for Healthcare Research and Quality.

WHO Expert Consultation. (2008). *Waist circumference
and waist-hip ratio.* Geneva, Switzerland: World Health
Organization.

Wright, M., Creed, P., & Zimmer-Gembeck, M. (2010).
The development and initial validation of a brief
daily hassles scale suitable for use with adolescents.
European Journal of Psychological Assessment, 26(3),
220–226.

Wright, L., & Leahey, M. (2009). *Nurses and families: A guide
to family assessment and intervention.* Philadelphia,
PA: FA Davis Co.

CHAPTER 5

Developing a Health Promotion-Prevention Plan

OBJECTIVES

This chapter will enable the reader to:

1. Identify the nine steps in the health planning process.
2. Discuss barriers to overcome in developing an individual and family health plan.
3. Describe strategies to increase the client's "ownership" of a behavior change plan.
4. Discuss strategies to ensure that the health plan is an interdisciplinary process.
5. Discuss barriers that hinder effective individual and family behavior change.
6. Describe how community-level plans and interventions influence individual and family health plans.

Clients must be active participants in planning and interpreting assessment data. Client collaboration with the nurse promotes positive perceptions of worth and affirms the ability of individuals, families, or communities to function on their own behalf to create conditions supportive of healthy lifestyles.

The role of the nurse is to *assist* clients with health planning rather than to *control* the process. The nurse and client develop a mutual understanding of the client's situation, including the following:

1. Health status
2. Current health-behavior patterns
3. Attitudes and beliefs that affect health and health-related behaviors
4. Expectations of important referent groups
5. Potentially available behavioral options
6. Social-ethnic-cultural background
7. Potential or actual barriers to health behavior change
8. Existing support systems for health-promoting behaviors

Developing a systematic plan for behavior change provides the client an opportunity to express purposeful ways to increase wellness and enhance life satisfaction.

Health planning is a dynamic process. Flexibility is critical to meet the changing needs of clients. The health promotion-prevention plan systematically lends direction but does not dictate goals or behaviors. The plan should be reasonable in terms of both demands on the client and the period allocated to accomplish desired health or health-related goals.

Knowledge, skills, and strengths of the client are critical components in the planning process. Capitalizing on current positive health practices creates a sense of competence or efficacy essential to successful behavior change. Together, the nurse and the client should assess the behaviors the client wishes to modify. The client can then discuss strategies for change that are likely to be most effective. The plan may need revisions to make behavior change a growth experience. The ultimate goal of health planning and implementation is to make health promotion and prevention a way of life for individuals, families, and communities.

Innovative developments in information technology increasingly personalize assessment and intervention protocols to the unique characteristics and needs of individual clients. In addition, modifications in electronic health records will enable clients to share their health promotion plan with multiple care providers. Nurses must be cognizant of the increasingly significant role of technology—health assessments/fitness applications for smart phones and tablets, as well as Web-based technology for health interventions, as they work with clients to develop and implement health promotion plans (Laustria, Cortese, Noar, & Glueckauf, 2009).

GUIDELINES FOR PREVENTIVE SERVICES AND SCREENINGS

The increased emphasis on disease prevention has resulted in helpful guidelines for the delivery of preventive services to individuals and families throughout the life span. These guidelines focus on clinical care to prevent specific conditions, such as HIV disease, or behavioral morbidity, such as substance abuse. The *Guide to Clinical Preventive Services* (Agency for Healthcare Research and Quality, 2012) recommends screenings as an important component of prevention. The value and benefits of age-specific periodic screenings based on gender and individual risk factors are available in the guidelines. Counseling clients about their personal health habits is one of the most important components of the health visit. Nurses in primary care settings should become familiar with available guidelines to ensure that their clients benefit from "state-of-the-science" preventive services, including the following:

1. *The Guide to Clinical Preventive Services* (Agency for Healthcare Research and Quality, 2012)
2. *Women: Stay Healthy at Any* Age (Agency for Healthcare Research and Quality, 2012)
3. *Men: Stay Healthy at Any* Age (Agency for Healthcare Research and Quality, 2012)

These guidelines are accessible on the Agency for Healthcare Research and Quality Web site.

Partnership for Prevention, a nonpartisan group, convenes the Commission on Preventive Priorities to rank evidence-based clinical preventive services recommended by the U.S. Preventive Services Task Force and Advisory Committee on Immunization Practices. They identify the clinical preventive services that have the greatest health impact and best cost value. It is a fact that high-value preventive care is widely underused, resulting in people who are less productive, incur high health care cost, and may have shorter lives. For example, increasing the number of people who use aspirin regularly to prevent health disease saves 42,000 lives annually. Health reform initiatives that use evidence-based preventive services as a primary goal are likely to result in a healthier population Preventive services that have the greatest health impact and best cost value are available on the AHRQ website as well.

The implementation of the Affordable Health Care Act partially addresses the cost barrier for many consumers. Insurers are required to cover preventive services such as blood pressure checks, cholesterol tests, colonoscopies, mammograms, and osteoporosis screenings at no cost to the consumer. New preventive and wellness resources for pregnant women, children, and seniors also are covered.

THE HEALTH-PLANNING PROCESS

The process for developing a health promotion-prevention plan includes nine steps that actively involve both the client and the nurse in the health-planning process:

1. Review and summarize data from assessment.
2. Emphasize strengths and competencies of the client.
3. Identify health goals and related behavioral change options.
4. Identify behavioral or health outcomes to indicate the plan's success from the client's perspective.
5. Develop a behavior-change plan based on the client's preferences and on the "state-of-the science" knowledge about effective interventions.
6. Reinforce benefits of change and identify incentives for change from the client's perspective.
7. Address environmental and interpersonal facilitators and barriers to behavior change.
8. Determine a period for implementation.
9. Formalize a commitment to behavior-change goals and provide support needed to accomplish them.

Review and Summarize Data from Assessment

During assessment, the nurse obtains a wealth of data from the client. The outcome of assessment activities includes information in a useful format and available in the following domains as a basis for planning and action:

1. Physical health status
2. Functional health patterns
3. Physical fitness
4. Nutritional status
5. Life stressors
6. Spirituality
7. Social support
8. Personal health behaviors
9. Family health practices
10. Environmental and community supports or constraints for health behaviors

During one or more clinic appointments or home visits, the nurse and client review the assessment summary. Both should retain either a hard copy or an electronic copy for continuing reference during the health-planning process. See Chapter 4 for a discussion of these assessment activities.

Emphasize Strengths and Competencies of the Client

Clients bring unique strengths to the health-planning task. Identifying, acknowledging, and reinforcing these strengths are critical to the process. Cultural beliefs, preferences, and current levels of knowledge and skills influence the choice of health practices and health behaviors. It is important to integrate existing cultural practices into the overall health plan to reinforce the client's sense of cultural and/or ethnic pride. Thus, the nurse and client should achieve consensus on areas in which the client is already taking informed and responsible health action as well as on areas for further development of self-care competencies. Health practices outside the mainstream health care system are often compatible with standard practices. For example, Native Americans often use tribal "medicine elders," or "medicine men," to prescribe self-care behaviors. Both traditional and nontraditional health care providers play important roles in the treatment and care of the client. When traditional and nontraditional health care providers cooperate, the client's belief system/culture mores are valued, and the client often has better outcomes.

Through teaching, guidance, and support, the nurse promotes existing competencies to enhance health practices. Self-care requirements and resources will vary according to the client's

---

Designed for: ___James Moore___

Home Address: ___714 George Street___

Home Telephone Number: ___222–3333___

Occupation (if employed): ___building services supervisor___

Work Telephone Number: ___445-6666___

Cultural Identification: ___African-American___

Birth Date: ___3/14/68___ Date of Initial Plan: ___1/15/2014___

Client strengths:	Satisfactory peer relationships, spiritual strength, adequate sleep pattern
Major risk factors:	Elevated cholesterol, mild obesity, sedentary lifestyle, moderate life change, multiple daily hassles, few reported uplifts
Nursing diagnoses: (derived from assessment of functional health patterns)	Diversional activity deficit; altered nutrition: more than body requirements; caregiver role strain (elderly mother)
Medical diagnoses: (if any)	Mild hypertension
Age-specific screening recommendations: (derived from *Guide to Clinical Prev. Services*)	Blood pressure, cholesterol, fecal occult blood, malignant skin lesions, depression
Desired behavioral and health outcomes:	Become a regular exerciser (3x/week), lower my blood pressure, weigh 165 lb

FIGURE 5–1 Example of an Individual Health Promotion-Prevention Plan

Personal Health Goals (1 = highest priority)	Selected Behaviors to Accomplish Goals	Stage of Change	Strategies/ Interventions for Change
1. Achieve desired body weight	Begin a progressive walking program	Planning	Counter-conditioning Reinforcement management Patient contracting
	Decrease caloric intake while maintaining good nutrition	Action (eating 2 fruits and 2 vegetables daily; using low-fat dairy products for last 2 months)	Stimulus control Cognitive restructuring
2. Decrease risk for hypertension-related disorders	Change from high- to low-sodium snacks	Contemplation	Consciousness raising Learning facilitation
3. Learn to manage stress effectively	Attend relaxation classes and use home relaxation tapes	Contemplation	Consciousness raising Self-reevaluation Simple relaxation therapy
4. Increase leisure-time activities	Join a local bowling league	Contemplation	Support system enhancement

FIGURE 5–1   Continued

age, gender, developmental stage, and health status. The self-care needs of families will vary by family composition, developmental stages of its members, and role demands. Although clients differ in their self-care and self-management competencies, it is important to emphasize each client's importance as the primary self-care agent. However, promoting individual responsibility for health does not negate the importance of changing the larger social infrastructure to make health-promoting options more available to groups and communities. Personal change and social change are both essential for effective health promotion and prevention.

Figure 5–1 presents a sample health promotion-prevention plan for an individual, and Figure 5–2 shows a family plan. In both plans, client strengths are emphasized.

Identify Health Goals and Related Behavior-Change Options

The next step in the planning process is to identify and prioritize personal or family health goals and review related behavior-change options. Systematically reviewing the range of changes that are possible to achieve health goals can assist clients in deciding the behavioral changes on which they will initially focus. Providing relevant options enables the client to prioritize behavior-change strategies. Clients need not feel guilty about their current health practices. During health counseling sessions, the nurse should create enthusiasm and excitement about growth in positive directions and the benefits of new health-related experiences.

Designed for (family name): ___The Marshalls___

Home Address: ___1718 Green Street___

Home Telephone Number: ___777-4444___

Occupations of Employed
Members of Household: ___Mother—Dental assistant___

Work Telephone Number: ___883-7777___

Family Form: ___One-parent family___

Cultural Identification: ___American___

Family Members: Position in Family	Birth Date	Occupation/ Student/Retired
Joan (Mother)	9/1981	Dental assistant
Dana (Daughter)	4/2001	Student
Tiffany (Daughter)	7/2004	Student
Eric (Son)	1/2006	Student

Date of Initial Plan: ___1/15/2014___

Family strengths:	Open communication patterns, intrafamily cooperation, healthy snacks consumed at home
Major risk factors:	Mother recently divorced, oldest daughter has driver's license, high life change for family, minimal family physical activity
Nursing diagnoses:	Family coping: potential for growth
Medical diagnoses for family members:	None
Desired behavioral and health outcomes:	Active family outings, avoidance of early sexual activity and binge drinking among adolescent family members, injury prevention for children, adjustment to new family status

FIGURE 5–2 Example of a Family Health Promotion-Prevention Plan

Family Health Goals (1 = highest priority)	Selected Behaviors to Accomplish Goals	Stage of Change	Strategies/ Interventions for Change
1. Healthy adjustment to single-parent family status	Realign family responsibilities	Action (divorced 3 mo)	Social liberation Family process maintenance Caregiver support
	Increase spiritual resources	Contemplation	Spiritual support Helping relationships
	Discuss life purpose and goals among family members	Planning	Self-reevaluation Self-esteem enhancement Anticipatory guidance
2. Develop more active family lifestyles	Plan active family outings (biking, recreation center)	Planning	Exercise promotion Environmental reevaluation Modeling
3. Foster healthy sexuality among preadolescent and adolescents	Provide age-appropriate information	Action	Anticipatory guidance Parent education: adolescent stage
	Enhance self-esteem through praise, expression of affection, and assistance with skill development	Maintenance	Self-esteem enhancement Helping relationships

FIGURE 5–2 Continued

| 4. Encourage adolescents to avoid alcohol use | Hold family meetings to discuss binge drinking, drinking and driving, use of nonalcoholic alternatives | Contemplation | Parent education: adolescent stage Self-responsibility facilitation Substance use prevention |

FIGURE 5–2 Continued

Many clients will place initially high priority on preventive behaviors for which the threat of illness is tangible and easily understood (see Chapter 2 for models of behavior change). Decreasing risk for specific chronic health problems fits the medical orientation to which most Americans are socialized.

Knowledge tailoring based on the client's readiness or interest level in reducing risk of a specific disease indicates that prevention is likely the most meaningful area for emphasis in early health planning. For example, a smoker may be concerned about lung cancer and seek assistance to help quit. Mastery of specific preventive measures often motivates clients to consider making additional lifestyle changes directed toward health promotion to experience a higher level of health and well-being (Allegante, Boutin-Foster, Ogedegbe, & Charlson, 2008; Kravitz et al., 2013).

Clients often give important emotional cues about the behaviors they wish to change. Examples of such cues include the following:

"I hate myself when I gorge on fattening foods!"
"I get mad at myself for being so uptight!"
"The only time our family is together is in front of the television."
"We need to stop eating at so many fast-food places."
"We are very critical of each other."
"We don't participate in physical activities together."

The more open an individual or family is in discussing health concerns with the nurse, the greater the probability of developing a meaningful health promotion-prevention plan. Areas that clients are most reluctant to discuss—such as marital relationships, human sexuality, spirituality, and family cohesiveness—are often the most crucial ones for behavior change. A "safe" climate ensures that personal health issues are open for discussion with assurance of confidentiality.

Identify Behavioral or Health Outcomes

Together, the nurse and client decide the desired health outcomes of the health promotion-prevention plan. Clear identification of outcomes both energizes and guides the client in changing or establishing new health behaviors. The client's perceptions about desired outcomes should guide the criteria used to evaluate the success of the plan and its implementation. "Have I reached my goal or made significant progress toward it?" is a critical question that the client must ask periodically to evaluate the relevance of the health promotion-prevention plan.

Research-based links between particular interventions and desired outcomes should be the basis of a plan. For example, integrating factors or strategies known to increase the likelihood of maintaining a healthy diet into the plan of persons wishing to address nutritional issues increases the likelihood of success. Examples include identifying smartphone and tablet applications on nutrition/diet, directing clients to interactive websites, or offering printed information. Clients often need assistance in setting realistic outcomes. For example, a behavioral goal of eating only at meal times may be easier to attain than a goal of losing a certain number of pounds. Weight reduction likely occurs if the plan is realistic, with tangible behaviors that are under the control of the client to reinforce and manage. Long-term successes that move clients toward their outcomes is the desired goal.

Develop a Behavior-Change Plan

A positive program of change results when the client takes "ownership" of behavior changes. Significant value-behavior inconsistencies may be exposed. Alternative actions that are both healthful and enjoyable should substitute for behaviors that are inconsistent with personal values. Many individuals and families prefer or value the American "lifestyle" (high-fat, high-sodium, and high-calorie foods) that are detrimental to health. Clarifying the value and meaning of health is important to do prior to developing an individual or family behavior-change plan (Allicock, Sandelowski, Devillis, & Campbell, 2008; see Chapter 1).

Clients should select, from the available options, behaviors that are appealing and that they are willing to implement. The client's priorities for behavior change will reflect personal values, activity preferences, cognitive and psychomotor skills, affective responses to the various behavioral options, expectations for success, and ease with which the selected behaviors can be integrated into one's daily lifestyle.

Appropriate strategies and interventions to facilitate individual behavior change are found in the nursing and behavioral science literature (Cameron, 2009; Kennett, Worth, & Forbes, 2009; Hall & Rossi, 2008; Williamson, Champagne, Harsha, Han, Martin, Newton, et al., 2008). As an expert in health care, the nurse can assist the client in gaining the behavior-change skills needed to adopt and maintain positive health behaviors.

Reinforce Benefits of Change

Reinforcement and reminders of the positive benefits of the desired change provide support for the client. A list of benefits, kept in highly visible places such as on the refrigerator, the bathroom mirror, the dashboard of the car, the computer, or smartphone, will serve as reminders to stay on target. Keeping health benefits in front of the client is a reminder that the behaviors in the health promotion-prevention plan are personally worthwhile and directed toward important life goals.

The benefits of change may include both health-related and non–health-related outcomes. Sensitivity to non–health-related benefits of change such as increased popularity or more time with friends is important, as these may be central to the client's motivation to engage in health promotion-prevention planning and implementation.

Address Environmental and Interpersonal Facilitators and Barriers to Change

The features of the physical environment and interpersonal relationships supportive of positive change bolster efforts to modify lifestyle. For example, social networks help counter barriers to change. Encouragement from family and friends helps the client to persist when change efforts are difficult, or other demands or preferences compete for attention. Individuals and families experience barriers to changing behavior. Although some obstacles are anticipated and their potential negative impact considerably weakened, others are not. When the client is aware of possible barriers and formulates plans for managing them, successful behavior change is more likely to occur.

Barriers to effective health behavior may arise from clients' internal conflicts, significant others, or the environment. Internal barriers to change include lack of motivation, fatigue, boredom, giving up, lack of appropriate skills, or disbelief that behavior is changeable. Family members may impose considerable barriers if they encourage continuation of health-damaging behaviors, or if they actively discourage attempts at behavior change.

Environmental barriers that may inhibit positive changes include unsafe neighborhoods, such as heavy traffic or high crime rate; lack of facilities to support positive behaviors, such as access to parks or grocery stores; and inclement weather. The nurse can assist both the client and the community to work to address environmental barriers, as they are major challenges confronting behavior change.

Determine a Time Frame for Implementation

To develop healthier behaviors, integrate them into one's lifestyle, and stabilize them takes time. Attempting to change or initiate multiple new behaviors simultaneously may result in confusion, discouragement, and even abandonment of the health promotion-prevention plan. Whether the client is attempting to reduce risk for chronic disease or enhance health, gradual change is desirable. Just as education for self-care must proceed at the pace of the learner, changes in behavior sequenced in reasonable steps as appropriate for the client will serve as a motivator to change.

A plan for implementation allows time to master appropriate knowledge and skills before a new behavior is implemented, For example, a warm-up before brisk walking or jogging may not be done if the client is not aware of appropriate warm-up exercises. The period for developing a particular behavior may be several weeks or several months. Many online programs and smartphone applications include reminders and data record keeping, are easy to manipulate and use, and can be shared with the nurse and/or other supporters.

Accomplishing short-term goals is important and needs positive reinforcement, as this provides encouragement to continue pursuit of long-term goals and desired outcomes. A meaningful plan requires that deadlines be set for accomplishing specific goals. Adherence to deadlines should be encouraged, with the time shortened or lengthened **only** to make the plan more conducive to permanent behavior change.

Formalize Commitment to Behavior-Change Plan

The client may be more motivated to follow through with selected actions if a formalized commitment follows one of these options:

1. Nurse–client contract agreements, as seen in Figures 5–3 and 5–4
2. Self-contracts, such as those shown in Figures 5–5 and 5–6

3. Public announcements to family members and friends of intentions to engage in new behaviors
4. Integration of new health behaviors into a written or online daily or weekly calendar
5. Purchase of necessary supplies (low-fat foods, exercise videos, music, audiotapes) and equipment (exercise bike, walking shoes)

Behavioral contracts contain specific information about (1) the change to be made, (2) how the change will be accomplished, (3) the individual or family members who are to engage in the change,

---

Nurse–Client Contract and Agreement

Statement of Health Goal: _____ Decreased feelings of stress and tension _____

I _____ Jim Johnson _____ promise to _____ use progressive relaxation _____
(Client)

_____ techniques upon arriving home from work each day _____
(Client Responsibility)

for a period of _____ one week _____ , whereupon,

_____ Kathy Turner _____ will provide (1) guest _____
(Nurse)

_____ coupon for 2 Coffees _____ (2) Complimentary message _____
(Nurse Responsibility)

on _____ Friday, March 7th _____ to me.
(Date)

If I do not fulfill the terms of this contract in total, I understand that the designated reward will be withheld.

Signed: _____
(Client)

_____
(Date)

_____
(Nurse)

_____
(Date)

FIGURE 5–3   Sample Nurse–Client Contract for an Individual Client

(4) the time frame for behavior change, and (5) the consequences of meeting or not meeting the terms of the agreement.

A *nurse–client contract* provides direction through the identification of mutual objectives and the responsibilities of each party. Contracts allow clients to participate actively by choosing goals that they want to accomplish realistically. Generally, the client is responsible for carrying out change

---

Nurse–Client Contract and Agreement

Statement of Health Goal: _____ *Improve eating habits* _____

We _____ *The Nichols* _____ promise to *eat two servings of*
　　　　　　　　　　(Family)

_____ *vegetables and two servings of fruit daily* _____
　　　　　　　　　　　　(Family Responsibility)

for a period of _____ *1 week* _____, whereupon,

_____ *Lana Buxton* _____ will provide _____ *guest passes* _____
　　　　　　　　(Nurse)

for Riverbanks Zoo _____
　　　　　　　　　　(Nurse Responsibility)

on _____ *Friday, April 11th* _____ to us.
　　　　　　　　　　　(Date)

If we do not fulfill the terms of this contract in total, we understand that the designated reward will be withheld.

Signed: _____
　　　　　　　　　　　　(Family Representative)

_____
　　　　　　　　　　　　(Date)

_____
　　　　　　　　　　　　(Nurse)

_____
　　　　　　　　　　　　(Date)

FIGURE 5–4 Sample Nurse–Client Contract for a Family

behaviors, whereas the nurse is responsible for providing information, training, counseling, and/or specific reinforcement rewards. The nurse bears the additional responsibility of providing helpful input and continuing feedback about the adequacy of performance of activities identified in the contract. It is critical that the nurse be consistent and conscientious in managing the reinforcement-reward contingencies of the contract. Failure to fulfill this commitment will alter the trust and confidence placed in the nurse.

In a nurse–client contract with a family, the agreement may be made for family members to walk, jog, or bicycle together two to three times each week, or to modify their nutritional practices, such as increasing vegetables at family meals. Engaged family members serve as important sources of encouragement, reinforcement, and reward for one another because of their continuing contact and emotional bonding.

Answers to the following questions determine the effectiveness of the contract:

Were the goals accomplished fully, partially, or not at all?

If failure occurred, what were the reasons?

Should the contract be rewritten to increase the probability of success?

Should the contract be renegotiated?

Should the contract be terminated?

Careful analysis of the contracting process and evaluation of subsequent outcomes will enable the nurse and client to design a contract that successfully moves the client toward desired health goals.

With a *self-contract,* the client is responsible for both the behavioral commitment and the reinforcement of identified behaviors. Self-contracting is an effective approach to enhancing one's control over behavior, thus creating a sense of independence, competence, and autonomy.

Self-Contract

Personal Health Goal: _____ *Change dietary habits* _____

I _____ *Doris Downs* _____ promise myself that I will ___ *follow* ___

_____ *the sample menus for a 1,200 calorie diet for breakfast, lunch, and* _____

_____ *dinner* _____ for a period of _____ *4 days* _____ ,

whereupon I will _____ *buy myself a new pair of earrings* _____

on _____ *Wednesday, June 8th* _____ .

Signed: _____

Date: _____

FIGURE 5–5 Sample Individual Self-Contract

Self-Contract

Family Health Goal: _____ *Get more exercise* _____

We, _____ *The Morrisons* _____ promise each other that we will ___ *go* ___

_____ *swimming at the "Y" once a week* _____ for a period of ___ *3 weeks* ___

We will then ___ *each buy an updated version of our favorite software* ___

on _____ *Friday, June 5* _____ .

Signed: _____

_____

_____

Date: _____

FIGURE 5–6 Sample Family Self-Contract

The client does not become overly dependent on the nurse for reinforcement. Instead, individuals may choose extrinsic sources for rewards such as tangible objects (new music app, cosmetics) or experiences (trip to visit a friend, take trip to the mall, telephone call to a friend), or intrinsic sources (self-praise, feelings of pride). Rewards selected should be highly desirable to have reinforcement value. The reward-reinforcement plan illustrated in Figure 5–7 provides examples of rewards and reinforcements.

Success in fulfilling contracts enhances the client's self-esteem and problem-solving abilities. The client gains increased confidence in meeting future health needs. In reality, the client must learn to manage a self-reward system to support new positive health practices.

Publicly announcing intentions to engage in a new behavior to family members and close friends is another way to increase one's commitment to a particular course of action. The positive expectations of family members or friends often enhance motivation to change behavior. Social media including Facebook, blogs, and other sharing online provide motivation and encouragement.

Integrating new behaviors into one's calendar is another important strategy necessary to incorporate them into daily routines; for example, exercise time scheduled during the lunch hour. The exercise appointment takes on importance, just as an appointment with one's friend or coworker does. Lack of time is a frequent excuse for being unable to follow through with newly adopted behaviors. Scheduling time to accomplish health behaviors enhances the probability of their occurrence significantly.

Purchasing necessary supplies and equipment is another strategy to help make a commitment to behavior change. Clients are more likely to follow through with the desired behavior if

Behavior: Learn to Use Progressive Relaxation as One Approach to Handling Stress

Component of Behavior	Reward or Reinforcement
Attend first class session at 9 AM Saturday at the County Health Department	Watch football game on TV in the afternoon
Use relaxation CD at home for 20 minutes of practice Sunday	Visit with my friend, John
Monday	Spend an hour bicycling with Leslie
Tuesday	Buy a new novel
Wednesday	Praise myself for practicing relaxation every day
Thursday	Invite Harry and Jim for dinner
Friday	Take my family to a movie
Attend second class session at 9 AM Saturday at the County Health Department	Take a juice break afterward with a class member
Practice relaxation techniques for 20 minutes providing my own cues rather than using the CD Sunday	Go for a short drive to enjoy the fall foliage
Monday	Spend 30 minutes reading my new novel
Tuesday	Buy myself my favorite cologne
Wednesday	Praise myself for persistence and successful practice
Thursday	Allow myself to stay in bed 30 minutes longer than usual
Friday	Go biking with the family
Keep my weekly record of relaxation practice	The nurse will provide a copy of *Relaxation Response* by Herbert Benson

FIGURE 5–7 Reward-Reinforcement Plan

they make a monetary investment. For example, people who have exercise equipment and exercise videos in their homes are more likely to be active than persons who do not.

THE REVISED HEALTH PROMOTION-PREVENTION PLAN

An established schedule for periodic review of the health promotion-prevention plan ensures the client of the importance of the plan. Revisions made during counseling sessions or online with both the client and the nurse contributing to the process increase commitment to the plan.

Impetus for changes in the plan may result from mastery of target behaviors, changes in client's values and priorities, or awareness of new options available to the client. Outdated plans fail to provide motivation or direction for change and thus become uninteresting and meaningless to the client. Periodic revisions and updates provide a systematic approach to assist the client in moving toward more positive health behaviors and a higher level of health.

COMMUNITY-LEVEL HEALTH PROMOTION-PREVENTION PLAN

Community-level plans and interventions may be the most effective way to engage members in improving their health. Important health concerns such as youth and family violence, substance abuse, unintended pregnancy in adolescents, and unintentional injuries may require broad-based planning and intervention. Evidence has validated the influence of the community's social and physical environments on the health of its members.

Wealth, access to health services, social inequity, race, and ethnicity are only a few of the factors taken into account when assessing a community to plan for behavior change. Low-income families and minority populations may perceive their participation in health services offered by the community as a series of trade-offs. For example, too much information may be seen as a source of additional stress, acceptance of services may result in a loss of control, and judgmental and intrusive agency staff may block free-flowing, open communication (Silverstein, Lamberto, DePaul, & Grossman, 2008). The nurse's roles as consultant to communities to implement community-based health plans and interventions include that of advocate for both the advantaged and disadvantaged citizens within the community.

CONSIDERATIONS FOR PRACTICE IN HEALTH PLANNING

Developing a plan to counsel clients about their health behaviors is a major responsibility of nurses in practice. The nurse must possess the skills necessary to guide clients to participate in developing a realistic, positive plan. Nurses with a working knowledge of current guidelines will ensure that information incorporated into the plan is accurate and up-to-date.

An interdisciplinary approach often is more effective in interpreting the assessment data and recommending appropriate goals. Support is critical during the change process, so the nurse must learn to identify family and other support systems for the client and to develop creative strategies to incorporate their support into the plan. The plan must be adapted to life span issues, gender, and cultural differences.

Knowledge of cultural issues is important to the design of a culturally sensitive, age- and gender-appropriate plan. Whenever possible, technology is also an important resource to incorporate in developing the plan. Interactive software that provides feedback on achieving outcomes increases motivation, as immediate results are available. Developing a health promotion-prevention plan is straightforward, but complex. Nurses must continually update their skills to assist clients in this important process.

OPPORTUNITIES FOR RESEARCH IN BEHAVIOR CHANGE

Nurses are in a pivotal position to address questions about planning for health promotion and prevention and to create new knowledge about the behavior-change planning process. Answers to the following questions will enhance the behavior-change process:

1. Does combining face-to-face and computerized feedback from the health assessment optimize one's level of motivation for health promotion planning?
2. What interventions are most effective to reinforce clients' positive health practices?
3. What are the most effective family strategies to promote change?
4. What is the relationship between behavior change and life stages?
5. What are the major barriers to implementing community intervention to improve the health of its members?
6. What types of community-based interventions are most effective in improving the health of special populations?

Summary

The health promotion-prevention plan provides individuals and families with a systematic approach to improve health practices and lifestyle. The client receives a paper or electronic health portfolio that contains a summary of the health assessment, the health promotion-prevention plan, and other relevant health records. It is imperative that clients have all the information and planning documents needed to follow through successfully with their desired behavior changes. Focusing on outcomes desired by the client will energize and direct implementation of the plan. Adjusting the plan as needed to ensure client success is vital to effective health-promoting care. Community-level plans that address broad-based health concerns support the efficacy and effectiveness of developing health promotion-prevention plans at the community level.

Learning Activities

1. Select a partner and develop an individual health plan for each person using the nine-step planning process. Evaluate your experiences and outcomes.
2. Develop a health plan for a family with teenagers using the nine-step planning process. Write a two-page summary of your experiences and outcomes.
3. Write a one-page summary of how community factors influence the individual and family planning processes you developed in Learning Activities 1 and 2.

References

Agency for Healthcare Research and Quality. (2012). *Guide to clinical prevention service, 2012*. Retrieved February 8, 2013, from http://www.ahrq.gov/clinic/pocketgd.htm

Allegante, J., Boutin-Foster, C., Ogedegbe, G., & Charlson, M. (2008). Multiple health-risk behavior in a chronic disease population: What behaviors do people choose to change? *Preventive Medicine, 46*, 247–251.

Allicock, M., Sandelowski, M., Devillis, B., & Campbell, M. (2008). Variations in meaning of personal core value: Health. *Patient Education and Counseling, 93*, 347–353.

Cameron, K. (2009). A practitioner's guide to persuasion: An overview of 15 selected persuasion theories, models and frameworks. *Patient Education & Counseling, 74*, 309–317.

Hall, H., & Rossi, J. (2008). Meta-analytic examination of the strong and weak principles across 48 health behaviors. *Preventive Medicine, 46*(3), 266–274.

Kennett, D., Worth, N., & Forbes, C. (2009). The contributions of Rosenbaum's model of self-control and the transtheoretical model to the understanding of exercise behavior. *Psychology of Sports and Exercise, 10*(6), 1–7.

Kravitz, J., Fiscella, K., Sohler, N., Romero, R., Parnes, B., Aguilar-Gaxiola, S., . . . Franks, P. (2013). Effects of tailored knowledge enhancement on colorectal cancer screening preference across ethic and language groups. *Patient Education and Counseling, 90*(1), 103–110.

Laustria, M., Cortese, J., Noar, S., & Glueckauf, R. (2009). Computer-tailored health interventions delivered over the Web: Review and analysis of key components. *Patient Education and Counseling, 74*(2), 156–173.

Silverstein, M., Lamberto, J., DePaul, K., & Grossman, D. (2008). "You get what you get": Unexpected findings about low-income parents' negative experiences with community resources. *Pediatrics, 122*(6): e 1141-8. doi:10.1542/peds. 2007-3587

Williamson, D., Champagne, C., Harsha, D., Han, H., Martin, C., Newton, R., et al. (2008). Louisiana (LA) health: Design and methods for a childhood obesity prevention program in rural schools. *Contemporary Clinical Trials, 29*, 783–795.

CHAPTER 6

Physical Activity and Health Promotion

OBJECTIVES

This chapter will enable the reader to:

1. List the benefits and risks of physical activity.
2. Describe strategies to develop a physically active lifestyle across the life span.
3. Describe the application of theories and models to promote physical activity.
4. Describe the relationship of built environments with active lifestyles in communities.
5. List the pros and cons of community interventions to promote physical activity.
6. Examine strategies for developing and implementing culturally appropriate physical activity interventions.

Regular physical activity is essential for healthy, energetic, and productive living. Modern life—with its automobiles, televisions, computers, mobile devices, video games, and low levels of physical activity in school and work environments—necessitates the commitment of significant leisure time to physical activity in order to gain health benefits. The rebranding of exercise to close the gap between values and behavior is essential if there is going to be a reversal of the growing sedentary lifestyles of most Americans. Physical activity must be integrated into everyday life, for example, parking a distance from your destination, using the stairs instead of the elevator or escalator, and being sensitive to the inclusion of physical activity in daily activities. The reader is encouraged to review the physiology of exercise to understand how the body reacts to, and benefits from, physical activity.

Physical activity is defined as any bodily movement produced by skeletal muscles that results in expenditure of energy and includes occupational, leisure-time, and routine daily activities. *Lifestyle physical activities* are those carried out in the course of everyday life that contribute to energy expenditure, such as climbing the stairs instead of taking the elevator. *Exercise* is a subcategory of physical activity performed during leisure time that is planned, structured, repetitive, and aimed at improving or maintaining physical fitness or health.

Physical fitness is a measure of a person's ability to perform physical activities that require endurance, strength, or flexibility and is determined by a combination of cardiorespiratory endurance (aerobic power), flexibility, balance, and body composition (U.S. Department of Health and Human Services [USDHHS], 2008a). The term *physical activity* is used in this chapter to encompass a broad range of activities that, if performed regularly, will improve health.

Maintenance of regular physical activity is dependent on personal and social motivation within the day-to-day environment. Family, peers, and the community play a powerful role in encouraging active lifestyles. Many individuals rely on the school or work environments to create programs to help them achieve their physical activity goals. Others cycle through periods of activity and inactivity, never establishing regular physical activity patterns.

Obesity is now one of the most serious and prevalent health problems in the United States. The alarming increase in the prevalence of overweight and obesity among children, adolescents, and adults is thought to be due to genetic influences, high-stress jobs, environmental influences, and primarily dietary and physical activity behaviors (Rauner, Mess, & Woll, 2013; Sallis, Floyd, Rodriquez, & Saelens, 2012). Despite evidence that physical inactivity is related to weight gain, a significant proportion of the U.S. population remains sedentary. Because of the central role of physical activity in health, this chapter focuses on strategies to increase physical activity for clients of all ages and racial, ethnic, and socioeconomic groups.

HEALTH BENEFITS OF PHYSICAL ACTIVITY

Regular physical activity contributes both to physiologic stability and high-level functioning and assists individuals in actualizing their physical performance potential. Research has demonstrated the health benefits of participating in *regular* physical activity. For example, the USDHHS Physical Activity Guidelines Advisory Committee rated the evidence of health benefits as strong, moderate, or weak for children and adolescents, and adults and older adults. The rating system was based on the type, number, and quality of published research, as well as consistency of findings across studies.

The rated health benefits of physical activity are shown in Table 6–1. The health benefits of physical activity can be seen in all ages and all ethnic and racial groups. Scientific evidence documents the role of physical activity in (a) reducing the risk of premature death, (b) managing chronic health problems, (c) improving cardiorespiratory and metabolic health, (d) decreasing the risks for overweight and obesity, and (e) preserving bone, joint, and muscle health.

In addition, *regular* physical activity improves or maintains physical function, lowers the risk for colon and breast cancer, and lessens the risk for depression and cognitive decline. Additional positive outcomes associated with physical activity are improved skin color, vibrancy, and sense of well-being.

Millions of Americans are at risk for a wide range of common mental health problems that might well be prevented or modified by active lifestyles. Regular physical activity can improve mental health, increase one's ability to do everyday tasks better, and serve as adjunct treatment in mental health disorders (Meng & D'Arcy, 2013; Zscucke, Gaudlitz, & Strohle, 2013).

Among children and adolescents, weight-bearing exercise is needed for normal skeletal development and attainment of peak bone mass. Regular physical activity increases strength and agility across all age groups, prevents falls among older adults, and increases their independence

TABLE 6–1 Health Benefits Associated with Regular Physical Activity

Children and Adolescents

Strong evidence

- Improved cardiorespiratory and muscular fitness
- Improved bone health
- Improved cardiovascular and metabolic health biomarkers
- Favorable body composition

Moderate evidence

- Reduced symptoms of depression

Adults and Older Adults

Strong evidence

- Lower risk of early death
- Lower risk of coronary heart disease
- Lower risk of stroke
- Lower risk of high blood pressure
- Lower risk of adverse blood lipid profile
- Lower risk of type 2 diabetes
- Lower risk of metabolic syndrome
- Lower risk of colon cancer
- Lower risk of breast cancer
- Prevention of weight gain
- Weight loss, particularly when combined with reduced calorie intake
- Improved cardiorespiratory and muscular fitness
- Prevention of falls
- Reduced depression
- Better cognitive function (for older adults)

Moderate to strong evidence

- Better functional health (for older adults)
- Reduced abdominal obesity

Moderate evidence

- Lower risk of hip fracture
- Lower risk of lung cancer
- Lower risk of endometrial cancer
- Weight maintenance after weight loss
- Increased bone density
- Improved sleep quality

Source: U.S. Department of Health and Human Services. (2008). *Physical activity guidelines for Americans.* Retrieved July 17, 2009, from http://www.health.gov/paguidelines

in activities of daily living in older adults and persons with disabilities. Physical activity maintains and enhances quality of life for all age groups (Chen & Lee, 2013; U.S. Department of Health and Human Services [USDHHS], 2008b).

POTENTIAL RISKS OF PHYSICAL ACTIVITY

Moderate intensity physical activity is associated with very low risk for adverse events. An overly aggressive approach to physical activity may exaggerate existing health conditions and put individuals, particularly older adults, at risk for untoward effects. See the Prescribing Physical Activity to Achieve Health Benefits section later in this chapter for definitions of moderate and aggressive physical activity.

If an individual has an undiagnosed heart condition and is habitually sedentary, strenuous physical activity *may* create arrhythmias or precipitate a cardiac arrest or myocardial infarction, although adverse events are not common. Individuals over 50 years of age, or with an existing chronic illness such as obesity or cardiovascular disease, should be evaluated medically before starting regular physical activity. Persons with cardiovascular disease or other chronic conditions must be cautioned to avoid activity at levels that are physiologically untenable or result in untoward symptoms. Recommendations for pre-exercise evaluation in older adults with diagnosed chronic cardiovascular disease include an exercise stress test and elimination of aerobic exercise programs (Elsamy & Higgins, 2010).

Overstressing muscles and joints may result in muscle soreness and joint pain. The risk of musculoskeletal injury increases with the total amount of physical activity. A program of gradually increasing physical activity is recommended, with emphasis on moderate activity for older adults. The benefits of appropriate physical activity far outweigh the potential risks.

Proper warm-up and cool-down is important for *any* physical activity. Warming up is important to increase blood flow to the heart and skeletal muscles, enhance oxygenation of tissues, and increase flexibility of muscles before physical activity. The warm-up period allows the heart rate and body temperature to increase gradually and the joints to become more flexible prior to initiating physical activity. Warming up can include activities such as slow walking, arm circles, leg exercises, or wall push-ups. The warm-up period should last about 7–10 minutes and be followed immediately by moderate or vigorous physical activity. A cooling-down period is essential after physical activity. It is important to take time to cool down for 5–10 minutes following physical activity because activity raises heart rate, blood pressure, body temperature, and lactic acid in the muscles. Cooling down allows the heart rate to decrease gradually and prevents pooling of blood in muscles, which can cause lightheadedness. It also helps eliminate lactic acid in muscles and maintains blood flow to and from the muscle. During the cool-down period, it is important to keep the lower extremities moving in activities such as slow walking, jogging, or cycling. At the end of the cooling-down period, the client's resting heart rate should be lower than 100 beats per minute.

GENETICS, ENVIRONMENT, AND PHYSICAL ACTIVITY

The interaction between genetics and the environment and their contribution to health has become a priority area of research. In a gene-environment interaction, the magnitude and direction of the effect that a genetic variant has on phenotype varies as the environment changes (Olden, 2009). In other words, the genetic risk can be modified by the environment, or the effect of the environmental exposure depends on the genetic background. It is now established that genes explain only a small number of complex diseases. Geographic differences in the incidence of disease, as well as differences in disease in immigrant populations, support the idea of a role for environmental influences, which includes lifestyles.

Gene–environment interactions have been studied to document the role of genetic factors in physical activity. In spite of the diversity in samples studied and assessment methods, these factors have accounted for 29 to 62% of the variation in daily exercise at the population level (Bryan, Burton, & Rowan, 2007). Various mechanisms have been proposed, including specific genes for motivation and maintenance of exercise, differential sensitivity to the mental health benefits of exercise, and genetic selection advantage for participating in physical activity (de Geus & de Moor, 2008). Tailored interventions to promote physical activity, based on individual genetic variations, will be needed as research unfolds.

Studies of twins and obesity research have shed light on the gene–environment interaction in physical activity. Although genetic factors are critical, environment is also an important contributor (Bergeman & Ong, 2007). Shared influences, such as social learning and parent role modeling, may offer potential mechanisms operating in the environment to promote physical activity.

Obesity is the result of genetic factors as well as environmental influences, such as overeating and physical inactivity (Giussani, Antolini, Brambilia, Pagani, Zuccotti, et al., 2013). Multiple genetic markers have been identified that increase susceptibility to weight gain, especially in an environment that promotes overeating and minimal physical activity.

PRESCRIBING PHYSICAL ACTIVITY TO ACHIEVE HEALTH BENEFITS

To achieve health benefits, medium and high levels of regular physical activity are essential. *Baseline activities* are the light-intensity activities of daily life, such as climbing stairs, standing, or carrying lightweight objects. People who do only baseline activity are considered inactive. Health-enhancing physical activity is activity that produces health benefits.

The 2008 Physical Activity Guidelines describe four levels of physical activity for adults: inactive, low, medium, and high (USDHHS, 2008a). Low levels of physical activity amount to activity less than 150 minutes per week. Medium physical activity refers to a range of 150–300 minutes of moderate-intensity physical activity a week, or 75–150 minutes of vigorous-intensity physical activity to obtain substantial benefits. A high level of physical activity is defined as more than 300 minutes of moderate-intensity activity a week.

A range of 500–1,000 metabolic equivalents (METs) of activity per week has been shown to provide substantial health benefits. The benefits show a dose-response relationship, in that 1,000 METs per week produce greater benefits than do 500 METs per week. A MET is the ratio of the rate of energy expenditure during an activity to the rate of energy expenditure at rest. One MET is the rate of energy expenditure at rest. Moderate-intensity activity is defined as 3–5.9 METs. Walking at three miles per hour is equivalent to 3.3 METs, so this is considered a moderate-intensity activity. Moderate-intensity activity is also defined as 40 to 59% of aerobic capacity reserve, where 0% of reserve is resting and 100% of reserve is maximal effort. Vigorous-intensity activities are considered 6 METs or greater. Running at ten minutes per mile is classified as vigorous activity, as it is a 10 MET activity. Vigorous activities are 60 to 74% of aerobic capacity reserve.

The American College of Sports Medicine includes frequency and duration—as well as intensity—in its guidelines and recommends 30 minutes of moderate-intensity activity five days a week, or a minimum of 20 minutes of high-intensity activity on three days a week (Garber, Blissmer, Deschenes, Franklin, Lamonte, Lee, et. al., 2011). Intensity (how hard), frequency (how often), and duration (how long) all make up the exercise prescription. However, research has shown that for health benefits, the total amount of activity (minutes of moderate intensity physical activity) is more important than any one component (USDHHS, 2008a).

The 30 minutes daily can be accumulated in 10-minute bouts. In comparing the health outcomes of 10-minute bouts (active lifestyle) to nonbouts (30-minute structured exercise), both approaches reduced cardiovascular disease risk factors equally well. The nonbout approach may be more appealing because people are more likely to adopt and maintain an active lifestyle that is more in line with their natural interests and tendencies, than to commit to a structured exercise program. The cost effectiveness of the active lifestyle approach compared to a structured exercise program is also an important consideration (Loprinzi & Cardinal, 2013).

Advanced practice nurses routinely counsel clients about physical activity and may be involved in determining exercise prescription and an active lifestyle model. They should be knowledgeable about MET equivalents. Likewise, graduates working in outpatient settings may be involved in helping explain MET equivalents to clients. Nurses report knowledge and confidence in some level of physical activity, but many acknowledge that additional education is needed to prescribe exercise programs (Grimslvedi, Ananian, Keller, Woolf, Sebren, & Ainsworth, 2012). Because the public is not familiar with METs and aerobic reserve, activity recommendations are more likely to be understood by the client if they are discussed in number of minutes needed per week and level of intensity.

The minimum number and range of minutes per week for activities of moderate intensity needed is straightforward. Adults should participate in at least 30 minutes of moderate-intensity activity on a minimum of five days a week for a total of at least 150 minutes. A *moderate-intensity* activity can be explained as a level of effort of 5 or 6 on a scale of 0 to 10, where 0 is the effort level when sitting and 10 is all-out maximal effort. This effort produces noticeable changes in heart rate and breathing. A *vigorous-intensity* activity is 7 or 8 on a 10-point scale, which produces large increases in heart rate and breathing. The general rule of thumb is that one minute of vigorous-intensity activity is equivalent to two minutes of moderate-intensity activity. A person doing moderate-intensity activity is able to talk but not sing during the activity, and a person who is doing vigorous intensity physical activity is only able to say a few words before pausing for a breath.

Another recommendation for daily physical activity in the past has been to walk 10,000 steps per day (Tudor-Locke, 2003). More recent research has indicated that moderate-intensity activity is equivalent to walking 3,000 steps in 30 minutes for five days each week or three daily bouts of 1,000 steps in ten minutes for five days each week (Marshall, Levy, Tudor-Locke, Kolkhorst, Wooten, et al., 2009). The authors concluded that moderate-intensity activity is equivalent to a minimum of 100 steps per minute. However, due to errors in using step counts as METs, this should be a general guideline only and a minimum number of steps per minute to see health benefits.

PROMOTING PHYSICAL ACTIVITY ACROSS THE LIFE SPAN

Interest in life span patterns of physical activity has been increased by the realization that many risk factors for cardiovascular disease, including obesity, high blood pressure, and elevated cholesterol, are evident in early childhood. Further, of the major modifiable risk factors for coronary heart disease (elevated cholesterol, smoking, hypertension, and inactivity), physical inactivity is most prevalent across the life span. Despite the evidence for the health benefits, more than half of the American population is not active enough to gain the physical and mental health benefits of physical activity.

Patterns of physical activity that begin early in life are likely to persist over time. While this presumption hasn't been proven or disproven, it is easier to develop positive physical activity patterns early in life rather than to change unhealthy behaviors after they are established habits (Cleland, Dwyer, & Venn, 2012). Lifestyle activity provides flexibility for increasing energy expenditure through altering patterns of daily activities such as walking to work or school, taking the stairs, and walking during lunchtime or after school or work.

Gender and type of physical activity influence motivation for exercise and should be considered in planning programs during adolescence. The 2008 Physical Activity Guidelines promote physical activity across the life span, beginning with age 6 years and older (USDHHS, 2008a). These guidelines are used in this chapter.

PROMOTING PHYSICAL ACTIVITY IN CHILDREN AND ADOLESCENTS

Regular physical activity has many immediate and long-term health benefits for children and adolescents. It improves cardiovascular fitness, increases bone mass, and enhances mental well-being. It is also associated with less obesity, hypertension, and cigarette smoking, which prevents the development of cardiovascular disease, diabetes, and other chronic diseases in adulthood (World Health Organization, cited 2013 March 10; Trost & Loprinzi, 2008).

However, a significant number of children and adolescents do not participate in the level of regular activity needed to achieve health benefits. In addition, the rise in childhood and adolescent obesity is alarming. In the past 30 years, the prevalence of obesity has more than doubled among children and more than tripled in adolescents (Bennette & Sothern, 2009). Although evidence indicates the trend is beginning to level in children of college-educated parents, the large number of obese children and adolescents across all socioeconomic levels warrants strategies for lifestyle change. Evidence consistently shows that only about a third of high school adolescents and about two thirds of children 9–13 years of age achieve the recommended amount of daily physical activity. Adolescent males are more physically active than adolescent girls, and whites are more physically active than Hispanics or African-Americans.

The long-term goal of physical activity research among youths is to design age-, gender-, and culturally appropriate interventions to promote lifelong physical activity. Pubertal changes (onset of menarche, changing patterns of body fat distribution) and social transitions (moving from elementary school to junior high school to senior high school) correspond to changes in sports participation and patterns of physical activity. Longitudinal studies are needed to identify changing activity patterns and design successful strategies to promote physical activity across childhood and adolescence.

Physical Activity and Gender

Physical activity patterns and related influences vary by gender across many studies. Gender differences are seen starting in adolescence. Boys report greater physical activity than girls in the preteen years and have been shown to increase their level of physical activity until about 11 years of age, plateau, and then decrease beginning about 13 years of age (Kahn, Huang, Gillman, Field, Austin, Colditz, et al., 2008). Girl adolescents increase their activity until 12 or 13 years and then decrease, similar to boys. Gender-specific factors are associated with the decline. For boys, changes in attitude toward physical education, perceived parental attitude about body shape and fitness, and risk behaviors (binge drinking and marijuana use) are associated with the decline.

For boys and girls, body mass index (BMI), self-esteem, perceived peer attitudes about physical activity, and parental attitude about physical activity are associated with the decline (Kahn, Huang, Gillman, Field, Austin, Colditz, et al., 2008). Research has consistently documented similar determinants and suggests that interventions should be implemented before the anticipated decline. Adolescent interventions also need to address modifiable individual, environmental, and parental factors.

Implementing Guidelines for Physical Activity

A minimum of 60 minutes or more of moderate or vigorous physical activity every day is recommended for adolescents and children (USDHHS, 2008a). Children and adolescents should participate in vigorous-intensity activities at least three days per week. Three types of activity are important: *aerobic, muscle-strengthening,* and *bone-strengthening* activities (see Chapter 4, Assessing Health and Health Behaviors). *Aerobic* activities increase cardiorespiratory fitness and include such things as running, hopping, skipping, jumping rope, swimming, dancing, and bicycling.

Muscle-strengthening activities in this age group are usually unstructured, such as climbing on playground equipment. Structured *muscle strengthening* activities for adolescents may include weight lifting. Activities that promote *bone growth* and *strength* include running, basketball, hopscotch, and jumping rope. Adolescents are more likely to engage in structured programs or play sports that provide aerobic benefits.

Physical activity should be age appropriate and enjoyable and should include a variety of activities. Sedentary and obese children may have difficulty performing physical activity for 60 minutes, so it is recommended that exercise begin gradually and increase 10% per week until the recommendation time is achieved (Bennette & Sothern, 2009). Developmentally appropriate activities are those that are suitable for the child's physical and cognitive development. A range of noncompetitive and competitive activities, age and ability appropriate, should be offered.

Interventions also should be aimed at decreasing sedentary behavior, such as limiting television and video game time to two hours daily. A review of studies using pedometers to promote physical activity in youth indicates that pedometers can be used successfully to promote physical activity in preadolescents and adolescents when used for self-monitoring (Lubans, Morgan, & Tudor-Locke, 2009). Examples of aerobic, muscle-strengthening, and bone-strengthening activities are shown in Table 6–2.

The physical inactivity level of preschoolers has followed the pattern for primary, secondary, and high-school students. In a seven-country study of preschoolers, only 54% of the children were sufficiently physically active (Espana-Romero, Mitchell, Dowda, ONeill, & Pate, 2013; Tucker & Gilliland, 2007). The amount of time spent in daycare, increase in screen viewing (television, video games, computers), and greater parental constraints in play places and safety concerns have resulted in a dramatic increase in sedentary behavior.

Physical activity habits begin to develop in preschool years, so this group also needs interventions to increase physical activity. The national physical activity guidelines do not include preschool children, ages 3–5 years. However, the National Association for Sports and Physical Education recommends 60 minutes of structured physical activity daily and at least 60 minutes of unstructured physical activity for preschoolers (National Association for Sport and Physical Education, 2009).

TABLE 6–2 Aerobic and Muscle- and Bone-Strengthening Activities

Type of Physical Activity	Age Group	
	Children	Adolescents
Moderate-intensity aerobic	• Active recreation such as hiking, skateboarding, rollerblading • Bicycle riding • Walking to school	• Active recreation, such as canoeing, hiking, cross-country skiing, skateboarding, rollerblading • Brisk walking • Bicycle riding (stationary or road bike) • House and yard work such as sweeping or pushing a lawn mower • Playing games that require catching and throwing, such as baseball, softball, basketball, and volleyball
Vigorous-intensity aerobic	• Active games involving running and chasing, such as tag • Bicycle riding • Jumping rope • Martial arts, such as karate • Running • Sports such as ice or field hockey, basketball, swimming, tennis, or gymnastics	• Active games involving running and chasing, such as flag football, soccer • Bicycle riding • Jumping rope • Martial arts such as karate • Running • Sports such as tennis, ice or field hockey, basketball, swimming • Vigorous dancing • Aerobics • Cheerleading or gymnastics
Muscle-strengthening	• Games such as tug of war • Modified push-ups (with knees on the floor) • Resistance exercises using body weight or resistance bands • Rope or tree climbing • Sit-ups • Swinging on playground equipment/bars • Gymnastics	• Games such as tug of war • Push-ups • Resistance exercises with exercise bands, weight machines, handheld weights • Rock climbing • Sit-ups • Cheerleading or gymnastics
Bone-strengthening	• Games such as hop-scotch • Hopping, skipping, jumping • Jumping rope • Running • Sports such as gymnastics, basketball, volleyball, tennis	• Hopping, skipping, jumping • Jumping rope • Running • Sports such as gymnastics, basketball, volleyball, tennis

Source: Centers for Disease Control and Prevention. Retrieved July 17, 2009, from http://www.cdc.gov/physicalactivity/everyone/guidelines/what_counts.html

Preschools are an important way to implement interventions because more than half of the children in the United States attend preschool. Only a limited number of studies have been done on this age group, and those that have been conducted show that when the preschooler, teacher, and parent are involved in the intervention, positive changes result (Goldfield, Harvey, Gratten, & Adamo, 2012; Williams, Carter, Kibbe, & Denniston, 2009). In addition, activity-friendly playgrounds that include balls, hoops, tricycles, and movable equipment tend to increase the physical activity in this age group, especially if accompanied by active supervision and structured physical activity (Cardon, Labarque, Smits, & de Buordeaudhuij, 2009).

Promoting Physical Activity in Families

Family-based activities are important in promoting a healthy lifestyle in children and adolescents. Parents' lifestyles influence adolescents' risk of developing active or inactive lifestyles as young adults (Crossman, Sullivan, & Benin, 2006). For example, parental obesity places male and female adolescents at greater risk for being overweight as adults. Parents influence their children's physical behavior as role models by being directly involved in activities with their children, offering encouragement and support, and providing opportunities and resources to engage in recreational sports and programs (Madsen, McCulloch, & Crawford, 2009).

Family-based programs encourage parents to change their behaviors and to be active with their children in relationship-building experiences. For example, weekend family bike outings and parent–child aerobic or recreational activities create opportunities for parents to be role models for active lifestyles.

Parental support is also needed for children to walk and cycle to school. Although the physical environment is important in the decision to walk to school, research indicates that parental support for walking is associated with increases in physical activity, especially among younger children (Hume, Timperio, Salmon, Carter, & Giles-Corti, 2009).

Interventions, including school-based programs, to increase physical activity behaviors in children and adolescents should target the entire family. A review of 14 clinical trials that involved parents in interventions to increase physical activity in youth found that programs need to engage parents directly in training and counseling (O'Connor, Jago, & Baranowski, 2009).

Family-based programs are often a major challenge, as parents may be difficult to reach and recruit due to their work commitments. Contacting families during organized activities is more effective than sending written materials home with the child. Telephone interventions with family members also show promise. Findings also indicate that the dosage of the intervention needs to be high enough to produce an effect. In other words, more-intensive programs may be needed to result in behavior change. Programs that involve the parent in physical activity have been successful in increasing time spent in physical activity by the child as well as the parents.

Childhood and adolescence are ideal periods in the life span to cultivate regular physical activity that can reap positive health benefits throughout life. Family involvement increases the health habits of the parents as well as the children. Restricting television screen time as well as computer gaming encourages physical activity among all the family members.

Promoting Physical Activity in Schools

Schools play a major role in promoting involvement of children in recreational activities that they can enjoy for a lifetime. By promoting physical activity on a daily basis, teaching the personal value of regular activity, and encouraging continuing involvement in moderate and vigorous activities both at school and at home, schools contribute to the goal of an "active" generation. Schools are an ideal setting because they have intense and continuous contact with most children ages 6–16 years. Teachers have an interest in health promotion; appropriate facilities (gymnasium, sports equipment, and playground) to promote activity are present; a structure with blocks of time available to train children (recess, lunch) is in place; and schools have the capacity to interact with the community-based activity providers (Trost & Loprinzi, 2008).

The time allotted for recess and physical education in public schools is minimal as schools try to meet obligations imposed by state and federal programs. Some states, for example, South Carolina, have enacted legislation requiring a minimum of physical education and physical activity in public schools. This action was in response to high rates of obesity among children and obesity-related diseases such as diabetes, hypertension, and heart disease (The Student Health and Fitness Act of 2005).

Physical activity can be promoted at break times or after school. Results of a meta-analysis that included 14 studies to promote physical activity indicate that after-school programs can improve physical activity levels (Beets, Beighle, Erwin, & Huberry, 2009). In a review of studies evaluating the effectiveness of programs to increase physical activity in schools, the results indicate that all of them increased activity levels (Zaga, Briss, & Harris, 2005). School-based programs are effective in increasing levels of physical activity, physical fitness, aerobic capacity, and time spent in moderate to vigorous activities. Based on the consistency of results, the U.S. Task Force on Community Interventions recommends that these programs should be adapted for all elementary, middle, and high-school students.

The most widely disseminated school-based programs are the Sports Play and Active Recreation for Kids (SPARKS) program and The Child and Adolescent Trial for Cardiovascular Health (CATCH). Both programs target physical activity behaviors, as well as behavior change skills and parental involvement. SPARKS has been disseminated in more than 300 schools, and CATCH has been disseminated in more than 1,800 schools in Texas (Trost & Loprinzi, 2008). Key reasons for sustainability of these school-based programs are strong support by the school principal, availability of adequate equipment, teachers who engaged in physical activity themselves, and availability of ongoing training (Owens, Glanz, Sallis, & Kelder, 2006).

Barriers to success include lack of resources—for example, large class size, inadequate number of physical education specialists, and inadequate school facilities. A major barrier to implementation in schools is placing physical activity as a low priority in the curriculum.

PROMOTING PHYSICAL ACTIVITY IN ADULTS AND OLDER ADULTS

Cardiovascular diseases (heart disease, stroke), type 2 diabetes, and cancer are the leading causes of illness, disability, and death among Americans and the most costly and preventable. Chronic diseases account for 70% of all deaths in the United States, and one third of the years of potential life lost before age 65. Heart disease and stroke account for almost one third of all deaths in the United States and are preventable.

Physical inactivity has consistently been shown to be associated with the risk of developing the major chronic diseases. Attention is being given to the fact that sedentary time (screen time at home and work, travel time, and watching sports) can account for the majority of an adult's waking hours. Adults who meet the 30-minute recommended physical activity for most days of the week, yet are sedentary for the remaining hours, risk serious adverse health consequences. The 30-minute physical activity recommendation (bout or nonbout) is not likely to be protective for those who spend a large amount of time in sedentary behaviors (Owen, 2012; see Figure 6–1).

Television screen time, but not reading and computer time, was found to be associated with increase in cardiovascular risk factors in a large Asian adult population (Nang, Salim, Wu, Tai, Lee, & Van Dam, 2013). Regular physical activity prevents or reduces the risk for cardiovascular diseases, as well as improves quality of life in adults and older adults. Physical activity in older adults protects against loss of mobility and increases functional independence through improved muscle mass, increased bone density, and cardiovascular fitness (SangNam, Smith, & Ory, 2012; Rosenburg, Kerr, Patrick, Moore, & King, 2009; World Health Organization, cited 2013 March 10).

The individual-focused theories and models discussed in Chapter 2 have been used to guide most of the adult physical activity research. Social cognitive theory, the transtheoretical model, the theory of planned behavior, the health belief model, and the health promotion model have all been used with limited success—along with social support theory, motivational interviewing, and relapse prevention theory. These theoretical models have focused on the cognitive, affective, and social influences on individuals, and although they have shown success, the amount of explained variance has remained low.

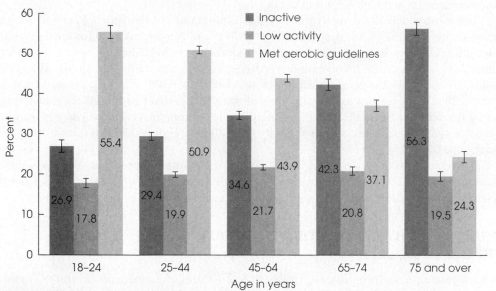

I 95% confidence interval.
Note: Estimates are based on household interviews of a sample of the civilian noninstitutionalized population.

FIGURE 6–1 Percentage of Adults Who Engaged in Leisure-Time Aerobic Physical Activity, by Level of Activity and Age: United States, Annualized, 2008–2010 *Source:* Schoenborn, C. A., Adams, P. F., & Peregoy, J. A. (2013). Health behaviors of adults: United States, 2008–2010. National Center for Health Statistics. *Vital Health Statistics, 10*(257). http://www.cdc.gov/nchs/data/series/sr_10/sr10_257.pdf

Researchers, practitioners, and policy makers see the value of paying attention to additional factors in the social and physical environment that also influence lifestyle behaviors and have implemented new approaches, such as social ecological theory, to guide health promotion interventions and policy initiatives. Social ecological models include intrapersonal, interpersonal, and environmental approaches that are interdependent in their effects on lifestyle behaviors. These models offer a greater likelihood of success, as they approach physical activity from the individual's perspective and include the social and physical forces operating in the environment that also influence health behaviors.

Several individual models, such as the health promotion model and the health belief model, include concepts such as barriers, facilitating conditions, and contextual factors. These concepts should be considered more broadly to account for environmental factors and their interaction with individual concepts in the models. Socio-ecological and other environmental models that explain individual behavior–environmental interactions are important to guide research and policy so as to develop, implement, and evaluate effective physical activity interventions.

Gender and Physical Activity

Evidence indicates that physical activity plays a role in the primary prevention of cardiovascular disease, diabetes, and some cancers in women, as well as in men (World Health Organization, cited 2013 March 10). However, women report less leisure-time physical activity than do men, as they spend more time in paid and unpaid working roles. Multiple family obligations decrease women's time for physical activity. Unmarried women generally are more active than married women with children at home.

In addition, leisure-time physical activity is influenced by role changes in women's lives— parenthood, employment, children leaving home, and retirement. The Baltimore Longitudinal Study of Aging found that a greater decline in total and high-intensity leisure-time physical activity is a predictor of all-cause mortality in men, but not in women (Talbot, Morrell, Fleg, & Metter, 2007). However, men and women of different races and cultures did not differ in the inverse dose-response relationship between leisure-time physical activity and the metabolic syndrome (Halldin, Rosell, deFaaire, & Hellenius, 2007).

African-American men and women did not show any significant difference in prevalence of metabolic syndrome and participation in physical activity, but age and marital status were strong predictors of metabolic syndrome with married women more likely to have metabolic syndrome (Bhanushali, Kumar, Karavatas, Habib, Daniel, & Lee, 2013).

In addition to the time barrier, other obstacles to engaging in physical activity have been consistently reported by women:

1. Lack of social support and encouragement to be physically active from family members or close friends and lack of child care may reinforce sedentary lifestyles (Hoebeke, 2008).
2. Low-income women report that exhaustion from completing the daily demands of child care and family and work responsibilities leaves little energy for themselves.
3. In some ethnic groups, cultural barriers exist, as physical activity may not be considered an appropriate activity for women.
4. Neighborhood safety issues and lack of facilities tailored to women's needs further impede adoption of active lifestyles (Morris, McAuley, & Motl, 2008).

All of these barriers should be considered in planning programs for women.

Implementing Physical Activity Guidelines

The 2008 Guidelines recommend that adults under age 65 years need to participate in at least 150 minutes each week of moderate-intensity aerobic (endurance) activity, or 75 minutes of vigorous-intensity physical activity each week in order to obtain substantial benefits for lowering one's risk of heart disease and stroke, type 2 diabetes, and depression (USDHSS, 2008a). As stated previously, the benefits are dose-related, so that 300 minutes per week results in additional benefits, which include lower risk for colon and breast cancer and prevention of weight gain. The activity should be performed at least three days a week to produce health benefits and can be performed in bouts of 10 minutes, which may be moderate intensity, vigorous intensity, or combinations of both.

Also recommended are muscle-strengthening activities to increase muscle fitness and bone strength. Muscle-strengthening activities include weight lifting, resistance bands, calisthenics, carrying heavy loads, and gardening. These activities should be done two days a week and will count if they work the major muscle groups at moderate- to high-intensity levels.

Inactive adults need to *begin slowly* and *gradually* increase the activity over a period of weeks to months. For example, they may begin with five minutes of slow walking several times a day and slowly increase each session. Initially, muscle-strengthening activities can be performed one day a week at a light- or moderate-intensity effort. Active adults can increase the number of minutes per week to exceed the minimum level or they can perform higher-intensity activities and do muscle-strengthening activities at least two days per week.

Structured programs have been successful with both adults and older adults. The Sedentary Exercise Adherence Trial (SWEAT2) promoted swimming and walking in sedentary women aged 50 to 70 years (Cox, Burke, Beilin, Sallie, & Saelens, 2008). Adherence and physical fitness were similar in both groups at six months, and increased physical fitness at six months was maintained at 12 months. Comparison of a home-based program support by telephone calls with structured, supervised weekly classes, and a control group resulted in similar improvements in the structured and home-based program at six months (Opdenacker, Boen, Coorevits, & Delecluse, 2008). However, at 12 months, the home-based group *maintained* physical activity levels compared with the structured group, providing support for lifestyle home-based programs in older adults.

Sedentary behavior increases with age, and older adults (aged 65 years and older) are the most sedentary group. However, aerobic and strength-building activities are essential for healthy aging, and older adults should be encouraged to develop or continue healthy lifestyle habits. The guidelines for younger adults also apply to individuals ages 65 years and older: a minimum of 150 minutes of moderate-intensity physical activity, 75 minutes of vigorous-intensity physical activity each week, or a combination of the two. All types of activities count, including walking the dog and taking an exercise class. Dog walking promotes physical activity, and research shows that dog walkers are less likely to be obese than are non-dog walkers (Coleman, Rosenberg, Conway, Sallis, & Saelens, 2008). The activities may be done in 10-minute bouts if performed at a moderate or vigorous intensity level. Supervision may be initially required for older adults so as to learn exercise at a moderate level of effort, especially for adults with low fitness levels.

Muscle-strengthening activities are also recommended for older adults. They should perform 8–10 exercises using resistance, such as weights, at 10–15 repetitions for each exercise, a minimum of two days a week. These exercises should be done at the same levels of intensity as aerobic activities: 5 to 6 on a 10-point scale for moderate intensity, and 7 to 8 for vigorous intensity.

Vigorous-intensity activities should be performed under supervision or by adults who have continued to be physically fit. Older adults at risk for falls also need to perform balance training three days a week. Examples of exercises in a balance program include walking backward, walking sideways, heel and toe walking, and standing from a sitting position. Tai Chi has been shown to prevent falls, so enrolling in one of these exercise classes is another option to improve balance. Pilates and Yoga, exercise programs that strengthen the core abdominal muscles, are other options for improving balance.

Adherence to home exercises as a part of a structured program intervention to prevent falls in persons over 60 is low. Individuals enjoy the socialization associated with the structured program and put less emphasis on follow-up at home. Adherence improves in interventions where there are telephone support and home visits (Simek, McPhate, & Haines, 2012).

Older adults consist of the young old (65–74 years), middle old (75–84 years), and very old (over 85 years), and the ability to be physically active varies over this age spectrum. Getting older adults to engage in an active lifestyle is particularly challenging, as evidenced by the fact that only 14 percent of adults aged 65 to 74 exercise and only 7 percent of those over 75 exercise regularly (Anderson-Hanley, Arclero, Brickman, Nimon, Okurma, Western, Mera, et al., 2012).

Barriers to physical activity are an important consideration for the elderly. Although work and family demands may lessen with age, convenience of facilities, cost, opportunities for physical activity with others, fear of resultant illness or injury, disability, and sensory impairment become more important. Concern about existing medical conditions may be a further deterrent to an active lifestyle. Environmental barriers, such as weather (extreme temperatures and precipitation), presence or quality of sidewalks, and lack of places to sit and rest while walking are concerns of older adults.

Many older adults also have misconceptions about physical activity, believing that it can be unhealthy. Barriers can be addressed by inclusion of an educational component with physical activity programs. Emphasis should be placed on reducing sedentary activity and increasing moderate activity, leaving vigorous activities for select older adults with appropriate fitness levels (Elsamy & Higgins, 2010). A stepwise program (additive approach) is also recommended to decrease the risks of injury and to gain experience and self-confidence performing the activities. Table 6–3 describes strategies for all adults to overcome the major barriers to physical activity.

Inactive adults and adults with chronic conditions should consult with their health care provider, who will assess their ability to participate in physical activity. Inactive adults should begin very slowly and increase activity gradually over a period of months. They should aim for 150 minutes a week. If an older adult who has a chronic condition is unable to meet the target goal of 150 minutes a week, even 60 minutes of moderate-intensity activity will produce some health benefits. Warm-up and cool-down activities are important.

Programs to increase physical activity in adults should be tailored to their interests, preferences, and readiness to change. Based on scientific evidence, the Guide to Community Preventive Services (Zaga, Briss, & Harris, 2005) recommends that programs teach the behavior skills needed to make leisure-time physical activity a daily habit. Other components of successful programs are setting goals for physical activity, monitoring progress, building social support, incorporating self-rewards for the new behaviors, and learning to problem solve to maintain change and prevent relapse. These programs can be delivered individually, in groups, or by telephone, mail, or computer.

Social support interventions have been successful, as they build, strengthen, and maintain social networks to promote physical activity (Kassavou, Turner, & French, 2013). These programs establish buddy systems and contracts or form walking groups. Group members or buddies

TABLE 6–3 Strategies for Overcoming Barriers to Physical Activity

Barrier	Strategies
Lack of time	Identify available time slots. Monitor your daily activities for one week. Identify at least three 30-minute time slots you could use for physical activity.
	Add physical activity to your daily routine. For example, walk or ride your bike to work or shopping, organize school activities around physical activity, walk the dog, exercise while you watch TV, park farther away from your destination, etc.
	Select activities requiring minimal time, such as walking, jogging, or stair climbing.
Social influence	Explain your interest in physical activity to friends and family. Ask them to support your efforts.
	Invite friends and family members to exercise with you. Plan social activities involving exercise.
	Develop new friendships with physically active people. Join a group, such as the YMCA or a hiking club.
Lack of energy	Schedule physical activity for times in the day or week when you feel energetic.
	Convince yourself that if you give it a chance, physical activity will increase your energy level; then, try it.
Lack of motivation	Plan ahead. Make physical activity a regular part of your daily or weekly schedule and write it on your calendar.
	Invite a friend to exercise with you on a regular basis and write it on both your calendars.
	Join an exercise group or class.
Fear of injury	Learn how to warm up and cool down to prevent injury.
	Learn how to exercise appropriately considering your age, fitness level, skill level, and health status.
	Choose activities involving minimum risk.
Lack of skill	Select activities requiring no new skills, such as walking, climbing stairs, or jogging.
	Take a class to develop new skills.
Lack of resources	Select activities that require minimal facilities or equipment, such as walking, jogging, jumping rope, or calisthenics.
	Identify inexpensive, convenient resources available in your community (community education programs, park and recreation programs, worksite programs, etc.).
Weather conditions	Develop a set of regular activities that are always available regardless of weather (indoor cycling, aerobic dance, indoor swimming, calisthenics, stair climbing, rope skipping, mall walking, dancing, gymnasium games, etc.).

Barrier	Strategies
Travel	Put a jump rope in your suitcase and jump rope.
	Walk the halls and climb the stairs in hotels.
	Stay in places with swimming pools or exercise facilities.
	Join the YMCA or YWCA (ask about reciprocal membership agreement).
	Visit the local shopping mall and walk for half an hour or more.
	Bring your mp3 player with your favorite aerobic exercise music.
Family obligations	Trade babysitting time with a friend, neighbor, or family member who also has small children.
	Exercise with the kids: go for a walk together, play tag or other running games, get an aerobic dance or exercise tape for kids (there are several on the market) and exercise together. You can spend time together and still get your exercise.
	Jump rope, do calisthenics, ride a stationary bicycle, or use other home gymnasium equipment while the kids are busy playing or sleeping.
	Try to exercise when the kids are not around (e.g., during school hours or their nap time).
Retirement years	Look upon your retirement as an opportunity to become more active instead of less. Spend more time gardening, walking the dog, and playing with your grandchildren. Children with short legs and grandparents with slower gaits are often great walking partners.
	Learn a new skill that you have always been interested in, such as ballroom dancing, square dancing, or swimming.
	Now that you have the time, make regular physical activity a part of every day. Go for a walk every morning or every evening before dinner. Treat yourself to an exercycle and ride every day while reading a favorite book or magazine.

Source: Centers for Disease Control and Prevention. Retrieved July 20, 2009, from http://www.cdc.gov/physicalactivity/everyone/getactive/barriers.html

provide motivational support, as well as companionship and encouragement to engage in regular leisure-time physical activities. Group facilitators provide encouragement and formal discussions to address barriers and other issues related to behavior change. Telephone calls to provide encouragement and monitor progress also are useful.

Promoting Physical Activity in the Work Site

An increasingly sedentary workplace, an aging workforce, and a rising rate of preventable chronic diseases make health promotion workplace programs a priority. Work sites are ideal places to promote healthy changes, as large numbers of employees are available for an extended period of time. Employers have multiple tools and resources with which to engage employees, such as department meetings, telephone or computer-based interventions, e-mail communication, signage on bulletin boards, and the ability to make policy and health benefit changes (Pronk & Kottke, 2009).

Health promotion programs in work settings are thought to help employees stay healthy, satisfied, and productive. Also important is the projected savings in health care costs and lost productivity. However, a meta-analysis of 29 studies examining physical activity or nutrition found that the workplace is a suitable environment for making changes in physical activity level, but the evidence that these changes can be maintained long term needs further study (Hutchinson & Wilson, 2012).

Scientific evidence supports the need to implement and test programs to promote leisure-time physical activities. Wellness programs that focus on nutrition and physical activity have been associated with a decrease in absenteeism and improvement in cardiovascular risk factors. The Worksite Opportunities for Wellness (WOW) promotes wellness through dietary and physical activity programs, pedometers, group exercise classes, weight-loss classes, and rewards. Differences in BMI and fat mass were noted between the intervention and control groups after 12 months (Racette, Deusinger, Inman, Burlis, Highstein, Buskirk, et al., 2009). However, improvements were observed with personalized health assessments and personalized reports without the intervention.

Get Moving, a website that promotes physical activity in sedentary employees, demonstrated improved physical activity in those participating in the program. Employees visited the website regularly to develop a personalized physical activity plan and to seek information and support. Technology continues to play a major role in improving the health of employees and has the potential to become the primary health promotion format in the workplace (Irvine, Philips, Seeley, Wyant, Duncan, & Moore, 2011).

The Move to Improve 12-month clinical trial, which was implemented at Home Depot work sites, resulted in physical activity increasing to 51% at the intervention sites, compared with 25% in the control sites (Dishman, DeJoy, Wilson, & Vandenberg, 2009). Participants exceeded the recommended 300 minutes per week of moderate to vigorous activity and 9,000 daily pedometer steps.

The findings of a worksite wellness program concluded that the employees who lowered their BMI also reported increased feelings of calmness, improved ability to cope with stress, and more physical energy (Merrill, Aldana, Garrett, & Ross, 2011). At year five, a health-promotion campaign and rearrangement of the environment to promote walking resulted in an increase in high-density lipoprotein cholesterol levels in middle-age employees (Naito, Nakayama, Okamura, Miura, Yanagita, Fujieda, et al., 2008).

In general, positive findings have been reported for physical activity programs; however, research continues to suffer from numerous barriers in the workplace. The most successful programs incorporate a socio-ecological approach, targeting the individual as well as the environment, and engage the organization (Kahn-Marshall & Gallant, 2012). Currently, employers can deduct the cost of on-site facilities from their taxes if the services are provided to benefit employees. If the services are outsourced, however, employees must pay income tax on this benefit (Wamp, 2009); thus, policy changes are needed to eliminate tax and other barriers for employers and employees.

PROMOTING PHYSICAL ACTIVITY IN PERSONS WITH DISABILITIES

Physical inactivity is particularly prevalent in persons with disabilities. Physical activity can improve functional capacity; reduce secondary conditions such as obesity, hypertension, and pressure sores; provide opportunities for leisure enjoyment; and improve the overall quality of life for persons with disabilities. The aim of physical activity in this population is to emphasize the importance of carrying out daily activities with a minimum of assistance. Physical activity recommendations for persons with disabilities are available at the National Center on Health, Physical Activity and Disability website.

INTERVENTIONS IN THE COMMUNITY TO PROMOTE PHYSICAL ACTIVITY

Interventions in the community to promote physical activity take place in schools, work sites, churches, and other community organizations, and these reach a larger group than do one-on-one interventions. These community-based programs focus on groups of individuals at the various sites. Community-level interventions focus on the entire population through mass media campaigns or by changing the physical or built environment.

Recently the term *whole community* has been used to describe community interventions that are based on social ecological approaches. Whole community interventions use participatory planning to develop strategies to intervene at the individual, social, environmental, and legislative levels (Mummery & Brown, 2009). Although individual factors, such as motivation, are important, it is well documented that community interventions require multiple intervention components, which include mass media, community activities to enhance social networks and social support, engagement with community members, participatory planning, and community partnerships.

Whole community approaches include (1) social marketing through local mass media, (2) other community strategies to raise awareness, (3) individual counseling, (4) engaging voluntary and nongovernment agencies, (5) working in specific settings, such as work sites and schools, and (6) environmental change strategies (Mummery & Brown, 2009).

Community-based approaches have been implemented to promote physical activity at all ages and socioeconomic groups with success. The Keep Minnesota Active clinical trial for adults aged 50–70 years successfully used a telephone- and mail-based activity maintenance intervention to promote maintaining physical activity at six months for participants in a large managed care organization (Martinson, Crain, Sherwood, Hayes, Pronk, & O'Connor, 2008). The Hartslag Limburg five-year community intervention program was successful in preventing age- and time-related unfavorable changes in walking and leisure-time activities, particularly among low socioeconomic status women (Weldel-Vos, Dutman, Verschuren, Ronickers, Ament, van Assema, et al., 2009).

Two physical activity programs, Active for Life and Active Living Every Day, were successfully translated into a wide range of institutions in community settings (Wilcox, Dowda, Leviton, Barlett-Prescott, Bazzarre, Campbell-Voytal, et al., 2008). Positive results were consistent across sites.

A multilevel walking intervention, implemented in a continuing care retirement community for adults over age 65, was successful in increasing walking in the intervention group. The multilevel intervention components included pedometers for self-monitoring, social support, changing perceptions about the environment, and counseling for goal setting (Rosenburg, Kerr, Patrick, Moore, & King, 2009).

The Guide to Community Preventive Services (Zaga, Briss, & Harris, 2005) recommends five evidence-based components that should be tailored to individual community needs:

- Community-wide media campaigns
- School-based physical education
- Individual adapted behavior change interventions
- Social support interventions
- Increased access to places for physical activity

Media campaigns should use television, newspapers, radio, and other media as appropriate. Social support interventions include organizing a buddy system, walking groups, or community physical activities, such as dances. Individual evidence-based interventions must be adapted for larger audiences. Interventions to increase access include work site programs and providing access to school playgrounds and gymnasiums (Zaga, Briss, & Harris, 2005).

Community-based physical activity programs must be evaluated to identify programs that are effective and can be recommended for practice. The CDC Physical Activity Evaluation Handbook recommends six steps in the evaluation process:

1. Engage stakeholders in the evaluation process.
2. Plan and describe the program.
3. Focus the evaluation.
4. Justify conclusions.
5. Gather credible evidence.
6. Disseminate the lessons learned.

Four community-wide walking programs were evaluated for program effectiveness. The evaluation plan included formative, process, and outcome evaluation strategies. The authors reported six major lessons learned from the evaluation process: (1) participatory planning is an essential first step; (2) it is important to coordinate media approaches and stay focused on the message; (3) knowing the media market is key; (4) organizers must be aware of the resources that will be needed to change; (5) having a community organizer who maintains links with stakeholders is critical; and (6) the sustainability of the program must be monitored (Reger-Nash, Bauman, Cooper, Chey, & Simon, 2006).

Community-based interventions are complex, require financial and human resources, and need time to be implemented and evaluated. Ongoing monitoring and evaluation using multiple sources of data is important. Also essential to evaluate is cost-effectiveness of community-based interventions. Seven physical activity interventions were evaluated for costs, health gains, and cost-effectiveness in a simulated cohort of healthy adults (Roux, Pratt, & King, 2009). All of the interventions included individually adapted behavior change, social support interventions, informational outreach activities, and the creation of access to places for physical activity. Cost-effectiveness ratios ranged from $14,000 to $69,000 per quality-adjusted life year (QALY) gained, relative to no intervention. All of the interventions were found to be cost-effective with gains in survival and health-related quality of life, supporting any of the seven programs to promote physical activity.

The overall value of community-based physical activity interventions versus individual physical activity interventions continues to raise questions. A meta-analysis of outcomes across 385 community based and individual physical activity interventions showed that the most effective interventions were behavioral instead of cognitive, face-to-face delivery instead of mediated (telephone or mail), and those targeting individuals instead of communities (Conn, Hafdahl, & Mehr, 2011).

The diverse nature of community-based lifestyle interventions is the major obstacle to comparing evaluation results. However, from a public health perspective, the opportunity to improve the health of the community supports the cost-effectiveness of most interventions (Montes, Sarmiento, Zarama, Pratt, Wang, Jacoby, et al., 2012).

Changing the Built Environment to Promote Physical Activity

Physical activity is considered the most place-dependent health behavior. Places hinder or facilitate physical activity on the basis of the presence or absence of a supportive infrastructure; in other words, some places are physically activity friendly, and others are considered physical activity unfriendly. Sallis classifies physical activity environments as a subset of physical environments, which encompass natural and built environments (Sallis, 2009).

Built environments include all spaces, buildings, and objects created or modified by people, such as homes, schools, workplaces, parks, and transportation systems. The regulations and policies that govern built environments also hinder or facilitate physical activity. For example, policy reform may need to occur to implement and maintain walking paths or recreational parks.

In the Institute of Medicine's (IOM) report, *Accelerating Progress in Obesity Prevention,* sustainable strategies for creating and/or enhancing access to green areas, rethinking community design, and increasing places and opportunities for physical activity are proposed to enhance the physical and built environments of our cities and towns (Institute of Medicine, 2012).

Neighborhood-built environments influence physical activity behaviors. In a study comparing two Alabama cities, the low socioeconomic status (SES) city had one public recreation area with monthly use fees ranging from $25 to $35 per month, whereas three of the four public facilities in the contrasting city did not charge a fee. The low-SES city also provided limited opportunities for physical activity (Bovell-Benjamin, Hathorn, Ibraim, & Bromfield, 2009). Moderate physical activity has also been shown to be higher in high-walkability neighborhoods compared with low-walkability ones (Sallis, Saelens, Frank, Conway, Slymen, Cain, et al., 2009). In addition, overweight/obesity was higher in low-walkability neighborhoods.

Walkability refers to the ability of individuals to walk to nearby destinations. Walking has been associated with access to an aesthetically pleasing neighborhood, convenient facilities, safe neighborhoods, and limited traffic. Neighborhood environments were compared in 11 countries for their relationship with physical activity (Sallis, Bowles, Bauman, Ainsworth, Bull, Craig, et al., 2009). The environmental variables included single-family houses or housing type, shops within walking distance, transit stop 10–15 minutes from home, sidewalks on most streets, bicycle facilities in or near neighborhoods, low-cost recreation facilities, and crime rate. Five of the seven variables were significant, with having sidewalks on most streets in the neighborhood being the most significant predictor of physical activity. In contrast, unsafe neighborhoods are barriers to physical activity.

Research supports the need to design activity-friendly communities to provide opportunities and facilities for families and their children to participate in leisure time physical activity. Additional research is needed to refine the indicators of activity-friendly communities and develop measures that can be used to design friendly physical activity environments.

Multiple sectors in the community play a role in promoting physical activity in the community (USDHHS, 2008a). Concerns about crime and safety involve law enforcement. Urban planners play a major role in designing activity-friendly communities, and the transportation sector plays a role in building pedestrian and bicycle paths for walking to school or work, or for leisure activities. Parks and recreation departments need to be involved to facilitate access to recreational facilities and playgrounds for all.

Ecological models have proven useful for guiding physical activity interventions. Rigorous evaluation of these community-level models across the multiple levels is complex, but is necessary to understand better the usefulness of multilevel interventions. Figure 6–2 shows the relationship among the aspects of the **individual level** (age, education, income); the **relationship level** (influence of peers, partners, and family); the **community level** including the physical

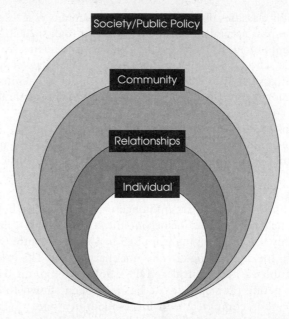

FIGURE 6–2   Social-Ecological Model   *Source:* Adapted from the Centers for Disease Control and Prevention, http://www.cdc.gov/violenceprevention/overview/social-ecologicalmodel.html

environment (residences and workplaces), sociocultural environment (health, economics), and institutional/organizational environment (workplace, schools); and the **society/public policy level** (educational and social policies). All of these factors determine an activity-friendly community (Kelly, Hoechner, Baker, Ramirez, & Brownson, 2006).

Objective indicators have been suggested for all of the domains, and measurement approaches have been described (Kelly, Hoechner, Baker, Ramirez, & Brownson, 2006). Although the model has undergone limited testing, it is a first step in evaluating ecological interventions for physical activity, and one in which multiple levels of change are implemented.

Designing Physical Activity Interventions for Diverse Populations

People of color and lower socioeconomic status report the lowest levels of regular physical activity and are most vulnerable to chronic conditions, such as cardiovascular disease and diabetes. In addition, inequality in environments also influences the ability in these groups to meet physical activity guidelines. People of color and those with low SES have less leisure time and energy to exercise, limited access to safe and affordable places to exercise, less support for regular physical activity, and are exposed to more stressful living conditions than are non-Hispanic whites (Lee & Cubbin, 2009). Living in impoverished neighborhoods is associated with depression, anxiety, anger, and apathy, which lead to increased stress and physical inactivity.

The built environment has a negative influence on physical activity in low-income communities. Low-income neighborhoods have fewer recreational facilities, and the ones that are available may be of lower quality and less likely to be maintained. Less money is spent on parks and open spaces in low-income communities of color than in affluent areas.

The amount of commute time is also a factor in leisure-time physical activity, especially for those who use public transportation. Long commute times leave little time for social interaction and physical activity after work. The process of changing environmental conditions in these communities is a challenge for individuals, local governments, and policy makers.

Cultural factors also must be taken into consideration in promoting physical activity in diverse populations. Cultures are not homogeneous, and subgroup variations in language, income, education, and acculturation also must be recognized. Gender socialization and role expectations also differ across cultures. Cultural beliefs and practices contribute to different patterns of activity across groups.

Racial/ethnic differences include variations in cultural attitudes as well as differences in geographic residence, degree of urbanization, family size, household composition, neighborhood characteristics, and degree of segregation. Cultural attitudes influence physical activity as well. Cultural values of automobiles and televisions as indicators of sufficient income promote inactivity. Physical activity may be seen as work in some groups, so leisure time is considered a time for sedentary activities.

Several factors should be considered in designing culturally appropriate programs for diverse populations, such as the community's history, the cultural values, and potential cultural barriers to physical activity, as every cultural group has historical events that have influenced it. Which cultural values are critical to incorporate in a physical activity intervention will impact the success of the intervention. For example, African-Americans generally value faith-based communities, so physical activities that are organized by churches, synagogues, mosques, and other religious communities are more likely to be well received and may result in more participation by the members.

Barriers may be environmental, interpersonal, financial, or legal. For example, transportation may not be available to reach safe walking paths. As mentioned in prior chapters, members of the target community must be engaged beginning with the planning stage. The integration of cultural values and strategies will minimize barriers in the activity plan and emphasize the community's strengths and resources to maximize their assets. All of these steps must be tailored to the diversity of cultural patterns and practices, including the group's history, beliefs, and preferences.

Examples of differences among underserved groups have been documented (Yancey, Ory, & Davis, 2006). African-Americans often value the *collectivist* versus the *individualist* approach. Physical activity programs may be more successful when (a) faith-based messages are used to present a positive ethnic identity, (b) physical activity participation is presented as an entitlement, and (c) prominent African-American athletes are shown as role models. Latino interventions are best focused on changing female perceptions of activity and linking group physical activity to traditional celebrations and intergenerational activities.

Native American tribes share several cultural concepts, including the oral tradition, intergenerational activities, and use of ceremonies for health. Native Americans also have norms about not telling others what to do, indicating that different strategies to increase physical activity are needed. In addition, many do not think physical activity is normal. Incorporating Indian music and pow-wow dances was done in one Native American "Celebrate Fitness" program to make activity a source of motivation and pride (Brown & Kraft, 2008).

Asians and Pacific Islanders value collectivism, intergenerational living, and respect for elders. Group physical activity participation, such as dance and martial arts, are potential interventions for this population.

A meta-analysis of exercise interventions and their impact on the health and behavior health of African-American, Hispanic, Native American, and Native Hawaiian adults found that physical activity increased and anthropometric measures improved when the intervention included supervised exercise (Conn, Phillips, Ruppar, & Chase, 2012) as opposed to unsupervised exercise programs. This finding supports the collectivist approach valued in these cultures.

In summary, physical activity programs should be built into the cultural practices of the community. The program should blend into community activities without changing social norms and community values. Also recommended are intergenerational approaches, which include children as well as elders. The preferences of the community are respected and incorporated into the program, and assets are emphasized. Programs should be flexible in accommodating the culture, offering choices to the extent possible. These steps empower diverse communities to take an active role in promoting the health of their members through physical activity.

Recommendations have also been suggested to address the built environment in low-income diverse communities (Floyd, Taylor, & Whitt-Glover, 2009). First, identify the most critical environmental needs and social variables. Second, determine how the environmental factors can be modified through policy, management, or programming changes, taking culture into consideration. Last, ensure adequate representation of community members using community-based participatory methods.

Stakeholders should be community members as well as members of community organizations. Involve stakeholders in all phases of development, implementation, and evaluation. These steps will help to ensure success in changing the built environment to positively influence physical activity in low-income communities.

CONSIDERATIONS FOR PRACTICE TO PROMOTE PHYSICAL ACTIVITY

This chapter emphasizes approaches for increasing physical activity as well as the barriers and strategies for overcoming barriers to physical activity. This information can guide nurses in counseling persons of all ages to adopt regular physical activity.

First, nurses must be positive role models and engage in healthy behaviors themselves. Although many in the public do not meet the recommended physical activity guidelines, they expect nurses to be healthy, and they notice when they are not fit. Nurses who need to increase their physical activity can start on a path toward a healthier lifestyle by identifying the barriers that prevent them from exercising and identifying practical strategies to overcome the barriers (Esposito & Fitzpatrick, 2011).

Inactive and sedentary people need to rethink the definition of exercise and build movement into both work and leisure behavior. An example would be taking the stairs instead of the elevator, then increasing the number of stairs each week; or parking a distance from work and shopping—both are small changes that can make a big difference. Motivation to change habits and engage in healthy behaviors requires commitment and a desire to live a healthier life. Nurses who embrace physical activity are more likely to be positive role models and teach the value of physical activity to their clients (Bruijn, 2011; Esposito & Fitzpatrick, 2011).

Within any given age, gender, or cultural group, nurses should start by assessing the client's level of physical activity. For example, when working with children, the nurse should assess patterns of physical activity; preferred activities; perceptions of barriers to being active; perceptions of self-efficacy; intentions to be active; availability of active parents, siblings, and friends; access to safe recreational facilities; and time spent outdoors.

Counseling should assist children and adolescents to select activities they enjoy and not focus solely on competitive sports. Children should be encouraged to engage in activities that can be carried into adulthood and are easily incorporated into their daily life year-round. Appropriate safety equipment should be used to prevent injuries, and youth should be counseled to avoid use of any anabolic steroids. By offering such simple recommendations to children and parents, nurses play a key role in promoting lifelong physical activity.

Adult clients should be asked about their physical activity habits at work, at home, and during leisure time to determine if these activities are sufficient to confer health benefits. Adults should be assisted in planning a program of physical activity that is medically safe, enjoyable, convenient, realistic, and structured to achieve self-selected goals. Routine monitoring, follow-up, and booster sessions are essential to assist clients in maintaining their exercise programs.

Home exercise programs may work for some adults, whereas for others structured programs may need to be offered at work sites or convenient community locations. Group activities may be particularly appealing to adults who prefer the social support and comradeship of group programs. For older adults, current health status, existing medical conditions, disabilities, fear of injury, and preferences need to be assessed.

Nurses should consider developing or using existing computer-based and mobile apps that tailor programs to optimize physical activity. Assessment and counseling should be followed up with mail, e-mail, text messages, or telephone calls at periodic intervals. Agencies may have Facebook pages that may be used to disseminate reminders, encouragement, and tips. Contacts should focus on providing appropriate strategies to increase or maintain activity and overcome any encountered barriers to being active.

The barriers and strategies outlined in Table 6–3 should be discussed with clients. Encourage clients to identify specific barriers to increasing their physical activity level and then commit to trying strategies to overcome them. Mobile apps are available to record data and set reminders. It is important to review contracts on a regular basis and adjust as needed.

The nurse should collaborate with the health care team to establish systems that will facilitate regular physical activity counseling for all clients. Physical activity components of health promotion and prevention systems should consist of (1) screening systems for assessing patterns of physical activity, (2) agency guidelines for physical activity counseling, (3) chart reminders for counseling at client visits, (4) relevant client education materials, and (5) follow-up protocols to reinforce interventions. When health care agencies systematize counseling protocols, physical activity counseling is much more likely to be an integral part of care by all health professionals.

OPPORTUNITIES IN PHYSICAL ACTIVITY RESEARCH

More research is needed to better understand how to tailor exercise programs to the needs of diverse populations. Particular focus should be placed on developing and testing interventions that help very young children accept physical activity as enjoyable and rewarding. Interventions to prevent the decrease in physical activity during adolescence also needs further study. Focusing on development of healthy behaviors rather than behavior change is critical; after behaviors are established in youth, they are highly resistant to change.

Additional suggestions for future research include the following:

1. Describe family and environmental influences during early childhood that promote or inhibit the development of physically active lifestyles.
2. Test multiple levels of the socio-ecological model to promote physical activity in low-income communities.
3. Test the effects of changing the built environment in rural communities on physical activity in older adults.
4. Develop and test strategies to promote the adoption and maintenance of physical activity for low-income sedentary women across the life span.
5. Investigate the interaction of genetic makeup, environment, and behavior on the adoption and maintenance of physical activity.
6. Test the long-term effectiveness of family interventions to increase physical activity for children and parents.
7. Test the effectiveness of changing national policies to promote physical activity on the health of the community.
8. Develop and test community-level measures to assess socio-ecological concepts and built environments.

Summary

Nurses, as key health professionals, must assume responsibility for using evidence-based knowledge so as to assist clients in developing lifelong habits of physical activity. Physical activity *must* be an integral part of everyday life in order to have optimum effects on health. Research findings promote focusing on multiple levels in the environment, as well as on individual behaviors, to promote leisure-time physical activity. Maintaining physical fitness can be enjoyable and rewarding for persons of all ages and contributes significantly to extending longevity and improving the quality of life.

Learning Activities

1. Conduct a self-assessment and design a physical activity plan for yourself. Identify barriers and strategies (refer to Table 6–3) you are likely to experience. Implement your plan for two weeks. Describe your successes and failures in a one-page summary.
2. Review the guidelines for promoting physical activity in children. Develop an exercise plan for a healthy child, 8 years of age. Tailor the plan to a sedentary child and describe steps and activities needed to reach the recommended activity guidelines.
3. Apply the recommended steps for physical activity programs for diverse populations to a low-income cultural group of your choice. Outline how you would ensure that the program is sensitive to gender (females), age (persons aged 65 years and over), and the cultural values of the community.
4. Develop a plan to promote physical activity for workers employed by an employer with 50 to 100 employees. Describe work site and leisure-time strategies to enable them to meet the national physical activity guidelines.
5. Find the percentage and estimated cost of obesity for all racial/ethnic groups in your region.

References

Anderson-Hanley, C., Arclero, P., Brickman, A., Nimon, J., Okurma, N., Western, S., Mera, M., et al. (2012). Exergaming and older adult cognition. *American Journal of Preventive Medicine, 42*(2), 109–119.

Beets, M., Beighle, A., Erwin, H., & Huberry, J. (2009). After-school impact on physical activity: A meta-analysis. *American Journal of Preventive Medicine, 36*(5), 527–537.

Bennette, R., & Sothern, M. S. (2009). Diet, exercise, behavior: The promise and limits of lifestyle change. *Seminars in Pediatric Surgery, 18*(3), 152–158.

Bergeman, C. S., & Ong, A. D. (2007). Behavioral genetics. In J. E. Birren (Ed.), *Encyclopedia of genontology* (2nd ed., pp. 149–160). New York, NY: Elsevier.

Bhanushali, C., Kumar, K., Karavatas, S., Habib, M., Daniel, M., & Lee, E. (2013). Association between lifestyle factors and metabolic syndrome among African-Americans in the United States. *Journal of Nutrition and Metabolism.* doi:10.1155/2013/516475

Bovell-Benjamin, A., Hathorn, C., Ibraim, S., & Bromfield E. (2009). Healthy food choices and physical activity opportunities in two contrasting Alabama cities. *Health & Place, 15,* 429–438.

Brown, L., & Kraft, M. (2008). Active living as an institutional challenge: Lessons from the Robert Wood Johnson Foundation's "Celebrate Fitness" program. *Journal of Health Politics, Policy and Law, 32,* 497–523.

Bruijn, G. (2011). Exercise habit strength, planning and the theory of planned behaviour: An action control approach. *Psychology of Sport and Exercise, 12,* 106–114.

Bryan, W. J., Burton, N. W., & Rowan, P. J. (2007). A transdisciplinary model intergrating genetics, physiological, and psychological correlates of voluntary exercise. *Health Psychology, 26*(1), 30–39.

Cardon, G., Labarque, V., Smits, D., & de Buordeaudhuij, H. (2009). Promoting physical activity at the pre-school playground: The effects of providing markings and play equipment. *Preventive Medicine, 48,* 335–340.

Chen, J., & Lee, Y. (2013). Physical activity for health: Evidence, theory, and practice. *Journal of Preventive Medicine and Public Health, 46*(Suppl 1), 51–52. Published online 10:396/pmph.2013.46.S.S1.

Cleland, V., Dwyer, T., & Venn, A. (2012). Which domains of childhood physical activity predict physical activity in adulthood? A 20-year prospective tracking study. *British Journal of Sports Medicine, 46*(8), 595–602, doi:10,1136/bjsports-2011-090508

Coleman, K., Rosenberg, D., Conway, T., Sallis, J., & Saelens, B. (2008). Physical activity, weight status, and neighborhood characteristics of dog walkers. *Preventive Medicine, 47,* 309–312.

Conn, V., Hafdahl, A., & Mehr, D. (2011). Interventions to increase physical activity among healthy adults: Meta-analysis of outcomes. *American Journal of Public Health, 101*(4), 751–758. doi:10:2105/AJPH.2010, 194381

Conn, V., Phillips, L., Ruppar, T., & Chase, J. (2012). Physical activity interventions with healthy minority adults: Meta-analysis of behavior and health outcomes. *Journal of Health Care for the Poor and Underserved, 23*(1), 59–80. doi:10.1353/hpu.2010.0032

Cox, K., Burke, V., Beilin, L., Sallie, J., & Saelens, B. (2008). Short and long-term adherence to swimming and walking programs in older women: The Sedentary Women Exercise Adherence Trial (SWEAT 2). *Preventive Medicine, 46,* 511–517.

Crossman, A., Sullivan, D., & Benin, M. (2006). The family environment and American adolescents' risk of obesity as young adults. *Social Science & Medicine, 63,* 2255–2267.

de Geus, E., & de Moor, M. (2008). A genetic perspective on the association between exercise and mental health. *Mental Health and Physical Activity, 1,* 53–61.

Dishman, R., DeJoy, D., Wilson, M., & Vandenberg, R. (2009). Move to improve: A randomized workplacc trial to increase physical activity. *American Journal of Preventive Medicine, 36*(2), 133–141.

Elsamy, B., & Higgins, K. (2010). Physical Activity Guidelines for Older Adults. *American Family Physician, 81*(1), 55–59.

Espana-Romero, V., Mitchell, J., Dowda, M., ONeill, J., & Pate, R. (2013). Objectively measured sedentary time, physical activity and markers of body fat in preschool children. *Pediatric Exercise Science, 25*(1), 124–37.

Esposito, E., & Fitzpatrick, J. (2011). Registered nurses' beliefs of the benefits of exercise, their exercise behaviour and their patient teaching regarding exercise. *International Journal of Nursing Practice, 17,* 351–356.

Floyd, M., Taylor, W. C., & Whitt-Glover, M. (2009). Measurement of park and recreation environments that support physical activity in low-income communities of color: Highlights of challenges and recommendations. *American Journal of Preventive Medicine, 36*(4S), S156–S160.

Garber, C. E., Blissmer, B., Deschenes, M. R., Franklin, B. A., Lamonte, M. J., Lee, I., Nieman, D. C., Swain, D. P. (2011). Quantity and quality of exercise for maintaining cardiorespiratory, muscloskeletal, and neuromoter fitness in apparently healthy adults: Guidance for Prescribing Exercise. *Medicine & Science in Sports & Medicine, 43*(7),1334–1359.

Giussani, M., Antolini, L. Brambilia, P., Pagani, M., Zuccotti, G., et al. (2013). Cardiovascular risk assessment in children: Role of physical activity, family history and parental smoking on BMI and blood pressure. *Journal of Hypertension,* Epub: 23425707.

Goldfield, G., Harvey, A., Gratten, K., & Adamo, K. (2012). Physical activity promotion in the preschool years: A critical period to intervene. *International Journal of Environmental Research and Public Health,* 9(4), 1326–1342. Published online April 16.

Grimslvedi, M., Ananian, C., Keller, C., Woolf, K., Sebren, A., & Ainsworth, B. (2012). Nurse practitioner and physician assistant physical activity counseling knowledge, confidence and practice. *Preventive Medicine,* 54(5), 306–308.

Halldin, M., Rosell, M., deFaaire, U., & Hellenius, M. (2007). The metabolic syndrome: Prevalance and association to leisure time and work related physical activity in 60 year old men and women. *Nutrition, Metabolism & Cardiovascular Diseases, 17,* 349–357.

Hoebeke, R. (2008). Low-income women's preceived barriers to physical activity: Focus groups results. *Applied Nursing Research, 21,* 60–65.

Hume, C., Timperio, A., Salmon, J., Carter, A., & Giles-Corti, B. (2009). Walking and cycling to school: Predictors of increases among children and adolescents. *American Journal of Preventive Medicine, 36,* 195–200.

Hutchinson, A., & Wilson, C. (2012). Improving nutrition and physical activity in the workplace: A meta-analysis of intervention studies. *Health Promotion International,* 27(2), 238–249.

Institute of Medicine. (2012). *Accelerating progress in obesity prevention: Solving the weight of the nation.* Washington, DC: IOM.

Irvine, A., Philips, L., Seeley, J., Wyant, S., Duncan, S., & Moore, R. (2011). Get Moving: A web site that increases physical activity of sedentary employees. *American Journal of Health Promotion, 25*(3), 199–206.

Kahn, J. A., Huang, B., Gillman, M. W., Field, A. E., Austin, S. B., Colditz, G. A., et al. (2008). Patterns and determinants of physical activity in U.S. adolescents. *Journal of Adolescent Health, 42,* 369–377.

Kahn-Marshall, J., & Gallant, M. (2012). Making healthy behaviors the easy choice for employees: A review of the literature on environmental and policy changes in worksite health promotion. *Health Education & Behavior, 39*(6), 752–776.

Kassavou, A., Turner, A., & French, D. (2013). Do interventions to promote walking in groups increase physical activity? A meta-analysis. *International Journal of Behavioral Nutrition and Physical Activity,* http://www.ijbnpa.org/content/10/1/18

Kelly, C., Hoechner, C., Baker, E., Ramirez, L., & Brownson, R. (2006). Promoting physical activity in communities: Approaches for successful evaluation of programs and policies. *Evaluation & Program Planning, 29,* 280–292.

Lee, R., & Cubbin, C. (2009). Striding toward social justice: The ecologic milieu of physical activity. *Exercise and Sports Sciences Reviews, 37,* 10–17.

Loprinzi, P., & Cardinal, B. (2013). Association between biologic outcomes and objectively measured physical activity accumulated in > 10 minute bouts and < 10 minute bouts. *American Journal of Health Promotion,* 27(3), 143–151.

Lubans, D. R., Morgan, P. J., & Tudor-Locke, C. (2009). A systematic review of studies using pedometers to promote physical activity among youth. *Preventive Medicine, 48,* 307–315.

Madsen, K., McCulloch, C., & Crawford, P. (2009). Parent modeling: Perceptions of parents' physical activity predict girls' activity throughout adolescence. *Journal of Pediatrics, 154,* 278–283.

Marshall, S. J., Levy, S. S., Tudor-Locke, C. E., Kolkhorst, F. W., Wooten, K. M., et al. (2009). Translating physical activty recommendations into a pedomoter-based step goal: 300 steps in 30 minutes. *American Journal of Preventive Medicine, 36,* 410–415.

Martinson, B., Crain, A., Sherwood, N., Hayes, M., Pronk, N., & O'Connor, P. (2008). Maintaining physical activity among older adults: Six months outcomes of the Keep Active Minnesota randomized controlled trail. *Preventive Medicine, 46,* 111–119.

Meng, X., & D'Arcy, C. (2013). The projected effect of increasing physical activity on reducing the prevalence of common mental disorders among Canadian men and women: A national population-based community study. *Preventive Medicine, 56*(1), 59–63.

Merrill, R. M., Aldana, S., Garrett, J., & Ross, C. (2011). Effectiveness of a workplace wellness program for maintaining health and promoting healthy behaviors. *Journal of Occupational & Environmental Medicine, 53*(7), 782–787. doi:10,1097/JOM.ObO13e318220c318220c2f4

Montes, F., Sarmiento, O., Zarama, R., Pratt, M., Wang, G., Jacoby, E., et al. (2012). Do health benefits outweigh the costs of mass recreational programs? An economic analysis of four Ciciovia. *Journal of Urban Health, 89*(1), 153–170. doi:10.1007/s11514-011

Morris, C., McAuley, E., & Motl, R. (2008). Neighborhood satisfaction, functional limitations, and self-efficacy influences on physical activity in older women. *International Journal of Behavioral Nutrition and Physical Activity.* http://www.ijbnpa.org/content/5/1/13

Mummery, W., & Brown, W. (2009). Whole of community physical activity interventions: Easier said than done. *British Journal of Sports Medicine, 43,* 39–43.

Naito, M., Nakayama, T., Okamura, T., Miura, K., Yanagita, M., Fujieda, Y., et al. (2008). Effect of a 4-year workplace-based physical activity intervention program on the blood lipid profiles of participating employees' health promotion (HIPOP-OHP study). *Atherosclerosis, 197,* 784–790.

Nang, E., Salim, A., Wu, V., Tai, E., Lee, J., & Van Dam, R. (2013, May 30). *Internatinal Journal of Behavioral Nutrition and Physical Activity.* doi:10.1186/1479-5868-10-70

National Association for Sport and Physical Education. (2009). *Active start: A statement of physical activity guidelines for children birth to five years.* Retrieved from http://www.NASPE.org

O'Connor, T., Jago, R., & Baranowski, T. (2009). Engaging parents to increase youth physical activity: A systemic review. *American Journal of Preventive Medicine, 37,* 141–149.

Olden, K. (2009). Human health and disease: Interaction between the genome and the environment. In H.Willard & G.Ginsberg (Eds.), *Genomic and Personalized medicine* (pp. 47–59). New York, NY: Elsevier.

Opdenacker, J., Boen, P., Coorevitis, N., & Delecluse, C. (2008). Effectiveness of a lifestyle intervention and a structured exercise intervention in older adults. *Preventive Medicine, 46,* 518–524.

Owen, N. (2012). Sedentary behavior: Understanding and influencing adults' prolonged sitting time. *Preventive Medicine, 55,* 535–539.

Owens, N., Glanz, K., Sallis, J., & Kelder, S. (2006). Evidence-based approaches to dissemination and diffusion of physical activity interventions. *American Journal of Preventive Medicine, 31*(4S), S35–S44.

Pronk, N., & Kottke, T. (2009). Physical activity promotion as a strategic corporate priority to improve worker health and business performance. *Preventive Medicine, 49*(4), 316–321.

Racette, S., Deusinger, S. S., Inman, C., Burlis, T., Highstein, C., Buskirk, T., et al. (2009). Worksite opportunities for wellness (WOW): Effects on cardiovascular disease risk factors after 1 year. *Preventive Medicine, 49*(2–3), 108–114.

Rauner, A., Mess, F., & Woll, A. (2013). The relationship between physical activity, physical fitness and overweight in adolescents: A systematic review of studies published in or after 2000. *Journal of Pediatrics and Child Health, 49*(2), 128–132. doi:10.1111/jpc.12082. Epub 2013 Jan 31.

Reger-Nash, B., Bauman, A., Cooper, L., Chey, T., & Simon, K. (2006). Evaluating community-wide walking interventions. *Evaluation and Program Planning, 29,* 251–259.

Rosenburg, D., Kerr, J., Patrick, K., Moore, D., & King, A. (2009). Feasibility and outcomes of a multilevel pace-based walking intervention for seniors: A pilot study. *Health and Place, 15,* 173–179.

Roux, L., Pratt, M., & King, A. (2009). Cost-effectiveness of community-based physical activity interventions. *American Journal of Preventive Medicine, 35,* 578–588.

Sallis, J. (2009). Measuring physical activity environments: A brief history. *American Journal of Preventive Medicine, 36,* S86–S92.

Sallis, J., Bowles, H., Bauman, A., Ainsworth, B., Bull, F., Craig, C., et al. (2009). Neighborhood environments and physical activity among adults in 11 countries. *American Journal of Preventive Medicine, 36,* 484–490.

Sallis, J., Saelens, B., Frank, L., Conway, T., Slymen, D., Cain, C., et al. (2009). Neighborhood built environments and income: Examining multiple health outcomes. *Social Science & Medicine, 68,* 1285–1293.

Sallis, J. F., Floyd, M. F., Rodriquez, D. A., & Saelens, B. E. (2012). Role of built environments in physical activity obesity, and cardiovascular disease. *Circulation, 125,* 729–737.

SangNam, A., Smith, M., & Ory, M. (2012). Physicians' discussions about body weight, healthy diet, and physical activity with overweight or obese elderly patients. *Journal of Aging and Health, 24*(7), 1179.

Simek, E., McPhate, L., & Haines, T. (2012). Adherence to and efficacy of home exercise programs to prevent falls: A systematic review and meta-analysis of the impact of exercise program characteristics. *Preventive Medicine, 55,* 262–275.

Talbot, L., Morrell, C., Fleg, J., & Metter, E. (2007). Changes in leisure time physical activity and risk of all-cause mortality in men and women: The Baltimore Longitudinal Study of Aging. *Preventive Medicine, 45,* 169–176.

Trost, S. G., & Loprinzi, P. D. (2008). Exercise-promoting lifestyles in children and adolescents. *Journal of Clinical Lipidology, 2,* 162–168.

Tucker, P., & Gilliland, J. (2007). The effect of season and weather on physical activity: A systematic review. *Public Health, 121,* 909–922.

Tudor-Locke, C. (2003). *Manpo-Kei: The art and science of step counting: How to be naturally active and lose weight.* New Bern, NC: Trafford.

U.S. Department of Health and Human Services (USDHHS). (2008a). *2008 physical activity guidelines for Americans.* Retrieved from http://www.health.gov./paguidelines.

U.S. Department of Health and Human Services (USDHHS). (2008b). *Center for Chronic Disease and Prevention.* Retrieved from http://www.cdc.gov/needphp/overview.htm

Wamp, Z. (2009). Creating a culture of movement: The benefits of promoting physical activity in schools and the workplace. American Journal of Preventive Medicine, 36(2S), S56–S57.

Weldel-Vos, W., Dutman, A., Verschuren, M., Ronickers, E., Ament, A., van Assema, P., et al. (2009). Lifestyles factors of a five-year community intervention program: The Hartslag Limburg intervention. *American Journal of Preventive Medicine, 37,* 50–56.

Wilcox, S., Dowda, M., Leviton, L., Barlett-Prescott, J., Bazzarre, T., Campbell-Voytal, K. et al. (2008). Active for Life: Final results from the tranlation of two physical activity programs. *American Journal of Preventive Medicine, 35,* 340–351.

Williams, C. L., Carter, B. J., Kibbe, D. L., & Denniston, D. (2009). Increasing physical activity in preschool: A pilot to evaluate animal trackers. *Journal of Nutrition Education and Behavior, 41,* 47–52.

World Health Organization. (cited 2013 March 10). *Global recommendations on physical activity for health.* http://who.int./dietphysicalactivity/factsheetrecommendations

Yancey, A., Ory, M., & Davis, S. (2006). Dissemination of physical activity promotion interventions in underserved populations. *American Journal of Prevention Medicine, 31*(4S), S82–S91.

Zaga, S., Briss, P., & Harris, K. (Eds). (2005). *The community guide to community services: What works to promote health?* New York, NY: Oxford University Press.

Zscucke, E., Gaudlitz, K., & Strohle, A. (2013). Exercise and physical activity in mental disorders: Clinical and experimental evidence. *Journal of Preventive Medicine and Public Health, 41*(Suppl 1), S1–S2.

CHAPTER 7

Nutrition and Health Promotion

OBJECTIVES

This chapter will enable the reader to:

1. Describe the U.S. Dietary Guidelines 2010 for healthy eating.

2. Describe MyPlate.

3. Discuss MyPlate's role in implementing the Dietary Guidelines 2010 for healthy eating.

4. Examine evidence-based factors that influence eating behaviors.

5. Describe the nutritional needs of infants and children, adolescents, and older adults.

6. Examine factors related to overweight/obesity and intervention goals in weight loss.

7. Examine interventions to motivate individuals to change eating habits and maintain weight loss.

Good nutrition is one of the primary determinants of good health. Two major risk factors responsible for the global increase in obesity and other noncommunicable diseases are an unhealthy diet and lack of activity. The role of nutrition has expanded from a focus on nutrients needed to feed populations, to its role in promoting health and preventing disease. The emphasis on healthy nutrition for children and adolescents is critical, as diet and eating behaviors that develop during these years tend to persist throughout life. Good nutrition is influenced by multiple factors, thus making successful promotion of optimal diets a challenge. Policy makers and health promotion experts acknowledge the need for population-based, multilevel changes, including multidisciplinary, culturally relevant approaches that target individuals and communities, as well as policies that are aimed at changing the food environment and food industry.

PROMOTING HEALTHY DIET AND NUTRITION

Chronic diseases, such as coronary artery disease, cardiovascular disease, cancer, diabetes, and obesity, account for about 63% of deaths (an increase of 3% over the 2002 reported figure), and almost half of the burden of disease worldwide (World Health Organization [WHO], 2008). A large percentage of these diseases could be avoided, as they are either begun or impacted by unhealthy nutrition in addition to other etiologies. Food choices are influenced by food preferences, portion sizes, and inactivity, as well as culture, socioeconomic status, advertising, the built (human-made) environment, and other "obesogenic" (unhealthy eating) factors (McKinnon, Reedy, Handy, & Rodgers, 2009). Understanding the national dietary guidelines and the MyPlate approach to healthy eating is instrumental in achieving dietary change.

Nutritional Health of Americans

The *obesity epidemic* is responsible for many of the health problems of Americans as well as the increasing cost of health care in America. In 2008, obesity-related health care costs in the United States were estimated to be $147 billion and were projected to increase to $175 billion in 2020. The medical costs per individual associated with obesity were $1,429 more than those of normal weight (Wang, McPherson, Marsh, et al., 2011).

The incidence of chronic disease in young people parallels the increase in the obesity rate in this population. Approximately 17% (12.5 million) of those aged 2–19 years are obese (Centers for Disease Control and Prevention, 2011a). By state, adult obesity prevalence in 2011 ranged from 20.7% in Colorado to 34.9% in Mississippi. The South had the highest prevalence of obesity (29.5%) with the Midwest reporting 29.0%, the Northeast 25.3%, and the West 24.3%. Due to an adjusted baseline for estimated state adult obesity prevalence by the Centers for Disease Control and Prevention (CDC), 2011 figures cannot be compared to estimates of previous years (Centers for Disease Control and Prevention, 2011b).

Americans rank prevention as the most important health reform priority. The shift of Americans' support of prevention over the past two decades is impressive, increasing from 45% in 1986 to 59% in 2009 (Trust for America's Health, 2009). Yet, obesity rates in adults and children have doubled and tripled, respectively, over the last 30 years, contributing to a higher incidence of chronic diseases and higher health care costs. Reversing the obesity epidemic is designated as one of ten key public health issues confronting America according to *A Healthier America 2013: Strategies to Move from Sick Care to Health Care in Four Years* (Levi, Segal, Fuchs Miller, & Lang, 2013).

Current evidence suggests that *distribution* of body fat may be more significant than *quantity* of fat, represented by the body mass index (BMI; Centers for Disease Control and Prevention, 2011c; Kragelund & Levine, 2005). Specifically, increased abdominal fat—measured by waist circumference and waist-hip ratio—has been associated with metabolic risk factors, even in high-risk individuals with a BMI below 30 (BMI greater than 30 is considered obese; WHO, 2008). Individuals with a large muscle mass, such as body builders, may have a higher BMI, but less fat. Both BMI and waist circumference have been shown to be clinically useful in identifying adolescents at risk for later cardiovascular disease onset (Messiah, Arheart, Lipschulz, & Miller, 2008).

However, in older adults, waist circumference is a more relevant measure, due to age-related changes in body size and composition that limit the usefulness of BMI in this population (Srikanthan, Seeman, & Karlamangia, 2009; WHO Expert Consultation, 2008). This finding is consistent with White and Black adult men and women younger than 65 years, in which waist-to-hip ratio had the strongest association with cardiovascular disease and mortality (Gelber, Gaziano, Orav, Manson, Buring, & Kurth, 2008; Reis, Aranta, Wingard, Macera, Lindsay, & Marshall, 2008).

Findings consistently indicate that waist circumference and waist-to-hip ratios are better predictors of risk than is BMI. Knowing one's waist circumference is a primary step in knowing one's risk of disease. However, BMI remains an important screening tool for excess body weight. It is important to keep in mind that BMI and waist measurements are indirect measures and are used—along with an assessment of lifestyle, the presence of other chronic diseases, other risk factors, and family history—to get a better picture of the individual's health risk.

Dietary Guidelines for Americans

The *Dietary Guidelines for Americans* are published every five years by the U.S. Department of Agriculture and U.S. Department of Health and Human Services and form the basis for federal nutrition policy. The guidelines offer dietary advice for Americans aged 2 years and older and include recommendations on reducing risks of chronic disease with good dietary habits. The *Dietary Guidelines for Americans 2010* focus on encouraging the consumption of fewer calories, improving education on food choices, and increasing physical activity while recognizing food preferences, cultural traditions, and customs of the diverse U.S. population.

A premise of the *Guidelines for Americans* is that food should be the primary source of nutrients that an individual needs to be healthy. Although dietary supplements and fortified foods may be useful sources for one or two nutrients, they cannot replace a healthy diet. The 2010 guidelines placed greater emphasis on individuals balancing calories with physical activity to manage weight, and reducing consumption of sodium, solid fats, added sugars, and refined grains; and increasing fruits, vegetables, whole grains, seafood, and fat-free and reduced-fat dairy products. Figure 7–1 shows typical American dietary intake in comparison to recommended intake levels or limits. As evident in Figure 7–1, there is much work to be done to change the excessive dietary intake of most Americans.

Two examples of eating patterns that are used to model the *Dietary Guidelines for Americans* are the U.S. Department of Agriculture Food Patterns (including vegetarian adaptations) and the Dietary Approaches to Stop Hypertension (DASH) eating plan. Originally developed to study eating patterns to prevent and treat hypertension, the DASH eating plan is a balanced plan consistent with the dietary guidelines. Both of these eating plans illustrate healthy ways to eat.

The *Dietary Guidelines for Americans* are used by policy makers, health care providers, nutritionists, and educators to develop educational materials and design and implement nutrition-related programs. Modifications are necessary to integrate the food preferences of different ethnic and racial groups, vegetarians, and other special groups. The guidelines are based on a 2000-calorie diet, but the recommended intake varies according to age, gender, and activity level. The recommendations are interrelated, and following all of them will improve nutritional outcomes. However, following just some of the recommendations also will have positive health outcomes. Key recommendations on balancing calories to manage weight are highlighted in Table 7–1, and food components to reduce are listed in Table 7–2.

The American Diabetic Association has published nutritional recommendations and interventions for the primary prevention of diabetes as well. Recommended changes for moderate weight loss for adults and adolescents at risk for type 2 diabetes include the following:

1. Reduction of calories and intake of dietary fats
2. Regular physical activity (30 minutes per day or 2.5 hours per week of aerobic exercise)
3. Encouragement of foods containing whole grains and a greater intake of low-glycemic index foods rich in fiber (at least 25 g of dietary fiber/100 kcal for women and 38 g for men daily)

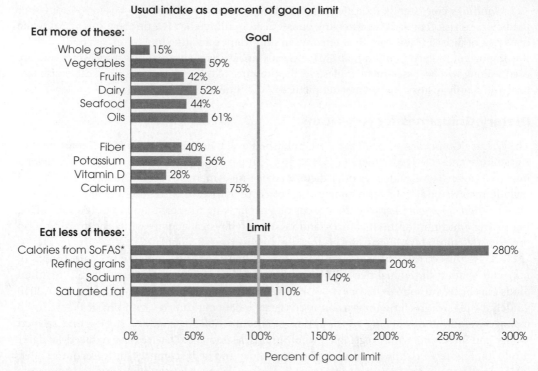

Usual intake as a percent of goal or limit

FIGURE 7–1   How Do Typical American Diets Compare to Recommended Intake?   *Source:* U.S. Department of Agriculture and U.S. Department of Health and Human Services. *Dietary Guidelines for Americans, 2010*. 7th Edition, Washington, DC: U.S. Government Printing Office, December 2010.

In addition, monitoring carbohydrates is a key recommendation for achieving glycemic control in persons with diabetes as well. Saturated fat should be limited to less than 7% of total daily calories with total fat intake to less than 25–35% of calories. Although there is insufficient evidence to suggest modifying usual protein intake, high-protein diets are not recommended because of their effect on kidney function, which is of major concern in both diabetes and hypertension. These guidelines are applicable to everyone who wishes to follow a healthy diet.

Some scientists suggest that dietary guidelines share some responsibility for the obesity epidemic in America. When dietary guidelines recommended that people eat less dietary saturated fat, sugar consumption increased, people doubled their caloric intake, and obesity increased. According to some scientists, the message should have been formulated to promote less caloric intake, reduce portion size, and increase physical activity (Marantz, Bird, & Alderman, 2008). However, as science has progressed, it is now evident that both saturated fat and calorie intakes

TABLE 7–1   Balancing Calories to Manage Weight

Key Recommendations

Prevent and/or reduce overweight and obesity through improved eating and physical activity behaviors.

Control total calorie intake to manage body weight. For people who are overweight or obese, this will mean consuming fewer calories from food and beverages.

Increase physical activity and reduce time spent in sedentary behaviors.

Maintain appropriate calorie balance during each stage of life—childhood, adolescence, adulthood, pregnancy and breastfeeding, and older age.

Source: U.S. Department of Agriculture and U.S. Department of Health and Human Services. *Dietary Guidelines for Americans, 2010.* 7th Edition, Washington, DC: U.S. Government Printing Office, December 2010.

are important—as is physical activity—so current guidelines address all of these components. Dietary guidelines are one important strategy to provide the best science-based information available to improve Americans' health.

MyPlate: A Visual Cue to Healthy Eating Habits

MyPlate translates the *Dietary Guidelines for Americans 2010* into messages that consumers can more easily understand and practice. MyPlate, shown in Figure 7–2, replaced MyPyramid as the government's primary food group symbol in 2010. MyPyramid was much maligned by many experts as vague and confusing to most Americans, heavily influenced by the meat and dairy industries, and based on out-of-date science (Harvard School of Public Health, accessed

TABLE 7–2   Foods and Food Components to Reduce

Key Recommendations

Reduce daily sodium intake to less than 2,300 milligrams (mg) and further reduce intake to 1,500 mg among persons who are 51 or older and those of any age who are African American or have hypertension, diabetes, or chronic kidney disease. The 1,500 mg recommendation applies to about half of the U.S. population, including children, and the majority of adults.

Consume less than 10 percent of calories from saturated fatty acids by replacing them with monounsaturated and polyunsaturated fatty acids.

Consume less than 300 mg per day of dietary cholesterol.

Keep *trans* fatty acid consumption as low as possible by limiting foods that contain synthetic sources of *trans* fats, such as partially hydrogenated oils, and by limiting other solid fats.

Reduce the intake of calories from solid fats and added sugars.

Limit the consumption of foods that contain refined grains, especially refined grain foods that contain solid fats, added sugars, and sodium.

If alcohol is consumed, it should be consumed in moderation—up to one drink per day for women and two drinks per day for men—and only by adults of legal drinking age.

Source: U.S. Department of Agriculture and U.S. Department of Health and Human Services. *Dietary Guidelines for Americans, 2010.* 7th Edition, Washington, DC: U.S. Government Printing Office, December 2010.

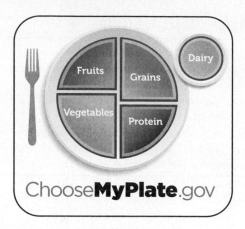

FIGURE 7–2 ChooseMyPlate.gov *Source:* U.S. Department of Agriculture and U.S. Department of Health and Human Services. *Dietary Guidelines for Americans, 2010*. 7th Edition, Washington, DC: U.S. Government Printing Office, December 2010.

May 11, 2013), so MyPlate was designed to replace MyPyramid. However, many countries around the world still use a pyramid to convey nutritional advice for its citizens. Many countries do follow the United States' leadership, but it remains to be seen whether other countries will change their nutritional model as a result.

The goal of the MyPlate symbol is to help consumers adopt healthy eating habits through a visual cue shown in Figure 7–2. A circle is divided into four brightly colored wedges representing vegetables and fruits (50%) and proteins and grains (25% each) with a smaller circle for dairy products. The logo shows proportions, not details, such as encouraging whole grains rather than refined grains, and that fish and beans are healthier choices than red meat. The consumer is encouraged to seek information from the USDA's website to learn how to eat a "healthy plate" at each meal.

The MyPlate website offers interactive tools and personalized recommendations to help individuals make changes to their diet. The website is an excellent teaching resource for nurses and health care professionals as well as the lay public, as it offers information for preschoolers (2–5 years), children (6–11 years), mothers, and the general population; information to develop a personalized plan; weight loss information; dietary analysis; and information that can be downloaded on tablets and smart phones. One can also follow MyPlate on Twitter.

Ethnic/cultural food pyramids include Latino/Spanish, Native American, and Asian, and these are available on the MyPlate website, as well as information on the Mediterranean diet. Special population pyramids include older adults, children, and vegetarians. The multiple options are intended to target diverse groups to encourage healthier meals by taking into account special needs and cultural backgrounds.

Issues in Undernutrition

Although the major problem in America is *over*nutrition, *under*nutrition is a problem in some segments of the population. Undernutrition has been documented in persons living below the poverty line, as well as children, adolescents, and the elderly.

Iron deficiency, the world's most common nutritional deficiency, is associated with multiple health problems. Chronic iron deficiency in childhood has an adverse effect on growth and development. Iron deficiency anemia is commonly caused by a decreased iron intake due to a diet insufficient in iron. The correction of iron deficiency accompanied by anemia is important to address developmental delays, impaired behavior, diminished intellectual functioning, and decreased resistance to infection (Trost, Bergfield, & Calogeras, 2006). Inadequate calcium intake in youth, another health problem caused by undernutrition, may result in failure to attain peak bone mass during the years of bone mineralization (up to age 20 years). This is thought to be a later predisposition for osteoporosis (Moore, Singer, Qureshi, Bradlee, & Daniels, 2012).

Eating disorders, such as anorexia nervosa and bulimia, are nutritional threats to the health of youth, particularly young white and Hispanic females, but these diagnoses are rare in black females. The incidence of anorexia and bulimia stabilized during the 1990s, and the occurrence of bulimia continues to decrease. A study of 10,000 U.S. adolescents between 13 and 18 years of age revealed that about 3 percent of them were affected by eating disorders (Swanson, Crow, LeGrange, Swendsen, & Merikangas, 2011).

Many of the physical complications of eating disorders are secondary to malnutrition, with osteoporosis and cardiac changes being significant problems (Winston, 2008). Promising prevention programs are reducing risk factors and eating pathologies, resulting in better outcomes (Marchand, Stice, Rohde, & Becker, 2011). *Under*nutrition is also a major problem in the elderly. In nursing home settings, the elderly may experience weight loss due to multiple issues, including loss of appetite and decreased ability to feed themselves. Undernourished nursing home clients, as defined by BMI (see Chapter 6), weight loss, and anthropometric measurements (see Chapter 6), require increased nutritional supplements to prevent recurring infections and premature death (Rahman, Simmons, Applebaum, Lindabury, & Schnelle, 2012). It is critical to access the nutritional status of the elderly and intervene to restore nutritional adequacy and healthy aging.

FACTORS INFLUENCING EATING BEHAVIOR

Making wise food choices is a cornerstone of good health. However, the multicausal nature of eating behaviors makes change a challenge, as eating behaviors are an integral part of individual, family, and community lifestyles. A strong cultural component adds to the difficulty of making modifications. Effective changes require consideration of all factors that influence eating behavior, the use of appropriate behavior-change strategies, and environmental and policy changes. Eating behaviors are influenced by multiple factors, including genetic-biologic, psychologic, socioeconomic, cultural, environmental, and health policy factors.

Genetic-Biologic Factors

Food intake and energy expenditure are controlled and kept in balance by complex neural systems. Humans have the ability to store a tremendous energy supply (fat) for later use. This ability has resulted in one of the major health risks for many human populations—obesity. The effectiveness of our neural system is seen in the body's ability to defend the lower limits of body weight by initiating external and internal nutrient-depletion signals, such as increased appetite, foraging, and stimulating the autonomic and endocrine systems to go into an internal energy saving mode.

The extra-hypothalamic brain structures that are responsible for reward, emotions, decision making, and choice (type of food intake) appear to assist the hypothalamus regulators in managing inadequate nutrition, but not overnutrition. The challenge is to understand why the neural system does not respond to overnutrition as it does to undernutrition. There are numerous regulatory mechanisms in the body, and their redundancy speaks to the biological importance of body weight regulation and to the futility of managing obesity without considering the neuro-regulatory determinants of energy balance.

Obesity, a complex disease characterized by disruption of the pathways between the brain and the gut that regulate hunger and satiety, is the excessive accumulation of fat in various organs involved in metabolism (Aronne, Nelinson, & Lillo, 2009). Heredity explains some of the variation in weight among individuals, indicating why some individuals gain weight and others do not. Researchers have identified at least 32 genes that are linked to obesity, and there is evidence of a genetic link to pediatric obesity. However, carrying an obesity-related gene does not necessarily predestine one to become obese, as carrying an obesity-associated gene is seen as just one risk factor in the overall obesogenic environment (Rhee, Phelan, & McCaffery, 2012). However, exposure to the food environment—such as the availability of fast food, takeaway meals, and convenience foods—makes people with genetic risk more susceptible to eating unhealthy foods.

Considerable research is underway to understand the physiological and cellular mechanisms that regulate energy balance and the events that converge and result in obesity. Multiple factors that regulate eating behaviors include specific hormones and genes. In the mid-1990s, the "ob" (obesity) gene was isolated from adipose tissue, and its protein product, leptin, identified. An adipocyte-derived protein hormone that circulates in the blood in proportion to whole-body adipose tissue mass, leptin is thought to serve as the signal to the brain to regulate the balance of food intake and energy expenditure (Morrison, 2008). Two possible mechanisms to explain metabolic and neural disorders of leptin are being investigated: leptin resistance, and central leptin insufficiency. Both hypotheses are under investigation to clarify the role of leptin and its contribution to energy balance. Evidence shows that increased leptin sensitivity protects against obesity, whereas loss of leptin sensitivity predisposes one to obesity, opening the doors for potential pharmacological interventions (Irving & Harvey, 2013, Schwartz & Baskin, 2013).

Epigenetics is a study of factors that can change the way genes respond without changing the genetic code itself. Single nutrients, toxins, behaviors, or environmental changes can stimulate a chemical that mobilizes a group of molecules—called a *methyl group*—that attaches to the control segment of a gene. The gene is either silenced or activated, altering its intended course of activity. Methylation has been described as like putting gum on a light switch—the switch isn't broken, but the gum blocks its function. Methylated genes can be demethylated through nutrients, drugs, and positive life experiences (Ptak & Petronis, 2008). The link between the environment and epigenetics is largely unexplored. However, some evidence shows that the environment and nutrition can influence the way the genes are controlled by DNA methylation (van Dijk, Molloy, Varinli, et.al, 2014). The "nature or nurture" debate is no longer valid, as environment and genes are inextricably linked.

The biologic changes of aging have a marked effect on eating behavior. A progressive loss of taste buds on the anterior tongue occurs with age, resulting in decreased sensitivity to sweet and salty tastes. In contrast, taste buds sensitive to bitter and sour increase with age. This taste distortion may result in decreased enjoyment of food and decreased intake of necessary nutrients by the elderly.

Changes in gastric secretions may result in limited absorption of iron, calcium, and vitamin B_{12} in the elderly. Decreased gastric mobility augments the need for foods high in fiber (fresh fruits, raw vegetables, whole-grain breads, and cereals) and increases the importance of water consumption to promote regularity in bowel evacuation. A decrease in basal metabolic rate also is associated with aging, often resulting in a decrease in caloric intake. Sensitivity to these changes in the elderly by the nurse can play a major role in improving the eating behaviors of older clients.

Psychological Factors

The most commonly performed human behaviors are eating, drinking, and making food choices. Although simple behaviors, they are determined by many factors—including individual, psychological determinants. In selecting foods Americans rate taste and price of food as more important than whether the food is healthy. Individual factors influencing eating, drinking, and making food choice decisions must be addressed among persons of *all* ages if healthy nutritional practices are to become a reality.

Affective processes (depression, low self-esteem, and lack of personal control over one's life) influence nutritional practices. Negative emotions (anger, frustration, fear, and insecurity) may also affect motivation to eat. Stress-related eating has been associated with weight gain. Emotions can decrease food intake in some individuals and increase food intake in others (van Strien, Cebolla, Etchemendy, Gutierrez-Maldonado, Ferrer-Garcia, Botella, & Banos, 2013). Increased food intake resulting from changes in emotional states provides comfort for many people. The emotion producing the change in food intake must be addressed before the behavior can be modified.

There are physical and social consequences of obesity stigma (see Table 7–3). Obese individuals often confront discrimination and stigma despite decades of science that suggest that obesity is a compelling social problem. The designation of obesity as a medical diagnosis by the American Medical Association may change this attitude over time; however, controversy surrounds this designation.

TABLE 7–3   Physical Health and Social Environmental Effects of Obesity Stigma

Physical Health Effects
• Depression
• Low self-esteem
• Negative body image
• Avoidance of physical activity
• Maladaptive eating behaviors
• Cardiovascular diseases

Social Environmental Effects
• Employment disadvantages
• Negative health care provider attitudes
• Blaming by family and friends
• Stereotyping by news media
• Educational disparities

Habits constitute another important determinant of eating behavior. A habit is a behavior that occurs often and is performed automatically or with little conscious awareness. Habits are performed so frequently that many cues within the environment serve as signals for the behavior. They often result in a psychological addiction to certain behaviors because they become a pervasive part of lifestyle. Such behaviors are known as *consummatory* because the response itself (eating) provides the reinforcement (Daily & Bartness, 2009). People may also become psychologically addicted to the consequences of habitual behaviors, such as the "energy spurt" experienced after the ingestion of highly refined sugars (doughnuts, sweet rolls, snack foods) or caffeine (sodas, coffee, energy drinks).

Often, individuals' perception of their weight and eating patterns differs from reality. Many people accept weighing more when the majority of the population is overweight and a shift in the social norm of what is normal weight occurs. Likewise, many diners have accepted larger food portions as the norm, unaware of the larger number of calories in their food portions, resulting in weight gain.

The public has varying beliefs about the causes of obesity. The majority of 1,139 adults surveyed believed that individuals were responsible for overeating that results in overweight and obesity (Fuemmeler, Baffi, Masse, Atienza, & Evans, 2007). Most respondents (66%) did not believe that obesity was caused by genes or a lack of knowledge of what constitutes a healthy diet. More women than men believed that the cost of healthy food is a factor in maintaining a healthy diet. Women were less likely than men to endorse the concept of "lack of willpower" as a contributing factor to overeating. The socialization processes and family responsibilities of men and women may influence gender differences, as men, more so than women, often believe that they have personal control over factors that affect their lives.

Socioeconomic and Cultural Factors

Sociological, economic, and cultural factors play dominant roles in eating behaviors and nutrition. People exist within a social and cultural context that shapes their eating behaviors and their access to healthy foods. Half of the 1,139 respondents in one study, regardless of gender, believed that society made it difficult for individuals to maintain a healthy weight. Within these groups, the likelihood exists that circumstances make it more difficult to manage weight. Many lower-socioeconomic-status individuals and racial/ethnic minorities believe that overeating and obesity are due in large part to societal influences. Other groups who believe society plays a major role in the increase in obesity are unemployed and unmarried individuals and older, retired persons who are overweight or obese (Dunn, Sharkey, & Horel, 2012; Fuemmeler, Baffi, Masse, Atienza, & Evans, 2007).

The relationship between socioeconomic position and consumption of fast foods suggests a possible reason for higher levels of obesity among individuals of low socioeconomic status and ethnic minorities. There are significant differences when comparing race and ethnic groups' knowledge of federal dietary guidance programs to that of non-Hispanic white Americans (who are more aware of federal dietary programs).

The regular consumption of fast food (high in fat, salt, and sugar; low in fiber) is associated with higher levels of overweight and obesity (Garcia, Sunil, & Hinojosa, 2012). Calorie consumption did not change before and after menu labeling in fast-food restaurants in New York. Lack of availability of grocery stores and access to healthy food (food desert) may contribute to the increased consumption of unhealthy foods (Burke, Froehlich, Zheng, & Glanz, 2012).

Ethnic minority populations are also more likely to experience higher exposures to environmental and psychological stressors associated with discrimination, economic security, and personal safety. Food may be used for coping with the day-to-day stressors. This type of unhealthy eating may result in the disposition of abdominal fat and risks for chronic diseases, as described previously in the chapter.

Ethnicity and culture also serve as important influences on eating behavior. Attitudes toward body size and shape are culturally defined, as well as traditional uses and meanings of foods. In addition, cultural traditions exist about which foods are harmful and protective, as well as how food relates to health. Food creates social interactions and conveys symbolic meanings across cultures. Ethnic foods are a source of pride and identity for many groups and may have deep emotional meaning for individuals because of an association with their country of origin, or because particular foods are associated with fond childhood memories.

Cultural factors may contribute to patterns of obesity in childhood and youth in many U.S. minority populations. Cultural wisdom may be strongly ingrained due to past economic deprivation, which led to a need to feast whenever food was available. High status and highly valued foods associated with survival are often red meats, sugars, and fatty foods. Larger body sizes have been associated with beauty, fertility, wealth, and power. In some cultures, overweight may be considered neutral or positive unless it is linked with a health problem, especially for women (Katz, 2012).

Suggestions for promoting healthy nutrition in diverse cultural communities include the following as well as those described in Chapter 12:

- Understand cultural beliefs about the interrelationship between food and health.
- Recognize how food consumption practices contribute to cultural identity.
- Assess the extent of acculturation to dominant-group nutritional behaviors.
- Offer clients nutrition or nurse consultants of similar ethnic backgrounds.
- Recognize nutritional attributes of ethnic foods.
- Reinforce ethnic nutritional practices that are positive.
- Provide information on nutrient values of ethnic foods to clients.
- Work with ethnic restaurants to offer healthy choices that are acceptable.
- Incorporate healthy ethnic food choices into work-site and school-site cafeterias.

Sensitivity to the difficulties that ethnic groups may have in identifying the contents of foods packaged in the United States and in understanding nutrition labeling is imperative. Inability to obtain familiar foods and trying to eat unfamiliar foods may be a source of frustration and distress. Language barriers and confusing mass media messages about nutritious foods often serve as barriers to good nutrition among members of varying ethnic groups. Improved access to consumer information is imperative so that members of ethnic groups can make informed decisions.

Environmental Factors

A population's preference for unhealthy diets and large portions is influenced by advertising, the food environment, and other obesogenic influences. Food and nutrition environments are believed to be major contributors to obesity and chronic diseases (Glanz, 2009). *Food environments* include home, school, work site, and neighborhoods. The *macro food environment* consists of food and agriculture policy, economics and pricing, and food marketing and advertising.

Obesogenic environments are all of the surroundings, opportunities, or conditions that promote obesity in individuals and populations (Saelels et al., 2012). Exposure to obesogenic environments is mediated by social, political, and economic factors. *Obesogenic food environments* include the production, distribution, and affordability of foods that contribute to obesity. The availability of fast foods, 24-hour takeaway, and home delivery has resulted in the consumption of fewer whole grains and more high-fat, high-sugar foods.

The *neighborhood environment* often is a promoter of obesity (Harrington & Elliott, 2009; Saelels et al., 2012). Obesogenic neighborhoods are those that discourage physical activity, have few parks and walking paths, and have a high concentration of fast-food places. Neighborhoods with walking trails, well-maintained sidewalks, and affordable recreational facilities, as well as access to supermarkets and health-related stores, promote healthy lifestyles, as compared to neighborhoods with only convenience stores and fast-food restaurants. Neighborhood disparities in access to food are of concern because of the potential influence on obesity. Neighborhood socioeconomic disadvantages may also play a role in an obesogenic environment as previously described. All of these factors reinforce the complexity of geography and eating behaviors.

For individuals to make healthy food choices, healthy food resources must be *accessible, available,* and *affordable* (Sharkey, 2009). The complexities of modern life make it difficult for many individuals to consistently maintain access to foods rich in important nutrients. "Food desert" is used to describe populated areas without adequate supermarkets or other outlets for healthy food choices. These same areas often have many fast-food options and convenience stores.

Cost of food is a critical consideration for many families, given the increasing numbers of families living at or below the poverty level. The cost of sources of complex carbohydrates (fruits, vegetables, and grains) may exceed that of highly refined sugar and grain products. Proteins also vary greatly in per-unit cost. An important responsibility of the nurse providing nutritional guidance to diverse populations is assisting families in identifying low-cost, high-nutrition options within their "choice" environments.

Seasonal variation in availability of foods such as raw vegetables and fresh fruits determines both accessibility and affordability. Seasonal patterns in the types of fruits and vegetables can be followed to maximize nutrient quality and lower cost. Use of frozen fruits and vegetables in their natural juices rather than canned foods during the off-season is recommended to decrease intake of sugar and salt. Home-frozen products are an important source of nutrients at reasonable cost.

Ease of preparation also plays an important role in food selection. Quick and effortless preparation techniques appeal to many families because of busy work schedules. In addition, attractiveness of prepared foods is an important consideration. Assisting the client in selecting nutritious foods that are quickly prepared and aesthetically appealing increases the likelihood of sustaining positive eating behavior.

Health Policy Factors

As science advances, new health regulations are implemented. For example, beginning in 2006, the Food and Drug Administration (FDA) required the labeling of the amount of "trans fat" per serving. The new regulations were added to the *Dietary Guidelines for Americans* to reflect the change. However, there was no coordinated effort to publicize the change, and the public only learned of the change through the mass media. Based on the sales immediately following the news coverage, the recommendations were heeded, as fewer products containing trans fats were purchased. However, this trend was short-lived, and after one week, sales of trans fat products reached pre-news levels (Niederdeppe & Frosch, 2009).

According to the Office of Food Additive Safety, trans fat intake did significantly decrease in 2012. This decrease was a result of (1) efforts to increase public awareness of its negative health effects, (2) required Nutrition Facts label changes, (3) the food industry's voluntary reformulation of foods, and (4) restriction of trans fat in food service outlets by some state and local governments (Doell, 2012).

Supersized fast foods, including sodas and larger serving portions of food, are under attack by some federal, state, and local governments as well as consumer groups. The lesson learned from the trans fat campaign was that including a well-planned and ongoing public awareness campaign will help to bring about sustained change. Individual responsibility for food selection and eating patterns balanced with mandates by governmental bodies and consumer groups will contribute to a healthier society.

In modern society, food additives are used to retard spoilage and prevent deterioration of quality, improve nutritional value, enhance consumer acceptability, and facilitate preparation. Laws require that labels of many products list the manufacturer, packer, and distributor, and the amount of each ingredient. Even when ingredients are listed, information on the products is often by itself insufficient to guide knowledgeable food selection. Not only are potentially carcinogenic additives used in the preparation of foods (nitrates in bacon), but unintentional food additives such as pesticides and other agricultural chemicals may appear in foods. Unfortunately, some of the synergistic, cumulative, and long-term effects of many additives will be determined only after years of use and exposure within human populations (Food and Drug Administration, 2011).

NUTRITIONAL NEEDS ACROSS THE LIFE SPAN

Infants and Children (0 to 8 years)

The caloric and nutrient intakes of children are critical for supporting growth and development. Infants, whose diet is primarily mother's milk or infant formula, consume 40% or more of their calories from fat that is appropriate during infancy. When children reach two years of age, however, they should be encouraged to consume a diet lower in total fat, saturated fat, and cholesterol than the usual American diet (36–40%) as a basis for lowering the risk for chronic diseases in later years. Diets of children two years of age and older should limit saturated fats to 10% of calories, total fats to 30% of calories, and dietary cholesterol to less than 300 mg/day (U.S. Department of Agriculture, 2010).

African-American children and children from low-income families appear to have diets least consistent with the national recommendations. When the diets of African-American children were examined separately, major sources of total dietary fat were franks, sausages, luncheon meats, and bacon, with whole milk a close second (U.S. Department of Agriculture, 2010).

A recent study showed that children whose families receive food stamps are just as likely to be overweight or obese as other low-income children. The Food Stamp Program, now known as the Supplemental Nutrition Assistance Program (SNAP), does not put any restrictions on the kinds of food that can be purchased under the program. Efforts to restrict purchases to healthy foods has been met with resistance by some participants, researchers, and policy makers who assert that more should be done to educate those participating in SNAP. Others suggest that the health of children is at risk and that SNAP funds should be used only for purchasing nutritious food (Pittman, 2013).

A healthy start for infants also means encouraging mothers to breast-feed or use iron-rich formulas for formula-fed infants. During pregnancy and lactation, mothers must maintain sufficient iron intake through iron-rich foods or supplements, as this increases the likelihood that the children will not be iron deficient during the early years of life (Centers for Disease Control and Prevention, 2011a).

The dietary habits of young children are profoundly affected by family food preparation and eating behaviors. Parental beliefs about good nutrition for children may not match health recommendations and thus may actually contribute to an unhealthy diet. Parents need to be taught appropriate food portion sizes for children, and monitor them at home and restaurants (Small, Lane, Vaughan, Melnyk, & McBurnett, 2013). Substituting 1% milk for whole milk, skim milk for low-fat milk, and reduced-fat cheese for whole-milk cheese would markedly decrease total fat intake. Not all children find the substitutes acceptable and not all are willing to consume them all the time. However, moderate changes in food consumption patterns result in favorable changes in dietary intake for most children.

The nutrition beliefs and practices of day care providers, other relatives, and preschool personnel have a significant influence on children in their care. Organized day care is an important setting for teaching nutrition and healthy behaviors, and concerns about food cost on the part of caretakers should not interfere with the provision of good nutritional meals. It is important that parents monitor the food provided in child care facilities until they are assured that healthy nutrition guidelines are followed (Ward, Benjamin, Ammerman, Ball, Neelon, & Bangdiwala, 2008).

Adolescents (9 to 19 years)

Adolescence is a period of biologic and social change. Body size, composition, functions, and physical abilities are changing rapidly. Undernutrition slows height and weight growth and may delay puberty. Among adolescents, minimal dietary requirements are those that maintain an optimal rate of pubertal development and growth. Adolescents, who are vigorously active, have increased energy needs. Thus, adolescents should consume diets providing more total nutrients than they consumed as young children.

Moderation is a good rule, as adolescents whose caloric intake is too high will gain weight, potentially leading to obesity. A caloric intake that is too low will result in loss of energy, weight loss, and, in the extreme, eating disorders that can lead to health problems and even premature death. Adolescents with chronic diseases such as type 1 diabetes have special nutrition needs, because absorption, metabolism, or excretion of particular nutrients may change as a result of both adolescent biologic changes and the disease.

In terms of fat intake, adolescents should be given dietary counseling to reduce total fat to less than 30% of calories per day with less animal fat, and cholesterol to less than 300 mg/day to lower risk factors for chronic disease. Because many adolescents consume fast foods at lunchtime or during the evening hours, selecting low-animal-fat fast foods is a significant challenge.

An example of a high-fat, fast-food meal is a double burger with sauce, milkshake, and French fries. The fat calories are 46% of the total calories in this meal. Because the goal should be less than 30% calories from fats, it is easy to see why consumption of such meals day after day increases the risk for cardiovascular disease and type 2 diabetes as early as adolescence.

There is accumulating evidence that this "risk" carries over into adulthood (U.S. Preventive Services Task Force, 2010).

Adolescent girls in the United States typically begin menstruating at 12½ years of age. Menstrual losses and increased physical activity increase the need for iron. Particular attention should be given to adequate intake of iron in the diet for women in general and, in particular, for very active young women. The mineral calcium helps to build strong bones. An adequate intake of calcium throughout childhood to age 25 years may reduce the risk of osteoporosis in later life. Young girls should learn to select foods that ensure adequate calcium, iron intake, and vitamin D (U.S. Preventive Services Task Force, 2010).

CDC data show that young men are the biggest consumers of added sugars, with one third of calories from added sugars coming from beverages. Most of the added sweetened food and beverages were consumed in the home and not at fast-food restaurants (U.S. Department of Agriculture, 2010). Efforts to reach young people about the importance of reducing intake of sugars and other empty calories are not succeeding. Increasing awareness of the need for good nutrition is important for overall adolescent health and performance. The challenge is to make nutritious food options appealing to adolescents who may eat primarily for taste, as do most Americans, rather than for good nutrition or health reasons. Peer support for healthy eating practices is critical during the adolescent years. Eating fast food, yet selecting lower-fat options, creates opportunities for adolescents to model good eating habits that may also influence their peers to make better food choices.

Pressure on fast-food establishments to offer healthier options will help create a supportive environment for healthy nutrition practices among adolescents. Schools are a vehicle for early health-promotion activities. School lunch programs are more carefully monitored than in the past, and because at-risk children are eligible for reduced or free breakfast and/or lunch, the nutritional status of these children has improved.

Efforts should continue to implement nutrition education, from preschool through grade 12. Efforts also should be made to integrate nutrition concepts throughout the entire curriculum, including courses in which they are not traditionally taught, such as math, chemistry, and history. Parents and guardians, critical to improving their children's nutritional status, must be included in efforts to improve the nutrition education of all students.

In 2010, the U.S. Preventive Services Task Force (USPSTF) updated its recommendation regarding weight management for overweight and obese children and adolescents to include behavioral and pharmacological interventions. Behaviorally based interventions are the first line of treatment, and pharmacological interventions are adjunct to behavioral interventions for severely obese adolescents (Whitlock, O'Connor, Williams, Bell, & Lutz, 2010). The Task Force chose not to comment on surgical interventions for obesity for this age group. The recommendation raises concerns about the state of the health of adolescents and their high risk for chronic health problems influenced by poor nutrition and poor eating habits.

Adults (19–50 years)

Many of the eating behaviors and patterns adults demonstrate are ones developed in childhood and adolescence, but caloric needs decrease when growth stops. This means that adults have less leeway for meeting nutritional requirements on a balanced diet to maintain health and a healthy weight.

Adulthood brings the stresses of family, career, and life responsibilities. Maintaining or improving health behaviors is critical during adulthood, as the health decisions made during

TABLE 7–4   Recommendations for Eating Patterns for Healthy Adults and Specific Population Groups

Key Recommendations	Recommendations for Specific Population Groups
Individuals should meet the following recommendations as part of a healthy eating pattern and while staying within their calorie needs.	*Women capable of becoming pregnant*[b]
	Choose foods that supply heme iron, which is more readily absorbed by the body, additional iron sources, and enhancers of iron absorption such as vitamin C-rich foods.
Increase vegetable and fruit intake.	
Eat a variety of vegetables, especially dark green and red and orange vegetables and beans and peas.	Consume 400 micrograms (mcg) per day of synthetic folic acid (from fortified foods and/or supplements) in addition to food forms of folate from a varied diet.[c]
Consume at least half of all grains as whole grains. Increase whole grain intake by replacing refined grains with whole grains.	*Women who are pregnant or breastfeeding*[b]
Increase intake of fat-free or low fat milk and milk products, such as milk, yogurt, cheese, or fortified soy beverages.[a]	Consume 8 to 12 ounces of seafood per week from a variety of seafood types.
Choose a variety of protein foods, which include seafood, lean meat and poultry, eggs, beans and peas, soy products, and unsalted nuts and seeds.	Due to their methyl mercury content, limit white (albacore) tuna to 6 ounces per week and do not eat the following four types of fish: tilefish, shark, swordfish, and king mackerel.
Increase the amount and variety of seafood consumed by choosing seafood in place of some meat and poultry.	If pregnant, take an iron supplement as recommended by an obstetrician or other health care provider.
Replace protein foods that are higher in solid fat with choices that are lower in solid fats and calories and/or are sources of oils.	*Individuals ages 50 years and older*
Use oils to replace solid fats where possible.	Consume foods fortified with vitamin B_{12}, such as fortified cereals, or dietary supplements.
Choose foods that provide more potassium, dietary fiber, calcium, and vitamin D, which are nutrients of concern in American diets. These foods include vegetables, fruits, whole grains, and milk and milk products.	

[a] Fortified soy beverages have been marketed as "soymilk," a product name consumers could see in supermarkets and consumer materials. However, FDA's regulations do not contain provisions for the use of the term soymilk. Therefore, in this document, the term "fortified soy beverage" includes products that may be marketed as soymilk.

[b] Includes adolescent girls.

[c] "Folic acid" is the synthetic form of the nutrient, whereas "folate" is the form found naturally in foods.

Source: U.S. Department of Agriculture and U.S. Department of Health and Human Services. *Dietary Guidelines for Americans, 2010.* 7th Edition, Washington, DC: U.S. Government Printing Office, December 2010.

this period greatly influence quality of life in the later years. *Dietary Guidelines 2010* provide the recommended eating patterns for adults (U.S. Department of Agriculture, 2010). Refer to Table 7–4 for key recommendations for healthy eating patterns for healthy adults, women during childbearing age, women who are pregnant or breastfeeding, and individual ages 50 years and older.

Older Adults (50 years and older)

Research on the nutritional needs of older adults is expanding rapidly as the American population ages. Aging is thought to alter nutrient requirements for calories, protein, and other nutrients as a result of changes in lean body mass, physical activity, and intestinal absorption. Although many older Americans maintain healthy eating patterns, for some, changing nutritional needs may be accompanied by deterioration in diet quality and quantity, jeopardizing nutritional status, quality of life, and functional independence.

Many elderly people skip meals and exclude whole categories of food from their diet because of reduced appetites, infrequent grocery shopping, lack of interest in cooking, and difficulties in chewing and swallowing. Consultation with health professionals is required if these individuals need supplementation. Self-medication may result in toxic levels of some multivitamin and mineral supplements. While the majority of older adults do take nutritional supplements, there is limited scientific support for health-related efficacy of these supplements. There is enough evidence to recommend not taking vitamins A, C, E, or antioxidant combinations for cancer or cardiovascular disease prevention (Buhr & Bales, 2009). Nurses must follow current research findings about nutritional supplements to safely advise the elderly.

Polypharmacy is common in older adults, so the interaction of food and drugs must be considered. The effects and absorption of medications can be altered by nutrients, foods, and other medicines. For example, crackers, dates, jelly, and other carbohydrates may slow down the rate of absorption of analgesics and limit their effectiveness in reducing pain.

Milk, eggs, cereals, and dairy products may inhibit the absorption of iron. Antibiotics such as tetracycline are less readily absorbed when milk, dairy products, or iron supplements are taken. Prune juice, bran cereal, and high-fiber foods may increase intestinal emptying time to the point where some drugs cannot be adequately absorbed. There is a need for further exploration of food–drug interactions that commonly occur among the elderly (Mallet, Spinewine, & Huang, 2007).

For individuals aged 65 years and older, recommended eating patterns lower in saturated fatty acids, total fat, saturated fats, and cholesterol help maintain desired body weight and lower the risk of cardiovascular heart disease (CHD). All of the risk factors for CHD, except cigarette smoking, are influenced by diet in some way. CHD is linked to nutritional patterns throughout life, with the damage manifest most frequently in middle-aged and older adults. Daily physical activity, along with a healthy diet to maintain adequate weight, can prevent premature mortality from heart disease and maintain vigor into old age (Fleg, 2012).

Essential components of the diets of older Americans generally are complex carbohydrates and fiber. Many elderly people have chewing and swallowing disorders that make eating fruits and vegetables difficult. Average daily fiber intake among the elderly is less than half of the recommended 20 to 35 grams. Health benefits attributed to fiber include proper bowel function, reduced risk of colon cancer, reduction of serum cholesterol, and improved glucose response. Six daily servings of whole grains are the recommended minimum for the elderly.

Energy requirements decline with reductions in body size, lean body mass, basal metabolism rate, and decreased physical activity. Because physical activity maintains muscle mass, it is highly desirable to keep physically active in later years. Diets of the elderly may also be deficient in protein along with calories as the result of an inability to chew meat or afford the cost of protein-rich foods. Infections, trauma, and other metabolic stresses may increase protein needs. Inadequate protein in the diet may lower resistance to disease and delay recovery from illness (Matte, 2010). See Chapter 4 for recommendations on assessing an elderly client's nutritional status.

Older adults with limited economic means should be assisted in selecting low-cost foods that meet recommended nutritional requirements. They may need guidance to learn to read label information to select and prepare foods that are easier to chew and swallow. Nutrition is integral to quality of life for the elderly, and thus, it is a primary area of focus for nurses who provide care to the elderly in primary care and long-term care settings.

PROMOTION OF DIETARY CHANGE

Altering nutrition education, the food environment, and food consumption patterns contributes to better nutrition and healthier lives. To alter nutrition patterns, all ages must be exposed to nutrition education through (1) mass media and Internet sources, (2) education at schools and work sites, (3) tailored self-help nutrition education packages, and (4) nutrition counseling in primary health care services. Information technology plays an increasingly larger role, so nutrition education approaches must be assessed to see if they are evidence-based and user friendly. Interactive computer nutrition programs, nutrition videos, social media, and healthy nutrition instant messaging are all important in broad-based nutrition education (Park, Nitzke, Dritsch, Kattelmann, White, Boeckner, et al., 2008).

Dietary information must evolve as scientific discoveries are made. Research is also needed to establish the effectiveness of interventions for low-income and ethnic minorities, children, and the efficacy of policy and environmental interventions. Despite the gaps in current knowledge, cumulative research findings support the basic advice: Take in fewer calories, eat less fat, move more, and eat more vegetables, fruits, and grains.

The food industry must be challenged to recognize its role in moving Americans toward a healthier society. Current legislation and regulation about the production and availability of food options influence cost and product development. Populations at school and work sites are captive and rely primarily on others to provide and prepare their food for a considerable part of the day, so the availability of healthy options from cafeterias and vending machines greatly affects nutrition behaviors. Furthermore, healthy food choices must have appeal in terms of taste and texture. Widespread research in the food production industry continues to create some food options that are both consistent with dietary recommendations and acceptable to the public. While marketing research plays an important role in supplying what the American public desires, food production research must also focus on how to provide more healthy food choices and how to motivate the public to increase intake of healthier foods. Every facet of food production, from the grower to the processor, has a part to play in the nutritional health of America.

INTERVENTIONS TO CHANGE EATING BEHAVIORS

Interventions are evidence-based strategies implemented to change unhealthy behavior(s). Most interventions target the individual and may occur in the home, school, organized child care centers, and work sites. Interventions also target populations such as churches, schools, and communities. Individual intervention formats include one-on-one, group, technology driven (telephone, Internet, and/or video), or combinations of these formats.

Individual targeted interventions to reduce obesity have had little long-term success. Preventing obesity in the population (population intervention) and helping overweight individuals prevent further weight gain (individual intervention) require new and different approaches. Intervention strategies for addressing change in dietary and eating patterns include the following:

- Increasing accessibility to nutrition information, education, counseling, and healthy foods in all settings and for all subpopulations
- Preventing chronic diseases associated with diet and weight, beginning in early childhood
- Strengthening the link between nutrition and physical activity in health promotion

Evidence-based interventions are necessary to continue to build the body of knowledge about nutrition and how to change eating behaviors. The U.S. Community Preventive Services Task Force created the *Community Guide* website as a free resource for sharing these evidence-based intervention programs for the benefit of health care professionals, policy makers, researchers, and others. The Task Force's findings are used to make recommendations for practice, policy changes, and future research.

The Task Force conducted systematic reviews of the evidence on nutrition and physical activity to determine the effectiveness of work site- and school-based interventions in preventing overweight and obesity. School- and work site-based interventions are the most potentially effective because children and adults spend most of their time in these respective sites.

School sites offer intensive contact with the majority of children and adolescents in America and are generally supportive of programs offered to improve students' health. Work sites provide access to approximately 65% of the population aged 16 years and older. Workers are accessible in a controlled environment with communication networks that facilitate employee participation. Facilities are also available to support interventions such as cafeterias, vending machines, and meeting spaces. A substantial proportion of calories are consumed at schools and work sites on a daily basis, making them ideal sites for dietary changes.

The Community Preventive Services Task Force recommends four strategies for school-based interventions aimed at weight control:

1. Include both nutrition and physical activity.
2. Incorporate additional time for activity during the school day.
3. Include noncompetitive sports such as dance.
4. Reduce sedentary activities.

Recommendations for work site interventions include combining instruction in better nutrition and eating habits with a structured physical activity program.

Comprehensive population-based interventions that address the interaction of multiple individual, social, and physical environmental factors are needed to bring about effective dietary change. However, the challenge is to develop interventions that are powerful enough to counteract the higher intake of calories and obesogenic factors in the environment for at-risk populations. The difficulty lies in identifying the set of interventions that would be effective in shifting the BMI distribution for a whole community.

One example of a set of interventions that focuses on one population is the Robert Wood Johnson Research Network to Prevent Obesity among Latino Children. *Salud America!* has developed a network of experts, community leaders, researchers, and others to work to reverse Latino childhood obesity. The programs and interventions include the children, family, school, church, and community to confront the increasing obesity problem in Latino children and the broader community (Robert Wood Johnson Foundation, 2013).

Population-based interventions must be complementary to individual-focused interventions. Population-based interventions address the health of the larger community, whereas individual interventions are tailored to the needs to specific individuals within the community. Population-based health interventions should promote healthy living for all, yet recognize and value the differences that exist in subpopulations. Individuals are responsible for their lifestyles; however, society has the ultimate responsibility for providing population-based interventions to improve the health of all.

RESEARCH-TESTED INTERVENTION PROGRAMS (RTIPs)

Research-tested intervention programs (RTIPs) move science into programs for people. These interventions have been reviewed by the Community Preventive Services Task Force and recommended based on meeting stringent criteria. Four RTIPs are presented as examples of strategies to promote better eating behaviors and improve health. They are New Moves (Neumark-Sztainer, Friend, Flattum, Hannon, Story, Bauer, et al., 2010); Strong Women-Healthy Hearts (Folta, Lichenstein, Sequin, Goldberg, Kuder, & Nelsom, 2009); Promoting Health Living: Assessing More Effects (PHLAME; Elliot et al., 2007); and Body and Soul (Resnicow et al., 2004).

New Moves—Preventing Weight-related Problems in Adolescent Girls in a Group Randomized Study

New Moves is a school-based program aimed at preventing weight-related problems such as obesity, inadequate physical activity, poor eating behaviors, unhealthy weight control practices, and body dissatisfaction in adolescent girls. The program consists of a physical education class, 5 days per week, 30 minutes each day, for approximately 16 weeks. Girls participate in physical activity 4 days a week, and nutrition and social support classes each 1 day per week. The physical activity classes are taught by physical education teachers for 3 days per week, and a community guest instructor for 1 day per week to expose the girls to fun activities such as dance, kickboxing, and hip hop. All the materials needed to implement this program can be found on the New Moves website.

Strong Women-Healthy Hearts

Strong Women-Healthy Hearts is a community-based intervention for sedentary, overweight, and obese women aged 40 or older designed to promote dietary habits and increase physical activity to reduce obesity. The intervention is an hour-long class, 2 days per week, for 12 weeks. Each class includes a physical activity session progressing to 30 minutes of moderate to vigorous aerobic exercise and a dietary session. The program is suitable for senior centers, assisted living centers, places of worship, and other settings where this population gathers. The program leader is required to attend an 8-hour training workshop.

Promoting Healthy Living: Assessing More Effects (PHLAME)

The PHLAME intervention promotes healthy eating, regular exercise, and appropriate weight among firefighters. Healthy eating is defined as five or more servings of fruits and vegetables each day and less than 30% of calories from fat. Peer-led, team-centered, scripted lesson plans are used in 11 team sessions (45 minutes per session) scheduled over one year. Sessions include nutrition, physical activity, and energy balance. The curriculum incorporates aspects of social-cognitive theory. The intervention is intended for professional firefighters and implemented in fire stations. Team materials cost approximately $25 per participant.

Body and Soul

The Body and Soul intervention offers a unique opportunity to increase fruit and vegetable intake among African Americans. The program includes three church-wide nutrition activities, one event with the church pastor, and one policy change, such as establishing guidelines for the type of food served at church functions. Lay counselors, who make at least two 15-minute calls to five participants, are given 12–16 hours of training. The program is suitable for implementation in home and church settings for African-American church members, aged 17–89 years. Implementation time varies based on length of church involvement.

STRATEGIES FOR MAINTAINING RECOMMENDED WEIGHT

Weight maintenance is a lifelong health goal to reduce the multiple health problems that result from obesity (see Tables 7–1 and 7–2). The physical basis for excessive weight gain is relatively simple and straightforward: Overweight and obesity result from an imbalance in energy because of too many calories and not enough physical activity. Weight management means balancing the number of calories consumed with the number of calories burned. Despite the multiple factors involved, diet and exercise are the cornerstones of prevention of overweight and obesity. Homes, schools, work sites, and the community must all work together to promote healthy eating and physical activity. Strategies to promote healthy eating habits and physical activity may be accessed at the National Institute of Diabetes, Digestive and Kidney Diseases weight control information network website. Strategies include the following:

- Choose sensible portions of foods lower in fat. Watch portion sizes.
- Learn healthier ways to make favorite foods.
- Learn to recognize and control environmental cues that make you want to eat.
- Have a healthy snack an hour before a social gathering.
- Engage in moderate-intensity physical activity for 30 minutes every day.
- Take a walk instead of watching television.
- Do not eat meals in front of the television.
- Keep records of your food intake and physical activity. Weigh yourself weekly.
- Pay attention to why you are eating.

STRATEGIES FOR INITIATING A WEIGHT-REDUCTION PROGRAM

Obesity is a global epidemic and continues to increase in the United States. It is estimated that two thirds of adults are either overweight or obese. As stated in previous chapters, overweight is defined as a BMI in the range of 25–29.9, and obesity as a BMI 30 or greater. Location of excess body fat also is important, as intra-abdominal fat is a risk factor for diabetes and cardiovascular disease. Obesity increases the risk of cardiovascular disease, type 2 diabetes, and other chronic diseases. The epidemic represents a public health crisis that requires primary and secondary prevention efforts to stop the escalating costs of managing chronic diseases associated with obesity as well as detrimental effects on quality of life.

Weight management is difficult and requires a lifelong commitment, making it a challenge for the individual and the health care provider. Individuals who are overweight or obese and desire to lose weight should consult a health care provider before starting an aggressive weight loss program. Consultation will assist with the type of dietary program to select. In addition, the health care provider will perform a health and family history, physical examination, BMI and waist circumference or hip-waist ratio measures, blood lipid and glucose analysis, and an electro-cardiogram or exercise stress test before beginning a weight-loss program. Careful assessment of current dietary habits is essential to develop an individualized, effective program.

Other questions to assist in the assessment include the following:

- Is the person strongly motivated to lose weight?
- Is the person willing or able to commit the time and financial resources needed?
- Does the person believe he or she can be successful in a weight loss program?
- Does the person understand the possible risks of weight loss interventions?
- Are weight loss goals realistic?
- What is the person's attitude toward physical activity?
- Does the person have a support system to facilitate weight loss?
- What are the potential barriers to successful weight loss?
- Has the person had past success in weight loss? If so, what worked? What did not work?
- What factors caused the person to relapse in the past?

Caloric reduction with attention to portion size, while maintaining adequate nutrient levels, adequate vitamins and minerals, and adequate fiber is the best way to achieve and maintain desired weight, in conjunction with a regular physical activity program. Radical changes in food consumption patterns are not recommended. It is important for clients to understand that even modest weight loss is beneficial.

Dietary preferences and the individual's ability to incorporate a particular diet into his or her daily routine should be taken into consideration when planning the type of dietary intervention. Dietary interventions include low carbohydrate, low fat, high protein, high fiber, and meal replacements. Meal replacement diets have become increasingly popular for those who do not have time to prepare meals and have difficulty controlling portion size. The meal substitutes are considered nutritionally well-balanced diets, and the result has been favorable with sustained weight loss for as long as four years. Very low-calorie diets should be avoided or undertaken under close supervision.

Behavioral management techniques refer to principles used to change an individual's behavior and lifestyle. The client must develop new skills to facilitate long-term change. These techniques have been shown to be an important component of weight loss programs (Hainer, Toplak, & Mitrakou, 2008). Behavioral modification techniques include self-monitoring, stress management, stimulus control, problem solving, rewarding behavior changes, cognitive restructuring, social support, and relapse prevention training. Learning to control daily food choices and physical activity is crucial to long-term success. Plannng and self-monitoring are considered to be two of the most useful behavioral management strategies. Planning meals for healthy dietary intake and time for physical activity and keeping records to assess one's progress give insight into personal behavior.

Although short-term change has been documented, it is much more difficult to maintain loss long term. A supportive approach with extended contacts has been shown to be effective in maintaining behavior change. Other strategies for long-term weight loss maintenance that have been successful include the following:

- Relapse prevention training to teach specific skills
- Telephone prompts to provide frequent contacts
- Peer/social support
- Extended behavioral therapy

Effective weight-loss programs for children suffer from many barriers, including lack of family motivation, financial costs, and lack of time. A meta-analysis of research interventions for children aged 4–18 years reported that the use of structured dietary and exercise regimens are effective in promoting weight loss. Diet, exercise, behavioral techniques, and parental involvement are all important in promoting the effectiveness of weight loss programs in this group. Parents should be included in the intervention, as they have control over the food purchased, meal planning and preparation, as well as model healthy eating (Whitlock, O'Connor, Williams, Bell, & Lutz, 2010).

Obesity in older persons is beginning to receive attention due to the increased prevalence of obesity in this population. A systematic review was undertaken to investigate the evidence of weight loss interventions in older adults (Bales & Buhr, 2008). Loss of lean body mass was noted in several studies. In general, the findings show benefits for osteoarthritis, physical function, and possibly type 2 diabetes and coronary heart disease. Results suggest that in persons aged 65 years and older, weight loss interventions should be considered on an individual basis with attention to the weight history and the medical conditions of the client. Resistance exercises should be part of all weight loss interventions for older adults.

CONSIDERATIONS FOR PRACTICE IN NUTRITION AND HEALTH

Health professionals are important role models for healthy eating and weight management. Nurses should not only advocate healthy diets for others, but also put the dietary guidelines into practice themselves as a part of their own commitment to a healthy lifestyle. Role modeling recommended eating patterns, as well as managing potential issues that undermine maintenance of positive nutritional practices, will indicate sincerity and commitment to good health practices that speak louder than words. The public expects health care professionals, especially nurses, to be healthy and to model positive weight and exercise habits.

The responsibility for monitoring the nutritional health of individuals, families, and the community is shared among all members of the health promotion team. Lack of commitment to positive dietary habits and good nutrition has resulted in a sizable population of children, adolescents, and adults who are overweight and/or obese. The chronic health problems that follow are costly in terms of resources and quality of life. Dietary counseling and education should be an integral part of nursing practice in all settings. Counseling and follow-up of clients who are at risk for or who are overweight or obese is a priority. Health teaching should begin with preschoolers, so that they learn healthy eating habits that can be sustained.

Opportunities should be created to engage clients and others in dialogue about their dietary practices and changes to improve their health. Studies show that talking with clients about weight control helps to promote behavior change. Many health professionals fail to do so due to limited office/clinic time and lack of training on how to talk to clients about weight. Nurses are in a position to influence other providers by speaking with clients caringly about their readiness to adopt healthier eating patterns and partnering with them to accomplish their goals.

School nurses and occupational health nurses must work with schools, workplaces, industry, and policy makers to improve the food choices in cafeterias and vending machines. Websites that focus on nutrition are a quick way to keep current on the latest research findings and practice guidelines. The nurse can help clients understand and select accurate information.

OPPORTUNITIES FOR RESEARCH IN NUTRITION AND HEALTH

The health consequences of overweight and obesity in America make research a priority to identify and test new strategies and treatments to reverse the trend. Research results indicate that the benefits of dieting interventions have had limited success for sustained weight loss. The role of physical activity as a treatment for obesity needs continued attention. Clinical trials that compare activity-only groups with diet-only and diet and exercise groups will help researchers better understand the role of physical activity in weight loss. Strategies to sustain weight loss also should be identified and tested. In addition, preschool interventions to promote physical activity and make healthy food choices need development, testing, and follow-up of long-term health outcomes. Measures of obesogenic environments and food environments should be developed that can be used to assess neighborhoods and communities. Multilevel approaches are needed to take into consideration the context of the individual. Community-level interventions must be carefully planned, implemented, and evaluated. Interventions that target ethnic and low-income communities and build on the existing community strengths and assets to bring about social change should be investigated. Interventions to increase the long-term effectiveness for family–child dietary pattern changes also are needed. It is no longer sufficient to focus solely on the individual to promote health food choices. The complexity of the multiple factors involved necessitates a multidisciplinary approach and the involvement of government officials and health policy makers (McKinnon, Reedy, Handy, & Rodgers, 2009; McKinnon, Tracy Orleans, Kumanyika, Haire-Josu, Krebs-Smith, Finkelstein, et al., 2009).

Summary

Lifelong patterns of health eating are needed to avoid the chronic health problems of overweight and obesity. Individual, social, and physical environmental barriers to changing eating behaviors must be addressed to facilitate lifestyles that promote healthy eating behaviors. Promoting good nutrition is a critical concern in prevention and health promotion and an important dimension of competent self-care.

Cultural and ethnic backgrounds influence eating behavior and must be accounted for in changing eating patterns. The individual, family, and community must all be part of nutritional interventions. Research has substantiated the complexity of factors that determine eating behaviors, and all of these determinants must be part of a strategy for successful change to occur.

Learning Activities

1. Compare your diet with the *Dietary Guidelines for Americans 2010* recommendations, and identify two modifications you are willing to make in your diet.
2. Use MyPlate to assist you in making the modifications you identified in Learning Activity #1.
3. Select, explore, and evaluate the nutritional information on two websites of your choice.
4. Engage an adolescent and an older adult in discussions to assess their knowledge and understanding of their nutritional needs. Assist them to develop a plan to overcome identified barriers to healthy eating.

References

Aronne, L., Nelinson, D., & Lillo, J. (2009). Obesity as a disease state: A new paradigm for diagnosis and treatment. *Clinical Cornorstone, 9*(4), 9–25: discussion, 26–29.

Bales, C., & Buhr, G. (2008). Is obesity bad for older persons? A systemic review of the pros and cons of weight reduction in later life older persons. *Journal of the American Medical Directors Association, 9*, 302–312.

Buhr, G., & Bales, C. (2009). Nutritional supplements for older adults: Review and recommendations—part 1. *Journal of Nutrition in the Elderly, 28*(1), 5–29. doi:10.1080/01639360802640545

Burke, L., Froehlich, R., Zheng, Y., & Glanz, K. (2012). Current theoretical bases for nutrition intervention and their uses. In A. M. Coulston (Ed.), *Nutrition in the prevention and treatment of disease* (3rd ed., pp. 141–155). New York, NY: Elsevier.

Centers for Disease Control and Prevention. (2011a). *Pediatric and pregnancy nutrition surveillance system.* Retrieved from http://www.cdc.gov/PEDNSS /pdfs/PED

Centers for Disease Control and Prevention. (2011b, January 13). *Adult obesity facts.* Retrieved May 5, 2013, from http://www.cdc.gov/obesity/data/adult.html

Centers for Disease Control and Prevention. (2011c, January 13). *Data and statistics.* Retrieved from Obesity and Overweight for Professionals: Children: Data at http://www.cdc.gov/obesity/data/childhood.html

Daily, M., & Bartness, T. (2009). Appetitive and consummatory ingestive behaviors stimulated by PVH and perifornical NPY injections. *American Journal of Physiology, 296*(4), R877–R892.

Doell, D. (2012). *Trans fat intake by the U.S. population.* Office of Food Additive Safety. Retrieved from http:// www.usfoodanddrugadministration/gov

Dunn, R., Sharkey, J., & Horel, S. (2012). The effect of fast-food availability on fast-food consumption and obesity among rural residents: an analysis by race/ethnicity. *Economics and Biology, 10*(1), 1–13. doi:10.1016/j.ehb. Epub 2011

Elliot, D., Goldberg, L., Kuehl, K., Moe, E., Berger, R., & Pickering, M. (2007). The PHLAME (Promoting Healthy Lifestyles: Alternative Models' Effects) firefighter study: Outcomes of two models of behavior change. *Journal of Occupational and Environmental Medicine, 49*(2), 204–213.

Fleg, J. (2012). Aerobic exercise in the elderly: A key to successful aging. *Discovery Medicine.* Retrieved from http://www.discoverymedicine.com/category /discovery-medicine/n0-070

Folta, S., Lichenstein, A., Sequin, R., Goldberg, J., Kuder, J., & Nelsom, M. (2009). The Strong Women-Healthy Hearts Program: Reducing cardiovascular risk factors in rural sedentary, overweight and obese middle and older women. *American Journal of Public Health, 99*(7), 1271–1277.

Food and Drug Administration. (2011). Retrieved from http://www.fda.gov/Food/IngredientspackagingLabeling /FoodAdditives

Fuemmeler, B. F., Baffi, C., Masse, L. C., Atienza, A. A., & Evans, W. (2007). Employer and healthcare policy interventions aimed at adult obesity. *American Journal of Preventive Medicine, 32*(1), 44–51.

Garcia, G., Sunil, T., & Hinojosa, P. (2012). The fast food and obesity link: Consumption patterns and severity of obesity. *Obesity Surgery, 22*(5), 910–918. doi:10.1007/ s11695-012

Gelber, R. P., Gaziano, J. M., Orav, J., Manson, J., E., Buring, J. E., & Kurth, T. (2008). Measures of obesity and cardiovascular risk among men and women. *Journal of the American College of Cardiology, 52*, 605–615.

Glanz, K. (2009). Measuring food environments. A historical perspective. *American Journal of Preventive Medicine, 36*(4S), S93–S98.

Hainer, V., Toplak, H., & Mitrakou, A. (2008). Treatment modalities of obesity. *Diabetes Care, 31*(S2), S269–S277.

Harrington, D., & Elliott, S. (2008). Weighing the importance of neighborhood: A multilevel exploration of the determinants of overweight and obesity. *Social Science & Medicine, 68*(4), 593–600.

Harvard School of Public Health. (accessed May 11, 2013). *Harvard School of Public Health.* Retrieved from The Nutrition Source: http://hsph.harvard.edu /nutritionsource/plate-replaces-pyramid

Irving, A. J. & Harvey, J. (2014) Leptin regulation of hippocampal synaptic function in health and disease. *Philosophical Translations of the Royal Society Biological Sciences, 369*, 20130155.

Katz, D. (2012). *Is obesity cultural?* Retrieved from http:// www.health.usnews.com/health-news/blogs/eat-run

Kragelund, C., & Levine, J. A. (2005). A farewell to body mass index? *Lancet, 306*, 79–86.

Levi, J., Segal. L., Fuchs Miller, A., & Lang, A. (2013). *A Healthier America 2013.* Trust for America's Health.

Mallet, L., Spinewine, A., & Huang, A. (2007). The challenge of managing drup interactions in elderly people. *The Lancet, 370* (9582), 185–191.

Marantz, P. R., Bird, E., & Alderman, M. H. (2008). A call for a higher standard of evidence for dietary guidelines. *American Journal of Preventive Medicine, 34*, 234–240.

Marchand, E., Stice, E., Rohde, P., & Becker, C. B. (2011). Moving from efficacy to effectiveness trials in prevention research. *Behaviour Research and Therapy, 49*, 32–41.

Matte, M. (2010). How many protein calories are required for the elderly? *Livestrong.* Retrieved from http://www .livestrong.com/article/285664

McKinnon, R. A., Reedy, J., Handy, S., & Rodgers, A. B. (2009). Measuring the food and physical environments: Shaping the research agenda. *Journal of Preventive Medicine, 36*(4 Suppl 1), S81–S85.

McKinnon, R. A., Tracy Orleans, C., Kumanyika, S. K., Haire-Josu, D., Krebs-Smith, S. M., Finkelstein, E., et al. (2009). Considerations for an obesity policy research agenda. *American Journal of Preventive Medicine, 36*(4), 351–357.

Messiah, S. E., Arheart, K. L., Lipschulz, S. E., & Miller, T. L. (2008). Body mass index, waist circumference and cardiovascular risk factors in aldoescents. *Journal of Pediatrics, 153,* 845–850.

Moore, L. L., Singer, M. R., Qureshi, M. M., Bradlee, M. L., & Daniels, S. R. (2012). Food group intake and micronutrient adequacy in adolescent girls. *Nutrients, 4*(11), 1692–1708. doi:10.3390/nu4111692

Neumark-Sztainer, D., Friend, S., Flattum, C., Hannon, P., Story, M., Bauer, K., et al. (2010). New moves—Preventing weight-related problems in adolescent girls: A group-randomized study. *American Journal of Preventive Medicine, 39*(5), 421–432. doi:10.1016/j.amepre

Niederdeppe, J., & Frosch, D. (2009). News coverage and sales of products with trans fat: Effects before and after changes in federal labeling policy. *American Journal of Preventive Medicine, 36*(5), 395–401.

Park, A., Nitzke, S., Dritsch, K., Kattelmann, K., White, A., Boeckner, L., et al. (2008). Internet-based interventions have potential to affect short-term mediators and indicators of dietary behaviors of young adults. *Journal of Nutrition Education and Behavior, 40*(5), 288–297.

Pittman, G. (2013). *Reuters Health.* Retrieved from htpp://www.reuters.com/article/2013/03/07us-kids-on-food-stamps-id

Ptak, C., & Petronis, A. (2008). Epigenetics and complex disease: From etiology to new therapeutics. *Annual Review of Pharmacology and Toxixology, 48,* 256–257.

Rahman, A. N., Simmons, S. F., Applebaum, R., Lindabury, K., & Schnelle, J. (2012). The coach is in: Improving nutritional care in nursing homes. *Gerontologist, 52*(4), 571–580.

Reis, J. P., Aranta, M. R., Wingard, D. L., Macera, C. A., Lindsay, S. P., & Marshall, S. J. (2008). Overall obesity and abdominal adiposity as predictors of mortality in U.S. white and black adults. *Annals of Epidemiology, 19,* 134–142.

Resnicow, K., Campbell, M., Carr, C., McCarly, F., Wang, T., Periasamy, S., . . . Stables, G. (2004). Body and soul. A dietary intervention conducted through African-American churches. *American Journal of Preventive Medicine, 27*(2), 97–106.

Rhee, K. E., Phelan, S., & McCaffery, J. (2012). *Early determinates of obesity: Genetics, epigenetic, and in utero influences.* doi:10.1155/2012/463850

Robert Wood Johnson Foundation. (2013). A research network to prevent obesity among Latino children. Retrieved from http://www.rwjf.org/en/research-publications

Saelels, B., Sallis, J., Frank, L., Couch, S., Zhou, C., Colburn, T., . . . Glanz, K. (2012). Obesogenic neighborhood environments, child and parent obesity: The neighborhood impact on kids study. *American Journal of Preventive Medicine, 42*(5), e57–e64.

Schwartz, M. W. & Baskin, D. G. (2014). Leptin and the brain: then and now. *The Journal of Clinical Investigation, 123*(6), 2344–2345.

Sharkey, J. R. (2009). Measuring potential access to food stores and food-service places in rural areas in the U.S. *American Journal of Preventive Medicine, 36*(4 Suppl 1), S151–S155.

Small, L., Lane, H., Vaughan, L., Melnyk, B., & McBurnett, D. (2013). A systematic review of the evidence: The effects of portion size manipulation with children and portion education/training interventions on dietary intake with adults. *Worldviews on Evidence-Based Nursing, 10*(2), 69–81.

Srikanthan, P., Seeman, T. E., & Karlamangia, S. K. (2009). Waist-hip ratio as a predictor of all-cause mortality in high functioning older adults. *Annals of Epidemiology, 19*(10), 724–731.

Swanson, S., Crow, S., LeGrange, D., Swendsen, J., & Merikangas, K. (2011). *Prevalence and correlates of eating disorders in adolescents: Results from the National Comorbidity Survey Replication Adolescent Supplement.* Retrieved from National Institute of Mental Health: www.nimh.nih.gov/news/science-news

Trost, L. B., Bergfield, W. E., & Calogeras, E. (2006). The diagnosis and treatment of iron deficiency and its potential relationship to hair loss. *Journal of the Academy of Dermatology, 54,* 824–844.

Trust for America's Health. (2009). *Americans rank prevention as most important health reform priority.* Retrieved from http://wwwhealthyamericans.org/report/70/prevention-survey-II

U.S. Department of Agriculture. (2010). *Dietary Guidelines for Americans.* Retrieved from http://www.health.gov/DietaryGuidelines

U.S. Preventive Services Task Force. (2010). Retrieved from http://www.uspreventiveservicestaskforce.org/recommendations

van Dijk, A. J., Molloy, P. L., Varinli, H., Morrison, J. L., Muhlhausler, B. S., & members of EpiSCOPE. (2014). Epigenetics and human obesity. *International Journal of Obesity, 1*-13. doi:10.1038/ijo.2014.34.

van Strien, T., Cebolla, A., Etchemendy, E., Gutierrez-Maldonado, J., Ferrer-Garcia, M., Botella, C., & Banos, R. (2013). Emotional eating and food intake after sadness and joy. *Appetite, 66,* 20–25. doi:10.1016/j. Epub

Wang, Y. C., McPherson, K., Marsh, T., et al. (2011). Health and economic burden of the projected obesity trends in the USA and the UK. *Lancet, 378*(9793), 815–825.

Ward, D., Benjamin, S., Ammerman, A., Ball, S., Neelon, B., & Bangdiwala, S. (2008). Nutrition and physical activity in child care: Results from an environmental intervention. *American Journal of Preventive Medicine, 35*(1), 352–356.

Whitlock, E., O'Connor, E., Williams, S., Bell, T., & Lutz, K. (2010). Effectiveness of weight management interventions in children: A targeted systematic review for the USPSTF. *Pediatrics, 125*(2), e396–e418. doi:10.1542/peds.2009-1955

WHO Expert Consultation. (2008). *Waist circumference and waist-hip ratio.* Geneva, Switzerland: World Health Organization.

Winston, A. P. (2008). Management of physical aspects and complications of eating disorders. *Psychiatry, 7*(4), 174–178.

World Health Organization (WHO). (2008). *The world health report—Primary health care.* Geneva, Switzerland: WHO.

CHAPTER 8

Stress Management and Health Promotion

OBJECTIVES

This chapter will enable the reader to:

1. Describe the relationship between stress and health.
2. Compare four approaches to assist patients to reduce stressful situations.
3. Contrast five psychological conditioning strategies to increase resistance to stress.
4. Examine three therapies to manage stress in individuals and groups.

Stress is of both theoretical and practical interest to nurses. The World Health Organization (WHO) Global Burden of Disease Survey estimated that the global impact of stress-related conditions would rise over the next decade so that by 2020, depression and anxiety disorders, including stress-related conditions, will be the second most prevalent health problem, second only to ischemic heart disease (World Health Organization, 1996). This estimate is on track, as conditions attributed to or made worse by stress account for more than three fourths of visits to health care professionals (Hogue, Sederer, Smith, & Nossel, 2010). With this high incidence of stress-related health problems, it is critically important for nurses to intervene and promote mental health through fostering stress resistance and overall resilience among individuals and families. Likewise, nurses must practice personal stress reduction and stress management, not only to maintain their own mental health, but also to intervene and promote healthy responses to their patients' stress.

Stress is the brain's response to any demand. Stress is an inevitable, unavoidable, human experience in any society, more so in a society characterized by rapid and accelerating change, and is not necessarily bad. All life events cause stress. Selye, a pioneer in stress research, defined stress as "the nonspecific response of the body to any demand made on it." The General Adaptation Syndrome (GAS), or "fight-or-flight" response, is the internal and external manifestations of stress (Selye, 1936). Chemicals and hormones released by the body in response to stress produce physiological changes such as increased pulse rate and respirations, muscle tension,

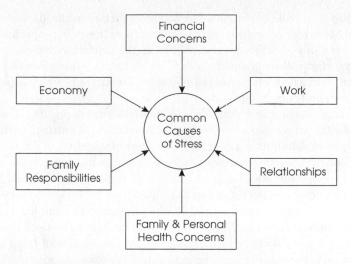

FIGURE 8–1 Causes of Stress

and increased brain activity—all functions aimed at survival. However, systems return to normal once the threat passes.

Stress in modern society tends to stem from psychological rather than physical threats (see Figure 8–1). The stresses of daily life consist of emotional threats such as being stuck in traffic, having disagreements with coworkers, and family problems. The frequency of these excessive or unnecessary stresses can cause these same lifesaving responses to lower immunity and decrease normal functioning of the digestive, excretory, and reproductive systems. People's responses to chronic stress differ; some experience digestive symptoms while others report headaches, irritability, sleeplessness, and depression. Over time, chronic stress can result in serious health problems that include heart disease, hypertension, diabetes, and other illnesses (see Figure 8–2).

Although Selye made major contributions to the general adaptation theory of stress and supported the idea of a relationship between prolonged stress and disease, the theory was not

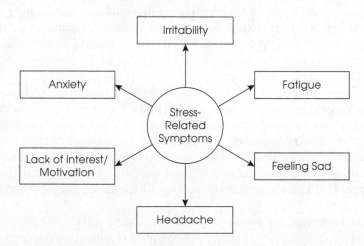

FIGURE 8–2 Symptoms of Stress

without limitations. The role of emotional or cognitive factors in the stress response was not accounted for in his model. All individuals experience stress; however, people interpret and react to it differently, resulting in differing vulnerabilities to the deleterious effects of stress. In addition, research has clarified the homeostasis concept by distinguishing between the conditions that are necessary to maintain the internal body systems for survival (*homeostasis*) and those that maintain balance in body systems (*allostasis*).

The goal of homeostasis and allostasis is to maintain internal stability. The differing reactions of individuals to stress led to a re-evaluation of homeostasis, contributing the terms *allostasis* and *allostatic load*. *Allostasis* is a continuous process of adapting in the face of potentially stressful events. When exposed to a stressor, the body responds by turning on a complex pathway for adapting and coping with physiologic and behavioral response (Sterling, 2012). The stressful event leads to the release of catecholamines (adrenalin), glucocorticoids (cortisol), and other hormones. The response returns to the baseline when the stressful event has ended or is under control, *unless exposure to an elevated level of stress continues over weeks and months.*

A continued elevated stress response results in *allostatic load,* with resultant vulnerability and dysfunction. *Allostatic load* reflects the cumulative negative effects of prolonged environmental and psychosocial stressors (McEwen, 2007) such as inadequate housing, excess calorie intake, smoking, and alcohol. In other words, how individuals cope with challenges over a lifetime influences allostasis, allostatic load, and resulting disease. Physiological indicators of allostatic load include (1) hypertension, (2) increased high-density lipoproteins (HDL) and total cholesterol, (3) increased glycosylated hemoglobin (HgbA1c) levels over time, and (4) increased urinary cortical excretion. *Cumulative stress* has the potential to predict risk for a variety of diseases, such as diabetes, cardiovascular disease, and cancer (Danese & McEwen, 2012; Gersten, 2008; Loucks, Juster, & Pruessner, 2008).

Stressors, or the causes of stress, are "environmental and internal demands and conflicts which tax or exceed a person's resources" (Lazarus & Folkman, 1984). Stress, the body's response to these stressors, involves the nervous, endocrine, and immunologic systems, which in turn affects all organ systems. Stressors viewed as challenging, stimulating, and exciting are desirable, whereas uncontrollable or emotionally distressing stressors are undesirable. Some individuals have "resistance resources" that enable them to successfully manage stressors and flourish, whereas others find the same stressors debilitating.

Coping strategies assist individuals in managing stress through learned and purposeful cognitive, emotional, and behavioral responses to stressors by either adapting to the environment or changing it (Lazarus, 1999). In the coping process, the ability to regulate emotions, behavior, and the environment is critical to successful adjustment. In other words, coping is behavior that uses available resources to manage stress situations.

Cognitive appraisal and coping constitute the stress-coping process. Cognitive appraisal consists of two phases: primary appraisal and secondary appraisal. The two phases are not mutually exclusive, in *primary appraisal,* the person questions whether there is potential harm or benefit to cherished commitments, values, goals, self-esteem, or to one's health and well-being. If an encounter is threatening, primary appraisal serves to reduce its significance for the person experiencing it (O'Connor, Arnold, & Maurizio, 2010). For example, if a person receives news that the results of a laboratory test are "abnormal," the person may discount the validity of the test.

In *secondary appraisal,* the person evaluates what coping options or behaviors are available to overcome or prevent harm, or to improve the prospects of a beneficial outcome. Various coping options include altering the situation, accepting it, seeking more information, or holding back from acting in an impulsive way. Primary and secondary appraisals converge to determine if the person–environment transaction is primarily *threatening* or *challenging* (O'Connor, Arnold, & Maurizio, 2010). *Reappraisal* results when a situation is relabeled a challenge or benign instead of a perceived threat.

Coping regulates stressful emotions (emotion-focused coping) and alters the person–environment relationship that is causing the distress (problem-focused coping). Both forms of coping occur in stressful encounters. The success of problem focused coping in large part may depend on the success of emotion-focused coping because heightened emotions are likely to interfere with cognitive activity necessary to manage effectively the stressors.

Problem-focused coping is likely to be dominant in encounters viewed as changeable, whereas *emotion-focused coping* often dominates in encounters viewed as unchangeable, with acceptance as the only recourse. Encounters involving threats to self-esteem are often the most difficult to resolve. These threats include the possibility of losing the affection of someone one cares about, losing self-respect or the respect of others, and appearing to be unethical or incompetent (Simpson, 2009).

Everyone experiences stress from time to time. Some people cope with stress more effectively and recover from stressful events more quickly than others recover. However, continued strain on the body from routine stress may lead to such diseases as heart disease, depression, obesity, or complicate other existing diseases. Of the many lifestyle events that affect the individual, none is more widespread than stress and stress-related conditions.

STRESS AND HEALTH

There are many ongoing unmet needs in providing care to individuals with stress-related problems. Stress can cause decreased life satisfaction, the development of mental disorders, the occurrence of stress-related illnesses (cardiovascular disease, gastrointestinal disorders, low back pain, headaches), and decreased immunologic functioning result from stress.

One of the major health problems in the world is cardiovascular disease. Long-term stress sensitizes arterioles to catecholamine, with even short-term stress responses causing overconstriction of the vessels and endothelial damage. Repetitive overconstriction may lead to hypertension, decreased myocardial perfusion, and arrhythmias (Epel, 2009).

Differential exposure to stress and negative life experiences—loneliness, poverty, low income, and subsequently, health and disease (Vimont, 2008)—can exact a toll and is a major contributor to socioeconomic health disparities (Lantz, House, Mero, & Williams, 2005). The lack of supportive relationships to deal with stresses can lead to psychological distress and depression.

Interestingly, there is some evidence that giving social support is more beneficial than receiving it. According to one study, individuals who reported giving support lived longer than those receiving support (Bacon, Milne, Shiekh, & Freeston, 2009). In other instances, the nature of interpersonal relationships may be detrimental to health. A meta-analysis of cohort studies showed a robust estimate of the positive effect of marriage on mortality that did not vary by gender, or between North America and Europe (Manzoli, Villari, Pirone, & Boccia, 2007). Both the absence of social relationships and the presence of social relationships serve as stressors that may have an impact on one's health. The quality of the relationship is the variant.

Psychoneuroimmunology examines the effects of social and psychological phenomena on the immune system as mediated by the nervous and endocrine systems. Both acute and chronic infections, as well as cancer, show an association with compromised immune functioning.

In a series of studies, male undergraduate college students with high heart-rate reactivity to stressors (mental arithmetic test with noise superimposed) were compared with low heart-rate reactors on neuroendocrine and immune responses to stressors. High reactors showed higher stress-related levels of plasma cortisol and increased natural killer (NK) cell lyses than did low reactors.

The finding that cortisol was elevated in high reactors is particularly interesting in view of the extensive literature linking cortisol with impaired functioning of the immune system. These findings suggest that individual variation in activation of the hypothalamic-pituitary-adrenocortical axis by brief psychologic stressors may explain why daily stressors have greater health consequences for some individuals than for others (Epel, 2009).

Results of a meta-analysis, conducted to evaluate evidence that psychological interventions affect the immune system, indicate only modest changes in the immune system. Research must address conceptual and methodological issues in order to determine if psychological interventions are effective in influencing changes in immune responses (Pace, Negi, Adame, Cole, Sivilli, Brown, et al., 2009). Clinical evidence suggests that central nervous system processes influence the immune system when psychological interventions are effective (Brydon, Walker, Wawrzyniak, Chart, & Stepto, 2009). A number of physiologic systems are highly responsive to life experiences and the psychological states that accompany them.

Further studies of varying human responses to stress are important as a basis for developing effective stress-management techniques, supporting healthy coping mechanisms, and restructuring faulty psychological defenses (Chrousos, 2008). Understanding the mechanisms that integrate our experiences into our biology relies on the emerging field of epigenetics.

Epigenetics, the study of developmental and environmental influences on the alteration of gene expression, is an attempt to describe how experiences such as stress, while not altering the DNA sequence, may modify DNA proteins, leading to enhanced or silenced expression of a specific gene. Twenty-one animal and human studies were reviewed that tested the relationship between psychological factors (stress, coping) and changes in DNA. The studies demonstrated causal relations between acute stress and DNA damage in animals and significant correlations between psychological factors and DNA changes in adults (Gridon, Russ, Tissarchondou, & Warner, 2006).

These findings, while limited, indicate that psychological factors may influence DNA integrity. The results are further evidence of the person–environment connection. The challenge is to determine whether stress management interventions can block stress-induced damage caused by environmental and experiential exposures, such as infections, toxins, and social interactions, and affect the genome throughout life (Nestler, 2012).

STRESS ACROSS THE LIFE SPAN

Children

Childhood is a critical period characterized by increased vulnerability to stressors. The prevalence of stress-related disorders in children appears to be increasing, although this increase may be due to changes in access to health care, resulting in more diagnoses, public perception, or changes in definitions of disorders. One positive finding in the final report of *Healthy People 2010* was that the proportion of children aged 4–17 years with mental problems who received care increased from 60% to 69% between 2000 and 2009 (Centers for Disease Control and Prevention, 2010, 2013).

Children experience stress and develop coping patterns early in life that often become lifelong coping patterns. Self-esteem, personality characteristics (temperament), gender, social support, parental child-rearing patterns, previous stressful experiences, and illness are factors related to stress in children. Stressors frequently identified by children include (1) feeling sick, (2) having nothing to do, (3) being alone, (4) family fighting, (5) not having enough money to spend, (6) being pressured to get good grades, and (7) feeling left out of the group (Ryan-Wanger, Sharrer, & Campbell, 2005; Ryan-Wenger, Wilson (Sharrer), & Broussard, 2013).

Problems caused by prolonged stress test children's stress-coping processes. Children with chronic illnesses, compared with well children, are less confident of their ability to handle problems and more often use ineffective coping skills (Walker, Smith, Garber, & Claar, 2007). Environmental and social stressors also place children at high risk and include the following:

- Personal safety concerns
- Community violence
- Prolonged poverty
- Increased availability of drugs
- Homelessness

The majority of children, regardless of their personal and environmental stressors, have a personal resiliency that enables them to overcome adversity and function well in spite of major stressors. *Family protective factors,* such as warm, close, supportive relationships among family members, and *environmental protective factors,* such as positive peer and adult role models, mediate the relationship between risk factors and healthy coping.

Personal resilience factors within children include (1) strong cognitive abilities and problem-solving skills, (2) easy temperament in infancy and adaptability in childhood, and (3) positive self-image. One or more of these factors, along with inclusion of family and environmental protective factors, contributes to the development of resilience in childhood (Ryan-Wenger, Wilson (Sharrer), & Broussard, 2013).

However, children who are more affected by stressful situations than are others can benefit from constructive coping techniques to enhance their well-being and health (Skybo & Buck, 2007). Untreated chronic stress in children may lead to mental health issues as well as chronic diseases. Recognizing the need to incorporate coping strategies into family, community, and school interventions is critical to ensure the physical and mental health of children at risk. See Chapter 4 for discussion of instruments to measure acute and chronic stress in children.

Adolescents

Adolescents experience many stressful situations. The most common stressors during the adolescent years are changes related to growth and development; family-related issues, such as quarrels and benign neglect; peer stressors, such as relationships across early and mid-adolescence; and academic concerns in high school-age youths.

Higher stress in early adolescence is associated with a range of risk-taking behaviors such as smoking, alcohol use, and sexual sensation experiences. Warning signs of stress-related disorders may be subtle and require careful observation on behalf of parents, friends, and health professionals. Symptoms include social withdrawal, anger, loss of appetite, changes in sleep patterns, persistent irritability, and changes in school performance.

Nurses can help adolescents avoid substance abuse and other risky behaviors by assisting them in learning effective stress-coping processes to apply across a variety of life circumstances. These processes include the following:

- Behavioral coping (information gathering)
- Decision making (problem solving)
- Cognitive coping (minimizing distress, focusing on the positive)
- Adult social support (talking with an adult)
- Relaxation (Hampel & Petermann, 2006)

See *Stress, Coping, and Adolescent Health* (Garcia & Pintor, 2013) and Chapter 4 for discussions of instruments for assessing adolescent coping skills.

Young and Middle-Age Adults

How an individual copes with stress does not change from childhood to adolescence to adulthood. Individuals use the same types of coping skills to manage the stressors identified with each developmental stage. However, as individuals age, they usually increase their use of problem-solving coping, and decrease the use of avoidance coping as compared with the preteen and adolescence years (Amirkhan & Auyeung, 2007).

Stress in America reported that young adults (18–33 years old) showed the highest levels of stress of any age group, with this age group reporting more diagnoses of anxiety disorders than other groups. They also reported that they frequently did not have the skills to deal with and manage their stress.

The stresses often experienced in young and middle age adulthood relate to establishing oneself in a productive career (job stability, income), nourishing long-term relationships in a dyadic unit, childbearing, and child rearing. Young adults desire to create a sense of self-identity as an independent, yet interdependent adult (American Psychological Association, 2012).

Adults who seek mental health care in primary care settings have fewer visits per year than do adults seen by specialists. Primary care is likely the only mental health care many clients receive, and currently few primary care providers routinely screen and treat stress-related problems and mental health disorders. The final report of *Healthy People 2010* did show that the objective to increase the number of primary care facilities providing treatment and/or referral for mental illness exceeded its goal by moving from a baseline of 62% to 74% (Centers for Disease Control and Prevention, 2010, 2013). However, many mental illnesses still go undiagnosed and/or untreated in primary care settings

Two new objectives added to the *Healthy People 2020* mental health area seek to reduce the proportion of persons who experience a major depressive episode and to increase depression screening by primary care providers. Nurses in primary care settings including schools, clinics, and work sites have a responsibility to promote and conduct early screening and intervention for mental illness and stress-related problems including depression (Centers for Disease Control and Prevention, 2010). See Chapter 4 for tools for assessing a person's vulnerability to stress and information on the Patient Health Questionnaire-2 (FPQ-2), a two-item scale to screen for depression in primary care.

Family responses to stressors occur in two stages: (1) adjustment during minor events that do not require major family changes, and (2) adaptation during major crisis events to restore balance and harmony in the family. This model can assist nurses in primary care settings in conceptualizing stressors and coping capabilities of families as a basis for assessment and intervention (McLain & Cashiff, 2008) and in understanding adjustment of mothers of children.

Constrained finances or arguments between spouses about how to spend limited income may markedly increase tension in the home. Single parents are particularly vulnerable to stress, as they may lack social support and also find that job demands leave them little time for parenting responsibilities. In the absence of authoritative parenting, children may get into difficulties that further stretch limited psychological resources of parents. Stress-management programs that address how to change the work and home environments to minimize stress and develop effective coping strategies best meet the needs of young and middle-age adults.

Older Adults

Although some sources of stress may abate in older adulthood, other stressors, particularly those resulting from loss, are more prevalent. The elderly are particularly vulnerable to negative life events such as the death of a spouse, death of a close family member, personal injury or illness, change in one's financial status, caregiving responsibilities, and retirement. Hassles of daily living may increase as a result of diminished sensory acuity, decreased dexterity and strength, and loss of flexibility. Cumulative stress along with depression can compromise immune function, leaving the elderly more vulnerable to acute and chronic infections and chronic disease (Trouillet, Gana, Lourel, & Fort, 2009).

In old age, we begin to see the increased morbidity and mortality associated with years of daily hassles and cumulative major life events, particularly when coping strategies have been ineffective. Systemic effects on the cardiovascular, gastrointestinal, neurologic, endocrine, and immune systems are increasingly apparent (Charmandari, Tsigos, & Chrousos, 2005). The elderly need to learn to use more productive coping strategies to maintain their health as resistance to disease decreases.

However, there is also evidence that the ability to manage stress seems to improve with age. Compared to younger age groups, older adults are more likely to be flexible and willing to compromise and adjust their expectations. They also report more willingness to express their feelings (American Psychological Association, 2012). Nurses, who are knowledgeable about the aging process and the capabilities of older adults, can help them manage the stressors they encounter more effectively and efficiently, which contributes to a healthier and more satisfying life for the elderly.

WORKPLACE STRESS

A major source of stress, and according to some, the greatest source of stress, is that created by the workplace. Low-to-moderate levels of stress in the workplace can generate positive performance; however, moderate-to-high stress levels result in negative performance. In addition to health-damaging effects of stress and mental illnesses, workplace stress leads to disability, absenteeism, and decreased productivity, all of which are very costly for businesses and industry (Milani & Lavie, 2007). Sources of work stress include the following:

- Lack of control over job environment or production demands
- Being "caught in the middle" between supervisors and customers
- Being underprepared for the job
- Lack of clarity about job expectations
- Unexpected transfers across departments or company locations

- Feeling trapped in a particular job
- Lack of positive relationships with coworkers

Stress often causes additional deterioration in performance and can further escalate already existing causes of stress and tension (Couser, 2008).

To help individuals manage stress and avoid its costly, health-impairing effects, it is essential to have incentives to encourage businesses and health care organizations to offer workplace programs. Changes in the work environment itself can reduce the incidence of stressful events. For example, instituting policies that provide flextime, job sharing, or child-care benefits or facilities can ease the stress on parents who must both maintain a job and also care for young children.

Low levels of stress at work can aid in protecting workers from job-related hazards, and ways to reduce stress include redesigning work assignments, creating pleasant workstations, instituting quality circles, and implementing participatory management styles. Job-related stresses are avoidable by becoming more aware of persons or experiences that create personal stress and minimizing contact to the extent possible.

Support at home can buffer work-related stressors, or the existence of additional stressors at home together with those at work may have a cumulative effect. Many employers are increasingly offering work-site stress-management programs. An analysis of client-centered stress management interventions in the workplace is available at the Centre for Stress Management.

Interventions that focus on the organization and the individual worker produce more favorable outcomes than do interventions that focus on one entity, suggesting that the best outcomes for reduction of stress in the workplace occur when a comprehensive framework guides the chosen interventions (Lamontagne, Keegel, Louie, Ostry, & Landsbergis, 2007).

APPROACHES TO STRESS MANAGEMENT

A holistic approach that integrates the mind and body has long characterized nursing; nurses understand the importance of the relationship between stress and health and stress and illness as a basis for assessment and nursing care. Nurses are in key positions to identify individuals and families that are not effectively coping. Through observation, active listening, and supportive decision making, nurses can help clients identify stressors and select strategies to manage stress in their lives. Assessment findings can direct the nurse to structure appropriate interventions and/or make referrals to assist clients in managing stressors *before* they exert health-damaging effects.

Each selected approach to stress management must be adapted to the culture of the individual and/or family because the success of the approach may well depend on its compatibility with cultural views and beliefs. For example, different cultures may or may not support the use of medications in treating stress-related problems. Selecting a stress management strategy requires the same caution; for example, people from Arabic-speaking countries generally support cognitive behavioral therapy because of its compatibility with their basic values and beliefs; what one does will have an impact in this life and the after-life (Elmasri, 2011). An important first step for the nurse to take in selecting a stress management approach is to investigate the individual and family's cultural background. (See Chapter 12 for further discussion about culturally appropriate interventions.)

Gordon describes a number of nursing diagnoses specific to problems in stress management (defensive coping, ineffective family coping, stress overload) in the functional health pattern category of Coping-Stress Tolerance Pattern. The first steps to managing stress are assessing the level of existing stress and the sources of stress (see Chapter 4) and then determining the appropriate interventions. The nurse must examine the effectiveness and safety of an intervention prior to using it in practice. Interventions for stress management should aim to achieve the following:

- Minimize the frequency of stress-inducing situations
- Increase resistance to stress (Gordon, 2009)

Interventions to Minimize the Frequency of Stress-Inducing Situations

Adaptation to externally imposed change is continuous. Nurses can assist clients in avoiding stressful situations by (1) changing their environment, (2) avoiding excessive change, (3) time control, and (4) time management.

CHANGING THE ENVIRONMENT.   In general, changing the environment to decrease the incidence of stressors is the "first line of defense." Widely held values and beliefs shape the environment in any society, and while changing the environment is the most proactive approach to minimizing the frequency of stress-inducing situations, it may be the most difficult.

Major changes in societal beliefs, values, and actions may be necessary if vulnerable populations are to experience less stress. Sexism, racism, and ageism create stress for selected groups, because of the devaluation of their status and lack of acknowledgment of their contributions to society. Discrimination directed at any group may result in decreased educational and employment opportunities, poverty, and personal devaluation. Racial disparities in disease rates are rooted in differences between races in exposure or vulnerability to pathogenic factors in the physical, social, economic, and cultural environments. Perceived discrimination is a stressor that does not vary based on the minority person's social status (Brondolo, Brady, & Pencille, 2009).

If a job change is required to decrease stress, make sure that the stress phenomena in the current job setting are not an inherent part of the new employment setting. Protective factors in the broader environment that can further decrease stress include (1) family characterized by warmth and cohesion, (2) cultural events and customs that promote identity, (3) supportive relationships with others outside the family, and (4) involvement in community structures such as churches and neighborhood organizations that promote competence and support.

When changing the environment is *not* possible, individual and family coping resources must come into play to reinterpret stress as a challenge and increase resilience against it. Every intervention or strategy to manage stress should be adapted to the individual and/or family culture.

AVOIDING EXCESSIVE CHANGE.   During periods of significant life change and resulting negative tension states, any additional unnecessary changes should be avoided. For example, if a family is experiencing the illness of one of its family members and a subsequent job loss, this may not be the time to consider geographic relocation, pregnancy, or any other change in lifestyle. Negative tension created by multiple changes is synergistic. Each time a distressing change occurs, the potency of previous change for upsetting stability is increased. Deliberately postponing changes that result in negative tension can help clients constructively manage unavoidable change, and postponement prevents the need for multiple adjustments at one point in time.

During periods of high or moderate stress, any changes in lifestyle should be self-initiated and should *challenge,* rather than *threaten,* the client. Increasing positive sources of tension that promote growth and self-actualization can offset the deleterious effects of negative tension. For example, learning to play tennis, to swim, or to dance may provide a distracting challenge to counterbalance potentially debilitating stress.

TIME CONTROL.   Time control is a technique to set aside specific time to adapt to various stressors. This period may be daily, weekly, or monthly and offer clients time to focus on a specific change and develop strategies for adjustment. Important goals or concerns require focus and critical actions. Encourage individuals to focus on managing time more effectively to prevent the stress that time shortages produce. This strategy reduces a sense of urgency, a high level of anxiety, and feelings of frustration and failure.

TIME MANAGEMENT.   The time management approach to stress management focuses on re-organizing one's time to accomplish those goals most important in life *within the time available*. Lack of time is a frequent reason for not participating in health-promoting activities, so teaching time management to clients contributes to their health and fitness. Time-pressured, high-anxiety clients are particularly in need of time-management skills.

A framework for time management is identifying and prioritizing goals. When clients identify time wasted on activities unrelated to personal goals, they can restructure how they spend their time. A frequent source of stress is overcommitment to others or unrealistic expectations of oneself. Time overload may be avoided by learning to say "no" to demands of others that are unrealistic or of low personal or family priority. *Overload* results in frustration and loss of satisfaction from the work accomplished because one seldom expends one's best efforts under strain and pressure.

An important approach to time management is to reduce a task into smaller parts. A task may appear overwhelming; however, accomplishment becomes feasible if the task is broken down into smaller segments. An example may be to learn several effective conditioning exercises before learning a complete conditioning routine, or developing skill with a conditioning routine before beginning a walk-jog activity. Breaking the routine down into component parts allows mastery and feelings of competence.

Individuals can avoid feelings of overload by delegating responsibilities to others and enlisting their assistance. Making use of *others'* skills provides freedom from the expectation of having to be "all things to all people." Another important aspect of time management is to reduce the perception of time pressure and urgency. Not all perceptions of time urgency are warranted; some are needlessly self-imposed. The client should differentiate between time urgencies that are valid and others that are needlessly created. One may avoid time urgencies by minimizing procrastination, as leaving tasks until the last minute often results in needless pressure and stress (Davis & Rob, 2008).

Interventions to Increase Resistance to Stress

Both physical and psychological conditioning increases resistance to stress. Physical conditioning for stress resistance focuses on *healthy behaviors,* such as exercise and good nutrition. Psychological conditioning focuses on (1) enhancing self-esteem, (2) enhancing self-efficacy, (3) increasing assertiveness, (4) setting realistic goals, and (5) building coping resources such as relaxation.

PROMOTING HEALTHY BEHAVIORS.   Exercise and eating a healthy and balanced diet are two positive stress management practices. Refer to Chapter 6, Physical Activity and Health Promotion, and Chapter 7, Nutrition in Health Promotion, for detailed discussions on exercise and nutrition. Physical activity positively relates to good mental health. In general, people who exercise regularly report feelings of well-being, whereas people who are inactive are twice as likely to be depressed. Although increased fatigue, anxiety, and decreased vigor can occur with over-training, in general, regular physical exercise contributes to good mental health (Ament & Verkerke, 2009). Exercise improves a person's mental and physical state and increases one's ability to combat stress.

A healthy and balanced diet contributes to good health and is especially important during periods of stress. Items to avoid during stressful periods include caffeine, alcohol, and tobacco. Overeating may provide immediate satisfaction, but it is only temporary. For others, chronic stress may depress the appetite, resulting in weight loss over time. Poor nutrition, regardless of the underlying cause, reduces one's ability to manage stress and maintain health.

ENHANCING SELF-ESTEEM.   Self-esteem is the value attributed to self or how one feels about oneself. A person's concept of his or her desirable and undesirable attributes, strengths and weaknesses, achievements, and success contributes to his or her self-esteem. Although self-esteem develops over time, studies have shown that the level of self-esteem may be changed.

One approach is positive verbalization. In this technique, clients identify positive aspects of self or personal characteristics that they value highly. They should also ask significant others to comment on their positive attributes. Each characteristic, one per day, is written on a 3 × 5 index card, which is placed in a conspicuous location and read several times a day. This technique helps clients to spend more time thinking about their positive attributes, and it decreases the amount of time spent in self-devaluation. Increased self-awareness of positive characteristics and their presence in conscious thought result in behavior that reflects positive attributes and generates more positive responses from significant others.

ENHANCING SELF-EFFICACY.   Mastery experiences help create a sense of competence to perform effectively and overcome obstacles, such as experiencing successful performance of a particular, valued behavior that provides positive messages regarding personal skills and abilities. Counseling clients to undertake tasks that are challenging, but from which they experience success rather than failure, can build a sense of competence. Self-beliefs about personal competency have wide-ranging ramifications affecting level of motivation, affect, thought, and action. Competence strengthens if an individual approaches situations with assurance and makes good use of the skills that they have. *Perceiving* oneself to be competent predicts performance better than does actual ability.

Persons with high levels of competency mentally rehearse *success* rather than *failures* at a task, set high goals, make a firm commitment to attain them, perceive more control over personal threats, and are less anxious in the face of day-to-day challenges. Highly competent persons also tend to be more assertive in accessing the support they need to optimize their chances of success (Folkman, 2009).

INCREASING ASSERTIVENESS.   Substituting positive, assertive behaviors for negative, passive ones increases one's personal capacity for psychological resistance to stress. *Assertiveness* is the appropriate expression of oneself and one's thoughts and feelings and results in greater personal satisfaction in living. Assertiveness is more constructive than aggression and is more effective than aggression in managing problems. Assertiveness enables individuals to share their perceptions and feelings with others in a way that facilitates rather than inhibits personal or group productivity. Nurses should encourage clients to use the following strategies to become more assertive:

- Make a deliberate effort to greet others and call them by name.
- Maintain eye contact during conversations.
- Comment on the positive characteristics of others.
- Initiate conversation.
- Express opinions.
- Express feelings.
- Disagree with others when holding opposing viewpoints.
- Take initiative to engage in a new behavior or learn a new activity.

Although it is possible for clients to become more assertive through the use of simple techniques, *very* passive and reserved clients might well benefit from more comprehensive assertiveness training provided by a competent instructor or counselor. The nurse may need to assist clients in locating such resources for personal development.

SETTING REALISTIC GOALS.   Clients must set realistic goals, including long- and short-term ones, to stay on course. Long-term goals set the direction for change, and short-term goals allow for immediate successes. Clients should set goals that can be attained within a reasonable period, and if the goals are met, it could reinforce the client's desire to continue to set health-promoting goals. Another useful rule is to plan to change only one behavior at a time.

The client can achieve desired outcomes through several approaches. As a result, lack of success in initial attempts to reach goals becomes much less ominous, because of the probability of success in achieving alternative goals that bring similar rewards or reinforcement. Remember, there are usually several ways to get to the same outcome.

BUILDING COPING RESOURCES.   Stress results when there is an *imbalance* between (1) appraised demands, and (2) appraised coping capabilities. Nurses should direct more attention to the *resource* side of the equation rather than the *demand* side. Coping resources are more predictive of reactions to stressors than the actual demands. General coping resources that have been identified as enhancing stress resistance include the following:

- *Self-disclosure:* Predisposition to share one's feelings, troubles, thoughts, and opinions with others.
- *Self-directedness:* Degree to which a person respects his or her own judgment for decision making.
- *Confidence:* Ability to gain mastery over one's environment and to control one's emotions in the interest of reaching personal goals.
- *Acceptance:* Degree to which persons accept their shortcomings and imperfections and maintain a positive and tolerant attitude toward others.
- *Social support:* Availability and use of a network of caring others.
- *Financial freedom:* Extent to which persons are free of financial constraints on their lifestyles.
- *Physical health:* Overall health condition, including absence of chronic disease and disabilities.

- *Physical fitness:* Conditioning resulting from personal exercise practices.
- *Stress monitoring:* Awareness of tension buildup and situations that are likely to prove stressful.
- *Tension control:* Ability to lower arousal through relaxation and thought control.
- *Structuring:* Ability to organize and manage resources such as time and energy.
- *Problem solving:* Ability to resolve personal problems.

After assessing the extent to which the various coping resources are present, the nurse assists the client in maximizing existing strengths and in developing additional resistance resources.

COMPLEMENTARY THERAPIES TO MANAGE STRESS

More than two thirds of the world's population uses complementary and alternative medicine (CAM), and 53 percent of Americans report use of CAM at some point in their lives. Among those who use CAM, only 58 percent discuss their use with their health care provider. Older Americans report higher use of complementary and alternative medicine than do other age groups (National Center for Complementary and Alternative Medicine, 2011).

Complementary therapies are diverse medical and health care interventions, practices, and products that are used alone, or with conventional medicine, to manage stress and stress-related illnesses. Complementary therapies used to manage stress include (1) self-regulation techniques such as mindfulness, (2) progressive muscle relaxation, (3) imagery, (4) acupuncture, (5) yoga, and (6) self-hypnosis. Tai Chi, herbal products, and dietary supplements also are used by many individuals to manage stress-related problems.

The goal of self-regulation techniques is to achieve a balance of physical, emotional, and spiritual factors in one's life. Mindfulness-based stress reduction (MBSR), progressive relaxation without tension, relaxation through imagery, and Breathe Away Stress in 8 Steps are interventions the nurse can use to assist clients in managing stress and stress-related problems.

Mindfulness-Based Stress Reduction (MBSR)

John Kabat-Zinn developed Mindfulness-Based Stress Reduction (MBSR) at the Massachusetts School of Medicine in 1979. MBSR is based on an early Buddhist teaching of being aware of everything in the present moment, without judgment (Kabat-Zinn, 2011). Mindfulness is about gaining awareness of your body, actions, feelings, and surroundings, deliberately giving your full attention to everything you are involved in from one moment to the next.

A meta-analysis of published and unpublished health-related studies using MBSR was conducted to determine the effectiveness of the intervention. Of the 60 research studies identified, only 20 met the criteria for inclusion in the meta-analysis. According to the meta-analysis, MBSR helped participants cope with a wide range of clinical and nonclinical problems (Grossman, Neimann, Schmidt, & Walach, 2004). A subsequent review substantiates the beneficial results for physical and mental health (Irving, Dobkin, & Park, 2009).

A systematic review of the effects of MBSR on sleep disturbances showed positive effects on sleep quality and duration, indicating a decrease in sleep-interfering cognitive processes (Winbush, Gross, & Kreitzer, 2007). Mindfulness training for older people with anxiety and depression resulted in very positive results, which were maintained a year later (Smith, 2006). Evidence supports the use of MBSR for decreasing mood disturbance and stress symptoms in people of all ages and diagnoses (Carmody, Reed, Kristeller, & Merriam, 2008; Mullaney, 2013; Smith, 2006; Winbush, Gross, & Kreitzer, 2007).

MBSR is a nonreligious, systematic procedure to develop enhanced awareness of moment-to-moment experiences of perceptual processes. Elements of the eight-week (2.5 hours per week) program include an emphasis on a non-goal orientation and a variety of meditation techniques, including body scan meditation, sitting and walking meditation, and Hatha yoga (Kabat-Zinn, 2011). Essential program components are daily practice and home study.

One way to experience an MBSR exercise is to try to become *mindful* while walking. Be aware of the inner chatter of the mind. Listen for the sound of your foot touching the ground, and feel the sensation while just being aware of what you are doing. Being mindful is active yet passive, as it can be done anytime or anywhere by simply focusing on what is happening in the present moment.

Progressive Relaxation without Tension

Clients may be taught how to relax without first tensing muscles. Relaxation through counting down is a frequently used strategy. The major advantage of this technique is that tension is no longer required. This is particularly important when elevations in blood pressure caused by prolonged or extensive muscle tensing are contraindicated. Deep relaxation without tension is the goal. Phrases that might be repeated to facilitate relaxation include the following:

- "I feel quiet."
- "I am beginning to feel quite relaxed."
- "My feet feel heavy and relaxed."
- "My ankles, my knees, and my hips feel heavy."
- "My hands, my arms, and my shoulders feel heavy, relaxed, and comfortable."
- "My neck, my jaw, and my forehead feel relaxed. They feel comfortable and smooth."
- "I am quite relaxed."
- "My mind is quiet."
- "My thoughts are turned inward, and I am at ease."
- "I can visualize and experience myself relaxed, comfortable, and still."

These phrases were suggested as a result of work in biofeedback at the Menninger Foundation. Such phrases result in physiologic imagery that decreases both sympathetic nervous system activity and tension in voluntary muscles.

Relaxation through the countdown procedure initially focuses on each muscle group used previously. The client is encouraged to relax each muscle group progressively as the count proceeds from 10 down to 1. When the client becomes skilled with this procedure, total body countdown is used, relaxing the entire body while silently counting down from 10 to 1. This procedure is particularly useful when facing stressful social situations. In 2–3 minutes, the skilled client can achieve total body relaxation while in a sitting position with eyes open and focused on a specific object. Mini-relaxation sessions several times throughout the day promote generalization of relaxation training to everyday life.

Relaxation through Imagery

Guided imagery is a stress-reduction intervention in which the interrelationship of the body and mind is used to influence physiological responses. This cognitive process uses the imagination to bring about positive mind/body responses and uses many senses, including sight, smell, taste,

and touch. The benefits of imagery include its influence on physiological responses of the autonomic nervous system that result in stress reduction. Research supports imagery as an effective
intervention for pain management and depressive disorders, and for changing health behaviors
(Apostolo & Kolcaba, 2009; Haase, Schwenk, Hermann, & Muller, 2005; Weydert, Shapiro, Acra,
Monheim, Chambers, & Ball, 2006). However, additional research is required to determine its
association with neuro-immunomodulatory effects (Telles Nunes, Rodriquez, Hoffman, Luz,
Filho, Muller, et al., 2007). Imagery plus progressive muscle relaxation is thought to be more
effective than imagery alone (Monone, Greco, & Weiner, 2008). See *Complementary Alternative
Therapies in Nursing* (Snyder & Lindquist, 2010) for further information and precautions in the
use of guided imagery.

Using imagery to relax requires passive concentration on pleasant scenes or experiences
from the past. Recalling the warmth of the sun, the feeling of warm sand, the sensations of a
gentle breeze, the vision of palm trees swaying, or the sounds of ocean waves may be comfortable
and pleasant for clients. Clients may vary in scenes or images that result in actual changes in
muscle tension. For some clients, visualizing specific colors, shapes, or patterns is as effective as
visualizing landscapes or scenes. If clients initially have difficulty in using imagery or visualiza-
tion for relaxation, the nurse may use one of the following techniques:

- Have the client, with eyes closed, visualize a particular room of his or her house (living
  room, bedroom, kitchen), focusing on colors, shapes, and specific objects. The client's
  mind should wander about the room, describing verbally what is seen in as much detail
  as possible.
- Have the client focus on a particular piece of clothing that is a personal favorite. The client
  should describe the color, texture, design, and trim on an article of clothing, and whether it
  feels soft, loose, fitted, light, or warm.

As individuals become more vivid in descriptions of concrete objects, their ability to
use less concrete imagery for purposes of relaxation will increase. Imagery is a highly useful
relaxation technique in many settings in which muscle tension or biofeedback equipment
would be obtrusive.

Breathe Away Stress in 8 Steps

Research shows that using relaxation strategies for as little as 10 20 minutes per day pays off in
many ways. Many stress-related responses are reduced or turned off when you move into the
relaxation response.

Dr. Herbert Benson, Harvard Medical School, developed this eight-step technique to
achieve a relaxed mental state. Relaxation is a skill that one learns, and it improves with practice.
To prepare for the relaxation activity you must maintain a sustained focus for your mind and
disregard everyday thoughts. Nurses will find this relaxation strategy beneficial for themselves as
well as for their clients. Nurses who take care of themselves are in a better position to be a role
model and advocate for their clients. This eight-step program is as follows:

1. Select a word or short phase or a group of words.
2. Find a private place where you will not be disturbed and sit in a comfortable position.
3. Close your eyes and begin to relax your muscles, beginning with the feet, and gradually
   moving up the body.
4. Breathe slowly and naturally. As you exhale say your selected word or phrase silently to yourself. You may say one word on inhalation and a different one on exhalation, if you choose.

5. When random thoughts invade your consciousness, acknowledge them and return to your breathing.
6. Continue focused breathing for 10–20 minutes. You may check the time but do not use an alarm.
7. When you are done, open your eyes, sit quietly, and do not stand up for at least one minute.
8. Practice this technique twice a day before breakfast and dinner. (*Harvard Men's Health Watch*, 2012)

The opportunity to help clients manage stress and pain through science-based interventions is well within the nurse's scope of practice. However, consultation with and/or referral to other professionals who specialize in complementary therapies is an opportunity for nurses to develop collaborative interdisciplinary relationships and referral networks.

Use of Medications

The use of prescription and over-the-counter medications to treat stress and stress overload is increasing rapidly. Due to the desire to respond quickly to stress-related problems, medications seem to be an easy solution. Drugs may *appear* to be an easy escape from stress, but their relief is usually temporary and can result in adverse side effects and dependency. The interventions of choice are stress management strategies, both psychological and physical. Drugs may be useful temporarily in conjunction with these strategies, but drug therapy alone is *not* likely to be successful in the long term.

CONSIDERATIONS FOR PRACTICE IN STRESS MANAGEMENT

Individuals who experience the same stressors often respond differently. Stress-related illnesses are very common and require appropriate interventions, or referrals to help the client manage stress before there are negative outcomes. The promotion and conduct of early screenings and developmentally specific interventions are necessary because children, adolescents, young adults, and older adults develop and use different coping strategies. Awareness of these differences ensures that the nurse intervenes at the appropriate time and with the appropriate strategy to achieve stress reduction. Although the stress management interventions discussed in this chapter are within the nurse's scope of practice, he or she should gain expertise in the use of them by working with an experienced provider and through study and practice. The rapidly growing field of stress research mandates that each practitioner stay current on the latest evidence-based practices.

OPPORTUNITIES FOR RESEARCH ON STRESS MANAGEMENT

Major advances in understanding the effects of stressors on the neuroendocrine and immune systems offer new possibilities for managing the brain–body interface in order to promote health. However, more research is needed to test stress-reducing interventions and their effect on these systems. The profile of stressors most likely to occur at different developmental stages and the best way to match stressors with targeted coping processes are priority research goals. A challenge is to discover how to build coping resources, resilience, and personal competence in the early childhood years so that patterns of successful adaptation manifest themselves throughout adolescence and adulthood.

Interventions that decrease environmental and family stressors for vulnerable populations also are priorities. Human tolerance for stress is finite, as people can manage only so much stress. The efforts of scientists from multiple disciplines are needed to learn more about the phenomenon of stress and its management.

Summary

This chapter presents a number of different approaches for assisting individuals and families in managing stress. Some of the suggested interventions are relatively unstructured, whereas others are more defined and complex. The client and the nurse should make collaborative decisions about the most appropriate interventions to use, taking into account the client's mental and physical health status. These decisions should also be based on the sources of stress experienced by the client and his or her general patterns of response to stressful events. The nurse must be aware of his or her own comfort level and expertise with stress-reducing interventions and refer clients to other health care providers when appropriate.

Learning Activities

1. Discuss the management of stress in children, young and middle adults, and the elderly.
2. Select one intervention to manage stress and develop a modified protocol for a client of a specific age.
3. Practice mindful walking, and describe your feelings, experiences, and sensations.
4. Practice the progressive relaxation without tension and Breathe Away Stress in 8 Steps techniques, using some of the suggested phrases until you feel comfortable saying them, and you identify a difference in your relaxation state.

References

Ament, W., & Verkerke, G. (2009). Exercise and fatigue. *Sports Medicine, 39*(5), 389–422.

American Psychological Association. (2012). *Stress in America*. Washington, DC: American Psychological Association.

Amirkhan, J., & Auyeung, B. (2007). Coping with stress across the lifespan: Absolute vs. relative changes in strategy. *Journal of Applied Developmental Psychology, 28*(4), 298–317.

Apostolo, J. L., & Kolcaba, K. (2009). The effects of guided imagery on comfort, depression, anxiety, and stress of psychiatric inpatients with depressive disorders. *Archives of Psychiatric Nursing, 23*(6), 402–411.

Bacon, E., Milne, D., Shiekh. A., & Freeston, M. (2009). Positive experiences in caregivers: An exploratory case series. *Behavioral and Cognitive Psychotherapy, 37*(1), 95–114.

Brondolo, E., Brady, V., & Pencille, M. (2009). Coping with racism: A selective review of the literature and a theoretic and methodology critique. *Journal of Behavioral Medicine, 32*(1), 64–88.

Brydon, L., Walker, C., Wawrzyniak, A., Chart, H., & Stepto, A. (2009). Dispositional optimism and stress-induced changes in immunity and negative mood. *Brain, Behavior, and Immunity, 23*(6), 810–816.

Carmody, J., Reed, G., Kristeller, J., & Merriam, P. (2008). Mindfulness, spirituality, and health-related symptoms. *Journal of Psychosomatic Research, 64*(4), 393–403.

Centers for Disease Control and Prevention. (2010). *Healthy People 2020*. Retrieved from: http://www.cdc.gov/ndhs/healthypeople2020

Centers for Disease Control and Prevention. (2013). *Final Report Healthy People 2010*. Retrieved from CDC: http://www.cdc.gov/nchs/data/hpdata2010

Charmandari, E., Tsigos, C., & Chrousos, G. (2005). Endocrinology of the stress response. *Annual Review of Psysiology, 67*, 259–284.

Chrousos, G. P. (2008). Stress and disorders of the stress system. *Nature Review Endocrinology, 5*(7), 374–381.

Couser, G. P. (2008). Challenges and opportunities for preventing depression in the workplace: A review of the evidence supporting workplace factors and interventions. *Journal of Occupational and Environmental Medicine, 50*(4), 411–427.

Danese, A., & McEwen, B. (2012). Adverse childhood experiences, allostasis, allostatic load, and age-related diseases. *Physiology & Behavior, 106*(1), 29–39.

Davis, M., & Rob, E. (2008). *The relaxation and stress reduction workbook* (6th ed.). Oakland, CA: New Harbinger Publications.

Elmasri, M. (2011). Mental health beyond the crises. *Bulletin of the World Health Organization, 89*(5), 326–327.

Epel, E. S. (2009). Psychological and metabolic stress: A recipe for accelerated cellular aging? *Hormones, 6*(1), 7–22.

Folkman, S. (2009). Questions, answers, and next steps in stress and coping research. *European Psychologist, 14*, 72–77.

Garcia, C., & Pintor, J. (2013). Stress, coping, and adolescent health. In V. Rice, *Stress, Coping, and Health* (2nd ed., pp. 254–309). Los Angeles, CA: Sage Publications.

Gersten, O. (2008). The path traveled and the path ahead for the allostatic framework: A rejoinder on the framework's importance and the need for further work related to theory, data, and measurement. *Social Science & Medicine, 66*, 531–535.

Gordon, M. (2009). *Manual of nursing diagnosis: Including all diagnostic categories approved by the North American Nursing Diagnosis Association* (12th ed.). St. Louis, MO: Mosby.

Gridon, T., Russ, K., Tissarchondou, H., & Warner, J. (2006). The relation between psychological factors and DNA-damage: A critical review. *Biological Psychology, 72*, 291–304.

Grossman, P., Neimann, L., Schmidt, S., & Walach, H. (2004). Mindfulness-based stress reduction and health benefits: A meta-analysis. *Journal of Psychosomatic Research, 57*(1), 35–43.

Haase, O., Schwenk, W., Hermann, C., & Muller, J. M. (2005). Guided imagery and relaxation in conventional colorectal resections: A randomized, controlled, partially blinded trial. *Diseases of the Colon & Rectum, 48*(10), 1955–1963.

Hampel, P., & Petermann, F. (2006). Preceived stress, coping, and adjustment in adolescents. *Journal of Adolescent Health, 38*(4), 409–415.

Harvard Men's Health Watch. (2012). Retrieved from Harvard Health Publications: http://www.health.harvard.edu

Hogan, M. F., Sederer, L. I., Smith, T. E., & Nossel, I. R. (2010). Making room for mental health in the medical home. *Preventing Chronic Disease, 7*(6), 1–5.

Irving, J., Dobkin, P. L., & Park, J. (2009). Cultivating mindfulness in health care professionals: A review of empirical studies of mindfulness-based stress reduction (MBSR). *Complementary Therapies in Clinical Practice, 15*, 61–66.

Kabat-Zinn, J. (2011). Some reflections on the origins of MBSR, skillful means, and the trouble with maps. *Contemporary Buddhism, 12*(1), 281–306.

Lamontagne, A., Keegel, T., Louie, A., Ostry, A., & Landsbergis, P. (2007). A systematic review of the job-stress intervention evaluation literature, 1990–2005. *International Journal of Occupational and Environmental Health, 13*(3), 268–280.

Lantz, P., House, J., Mero, R., & Williams, D. (2005). Stress, life events, and socioeconomic disparities in health: Results from the Americans' Changing Lives study. *Journal of Health and Social Behavior, 46*(3), 274–288.

Lazarus, R. S. (1999). *Stress and emotion: A new synthesis*. New York, NY: Springer.

Lazarus, R. S., & Folkman, S. (1984). *Stress, appraisal, and coping*. New York, NY: Springer.

Loucks, E. B., Juster, R. P., & Pruessner, J. C. (2008). Neuroendocrine biomarkers, allostatic load, and the challenges of measurement: A commentary on Gerstein. *Social Science & Medicine, 66*, 525–530.

Manzoli, L., Villari, P., Pirone, G., & Boccia, A. (2007). Marital status and mortality in the elderly: A systemic review and metanaylsis. *Social Science & Medicine, 64*(1), 77–94.

McEwen, B. S. (2007). Stress, homeostatis, rheostasis, allostatic and allostatic load. In G. F. (Ed.), *The Encyclopedia of Stress* (2nd ed., pp. 557–561). San Diego, CA: Academic Press.

McLain, R., & Cashiff, C. (2008). Family stress, family adaption and psychological well-being of elderly coronary artery bypass grafting patients. *Dimensions of Critical Care Nursing, 27*(3), 125–131.

Milani, R., & Lavie, C. (2007). *Stopping stress at its origins*. doi:10.1161/01.HYP.0000255016.24162.1f

Monone, N., Greco, C., & Weiner, D. (2008). Mindfulness meditation for the treatment of low back pain in older adults: A randomized controlled pilot study. *Pain, 134*, 310–319.

Mullaney, A. (2013). *Training*. Retrieved from http://trainingmag.com/content/mindfulness-and-training-take-breath

National Center for Complementary and Alternative Medicine. (2011). *Complementary and alternative medicine dialogue lacking between patients and providers*. Bethesda, MD: National Institutes of Health.

Nestler, E. J. (2012). Stress makes it molecular mark. *Nature, 490,* 171–172.

O'Connor, M., Arnold, J., & Maurizio, A. (2010). The prospect of negotiating: Stress, cognitive appraisal and performance. *Journal of Experimental Psychology, 46*(5), 729–735.

Pace, T. W., Negi, L. T., Adame, D. D., Cole, S., Sivilli, T., Brown, T., et al. (2009). Efffect of compassion mediation on neuroendocrine, innate immune and behavioral responses to psychosocial stress. *Psychoneuroendocrinology, 34*(1), 87–98.

Ryan-Wanger, N., Sharrer, V., & Campbell, K. (2005). Changes in children's stressors over the past 30 years. *Pediatric Nursing, 31*(4), 282–291.

Ryan-Wenger, N., Wilson (Sharrer), V., & Broussard, A. (2013). Stress, coping, and health in children. In V. H. Rice (Ed.), *Handbook of stress, coping, and health: Implications of nursing research, theory, and practice* (pp. 226–253). Los Angeles, CA: Sage Publications.

Selye, H. (1936). A syndrome produced by diverse nocuous agents. *Nature, 138,* 32.

Simpson, E. A. (2009). Stressful life events, psychological appraisal and coping style in postmenopausal women. *Maturitas, 63*(4), 357–364.

Skybo, T., & Buck, J. (2007). Stress and coping responses to proficiency-testing in school-age children. *Pediatric Nursing, 33*(5), 413–418.

Smith, A. (2006). "Like waking up from a dream": Mindfulness trainig for older people with anxiety and depression. In R. A. Baer (Ed.), *Mindfulness-based treatment approaches, clinician's guide to evidence base and applications* (pp. 199–215). Boston, MA: Elsevier.

Snyder, M., & Lindquist, R. (Eds.). (2010). *Complementary alternative therapies in nursing* (6th ed). New York, NY: Springer.

Sterling, P. (2012, April 12). Allostasis: A model of predictive regulation. *Psychology & Behavior, 106*(1), 5–15.

Telles Nunes, D., Rodriquez, A., Hoffman, F., Luz, C., Filho, A., Muller, M., et al. (2007). Relaxation and guided imagary program in patients with breast cancer undergoing radiotherapy not associated with neuroimmunomodulatory effects. *Journal of Psychosomatic Research, 63*(6), 647–655.

Trouillet, R., Gana, K., Lourel, M., & Fort, I. (2009). Predictive value of age for coping: The role of self-efficacy, social support satisfaction and perceived stress. *Aging and Mental Health, 13*(3), 357–366.

Vimont, C. (2008, Winter). How to fight stress and ward off illness. *Medline Plus, 3*(1), 5–6.

Walker, L., Smith, C., Garber, J., & Claar, R. (2007). Appraisal and coping with daily stressors by pediatric patients with chronic adominal pain. *Journal of Pediatric Psychology, 32*(2), 206–216.

Weydert, J., Shapiro, D., Acra, S. Monheim, C., Chambers, A., & Ball, T. M. (2006). Evaluation of guided imagery as treatment for recurrent abdominal pain in children: A randomized controlled trial. *BMC Pediatrics, 6*(29) 1–23.

Winbush, N. Y., Gross, C. R., & Kreitzer, M. J. (2007). The effect of mindfuness-based stress reduction on sleep disturbance: A systematic review. *Explore, 3*(6), 585–591.

World Health Organization. (1996). The global burden of disease. In C. H. Murray, *A comprehensive assessment of mortality and disability from diseases, injuries, and risk factors in 1999 and projected to to 2200* (pp. 247–293). Cambridge, MA: Harvard School of Public Health.

CHAPTER 9

Social Support and Health

OBJECTIVES

This chapter will enable the reader to:

1. Differentiate between social networks, social integration, and social support.
2. Describe the components of an individual's network system to consider in a social systems review.
3. Discuss the major types of social support to include in a social systems review.
4. Discuss the role of virtual communities in social support.
5. Describe the role of social networks and social support in the promotion of health.
6. Discuss strategies to enhance social support systems.

Understanding the social context in which individuals live and work is critically important in health promotion. In human interactions, individuals and groups both give and receive social support, a reciprocal process and interactive resource that provide comfort, assistance, encouragement, and information. Social support fosters successful coping and promotes satisfying and effective living. The amount and type(s) of social support needed fluctuate across the life span and across situations. Individuals and families usually call on personal resources first to cope with unanticipated, difficult, or threatening circumstances. Contacts with others in the support system may be initiated when self-reliance fails. All individuals need a system of sustaining support to realize their full potential. However, it is important to note that some may choose not to ask for or accept support, or that support may also be a source of distress rather than of comfort. The multiple dimensions of social support have been explored, defined, and measured in various ways. In addition, the relationship between social support and health has been studied extensively. Social support is considered to be a person–environment interaction that decreases the occurrence of stressors, buffers the impact of stress, and decreases physiologic reactivity to stress.

Much of our understanding of the relationship between social support and health has come from multiple disciplines. Continued advances in our understanding of the mechanisms by which social support affects mental and physical health are essential to promote mental, social, and physical well-being. Relationships among social support, health behaviors, and health are addressed in this chapter. In addition, the role of the nurse in assisting clients to assess, modify, and develop effective social support systems to meet their needs is described.

SOCIAL NETWORKS

Although the terms *social networks, social integration,* and *social support* are often used interchangeably and are overlapping, they are not the same (Gottlieb & Bergen, 2010). *Social networks* refer to the web of social relationships or social ties that surround an individual and the characteristics of those ties. *Social integration* is the degree of involvement or participation in the social network, and *social support* is considered the qualitative, or perceived, functional component. A social network is made up of persons an individual or family knows and interacts with. These interactions may occur frequently or infrequently and may include varying numbers of individuals.

Social integration is the extent to which individuals participate in their social environment at different levels (Gottlieb & Bergen, 2010). The converse of social integration is social isolation or the lack of contact with family, friends, and others in the social network.

Social support refers to resources within the network that are sensed as being available and helpful (perceived support) or are actually provided (received support). The social support system for any given individual or family is usually much smaller than the social network or number of contacts.

Characteristics of social networks have been described in various ways. These characteristics or network properties usually include network *size* or the actual number of people in a network, density or the extent to which network members know each other, network *composition* or *type* (family, relatives, friends, religious organizations, work, etc.), and *frequency of contact* with network members. These characteristics are common assessment measures of social networks. Frequently cited characteristics, including duration, reciprocity, and strength are described in Table 9–1. The connections and contacts with others in one's social networks are considered one's social ties (Thoits, 2011). They have been organized into a typology along three dimensions: network, location, and resources (Moren-Cross & Lin, 2006). Network characteristics include density, size, homogeneity, and demographics. Location characteristics include degree, strength of tie,

TABLE 9–1   Characteristics of Social Networks

Characteristic	Measure
Size	Actual number of persons in network
Density	Extent individuals are connected or know each other
Contact	Amount of interaction with network members in a specified time
Type	Specific relationship to network member, such as family member, friend, etc.
Duration	Length of time individual has known network members
Reciprocity	Degree of exchange in relationship with network members
Strength	Extent to which network ties are voluntary or obligatory

Source: Adapted from Uchino, B. N. (1972). *Social Support & Physical Health,* New Haven: Yale University Press, page 12.

frequency, duration, and reciprocity. Resource characteristics include social capital, which refers to resources embedded in the network. The most commonly studied network characteristics are network size, frequency of interactions with network members, and composition of network.

Social network is not a static concept, as its structure changes across the life span. The nature of an individual's relations can be depicted using a hierarchical mapping technique that has three progressively enlarging concentric circles around an inner circle. The inner circle consists of closest, intimate relationships, such as family and longtime friends. Individuals in the middle circle may be close relatives, friends, and neighbors. The outer circle reflects contacts that are somewhat close, such as coworkers. Throughout the life span, the middle and outer circles are more likely to change, whereas the inner circle tends to be more stable. Inner circle members are difficult to replace, and when they are no longer available, there may be a sense of grief and loss.

Social networks are important as they determine the availability and adequacy of social support, which has been linked to health outcomes. The size of the network is thought to be a major component in social support. However, the types of persons in the network who provide the support, not the network size, have been associated with satisfaction. For example, voluntary social network ties, such as friends and church membership, may be more important for well-being than obligatory social network ties such as family, because one usually chooses network ties that are rewarding. Social networks also promote social participation, providing opportunities for companionship and promoting a sense of belonging. This connectedness helps shape activities and behaviors that individual engages in, such as health behaviors.

SOCIAL INTEGRATION

Social integration, the extent of close family and friends and community ties, has two components: a behavioral component, or the extent of actively engaging in multiple social activities and relationships; and a cognitive component, the extent of a sense of community and identification with one's social roles. Socially integrated individuals have been reported to live longer than those who are less integrated into their networks. This is thought to be due to less social isolation and a sense of meaning in life. Social isolation, on the other hand, has been associated with an increase in morbidity and mortality, although the mechanisms are still being studied (Yang, McClintock, Kozloski, & Li, 2013).

SOCIAL SUPPORT

The functions provided by social relationships are considered social support. *Social support* can be defined as a network of interpersonal relationships that provide psychological and material resources intended to benefit an individual's ability to cope. Social support may be perceived (emotional support) or tangible (supportive acts). Social support is usually described as four broad categories: emotional, instrumental, informational, and appraisal support. Emotional support refers to the demonstration of caring, empathy, love, and trust. Instrumental support includes tangible support or actions, including help obtaining goods or services. Informational support refers to advice provided as well as personal information or suggestions offered. Last, appraisal support refers to the provision of affirmation or constructive feedback. The type of support that is beneficial at any given time may differ, depending on the nature and the situation. For example, emotional support may help in a crisis circumstance, whereas informational support may be more useful in assisting individuals to understand how to learn specific tasks, such as the preparation of nutritious meals. Appraisal or affirmation support may help individuals realize their own strengths and potential.

Social support must be viewed within the context of social relationships. This requires knowledge of cultural characteristics that shape receiving and giving support. Cultural boundaries define the various subgroups of American society, such as African Americans, Asian Americans, Hispanics–Latinos, and Native Americans. Within these cultural boundaries, social support operates uniquely within each social context. For example, religious support plays a unique role for African Americans in promotion of health behaviors (Debnam, Holt, Clark, Roth, & Southward, 2012; Wilcox et al., 2013). Hispanic–Latino Americans and Asian Americans are similar in that the core of their social support systems is the family, which includes close and distant kin. Asian Americans have rules regulating gender hierarchies (patrilineage) and respect for older adults and may use shame and harmony in giving and receiving support. In the Native American culture, social support is less well understood, as the term is not defined in many tribal languages. However, Native Americans live in relational networks that foster mutual assistance and support, and the extended family is a core feature of their network. The social structure reinforces an individual's sense of belonging; however, the high-density networks can also exert conformity pressures and social obligations that may promote and even normalize health-damaging behaviors.

Although many similarities in social support exist among the various American cultures, the influence of the sociohistorical context differs greatly across different populations. Culturally sensitive theoretical views are needed to understand the role of social support as well as gender and life span differences in these populations.

Several social support systems relevant to health have been identified and described: natural support systems (families), peer support systems, religious support systems, professional support systems, and organized self-help support groups not directed by health professionals. In most instances, the family remains the primary support group.

Professional helpers, who have a specific set of skills and services, offer clients a different type of support system. Questions have been raised about the effectiveness of their role in social support. Although professionals have access to information and resources that might not otherwise be available, they are seldom the first source of help for an individual. Initially, family and close friends or peers are sought for advice and support. Health professionals are rarely included as members of an individual's social network. They become the support system only when other sources of help are unavailable, interrupted, or exhausted. Professionals usually are unable to provide support over long periods of time. In addition, these relationships are not characterized by reciprocity; they usually involve a power differential and offer limited empathetic understanding due to lack of intimacy. In spite of these limitations, professional helpers have a role to play in offering short-term emotional and appraisal support as well as informational support.

All support systems of an individual or family are synergistic. In combination, they represent the social resources available to facilitate stability and actualization. Various systems are dominant at different points in the life cycle, depending on stage of development and the stressors or challenges at hand. For example, in preadolescence and early adolescence, parents are the greatest source of support. The network shifts to a greater reliance on peers for lifestyle choices during middle adolescence with a decreased perception of parental support. Friends remain dominant in young adults. The family network and friends are important sources of support for the elderly.

Functions of Social Support Groups

The primary functions of social support groups are to augment personal strengths of members and promote achievement of life goals. The functions of social support groups in promoting health can be conceptualized in four ways, as depicted in Figure 9–1.
Social groups contribute to health as follows:

1. Creating a growth-promoting environment that supports health-promoting behaviors, self-esteem, and high-level wellness;
2. Decreasing the likelihood of threatening or stressful life events;
3. Providing feedback or confirmation of an individual's actions; and
4. Buffering the negative effects of stressful events.

Support groups function to share common social concerns, provide intimacy, prevent isolation, respect mutual competencies, offer dependable assistance in crises, serve as a referral agent, and provide mutual challenge.

Social support groups offer insight about the unique role of social support in reducing stress. They provide a strong sense of community, nonjudgmental acceptance, and invaluable information, which empowers individuals to gain control over life. The type of group leader (professional or peer) does not matter, as long as the group provides a supportive environment, a sense of belonging, and meets an individual's perceived needs.

Family as the Primary Support Group

The family is the primary context for learning to give and receive social support. Family cohesion, expressiveness, and lack of conflict are reflected in the supportive behaviors that family members provide to one another. Low family support and poor child–parent interactions influence the life course trajectories of young people. Family stressors, such as unemployment, welfare dependence, change in family structure (as a divorce), crime, and substance use can decrease family cohesion and increase conflict and adolescent behavioral and mental problems (Luecken, Kraft, & Hagan, 2009).

Family social support exerts complex effects on the physical and mental health of its members. The classic Alameda County, California, study provided initial information about the association of social networks, social integration, social support, and mortality (Berkman & Syme,

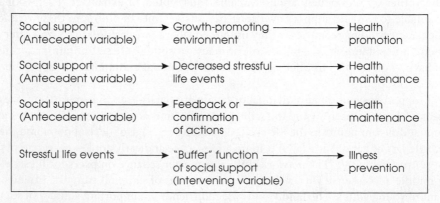

FIGURE 9–1 Possible Impact of Social Support on Health Status

1979). Men who are single or widowed have continued to consistently show higher mortality rates than have married men. Depressive symptoms have been associated with an adverse family environment that offers low levels of social support. Men who remain socially isolated after losing their partners are at higher risk of developing symptoms of chronic depression, whereas having supportive relationships has been associated with a decreased risk. Having a marital partner or socially supportive relationships reduces psychological distress.

Instrumental support has positive effects throughout the life span. Using the well-known convoy model (Antonucci, Ajrouch, & Janevic, 2003), two aspects of social support networks—a greater proportion of kin and the presence of family members in the inner circle—significantly reduce distress. The interplay between family stressors and family support is depicted in Figure 9–2.

Within families, both positive and negative interactions occur. Negative interactions can be viewed as stressors, whereas positive, helpful interactions constitute support. Positive emotional bonds with its social network buttress the family's competence and effective functioning. For example, in the longitudinal East London RELACHS study, low levels of family support were associated with depressive symptoms in an ethnically diverse population of adolescents (Khatib, Bhui, & Stansfeld, 2013).

Social support is unequally distributed and varies by socioeconomic status. Neighborhood stressors, such as abandoned buildings, litter and graffiti, physical decay, and absence of green space, have been associated with poorer mental health (Mair, Diez Roux, & Morenoff, 2010). Neighborhood poverty has consistently been associated with poor mental and physical health status (Kim, 2010). Persons living in disadvantaged neighborhoods may lack social networks and supportive relationships. Neighborhood poverty prevents the formation of supportive relationships due to distrust, fear, and self-imposed social isolation. However, if supportive social relationships exist, they may buffer the effects of neighborhood disadvantage and provide critical resources for day-to-day survival (Keene, Bader, & Ailshire, 2013). Impoverished women are especially vulnerable and less able to nurture children due to multiple issues. Many rely on minor children for support, which may result in worse well-being for the children and poor outcomes for the mother. Burdening the children decreases their well-being, which

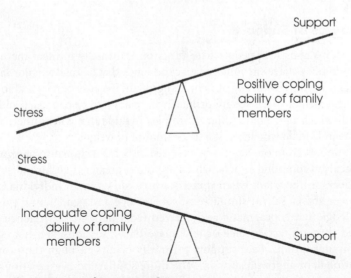

FIGURE 9–2 Family as a Source of Support or Stress

becomes an additional stressor for the mother. These findings support the need to help persons with low socioeconomic status explore alternate networks for social support, such as local organizations. Special attention to social support resources for persons with lower socioeconomic status is critical.

Community Organizations as Support Groups

Characteristics of a community and its organizations have a direct bearing on the level of well-being of individuals and families who reside in it. The quality of social interaction and the life experiences of residents contribute positively or negatively to health. Stability within a community tends to promote close-knit ties among residents that mitigate the effects of crises on community members. Stable communities are characterized by value similarity, mutual assistance, shared trust, and concern for members.

Organized religious support systems, such as churches, temples, mosques, or other religious meeting places, constitute a support system for individuals, as congregations share similar value systems, a common set of beliefs about the purpose of life, and a set of guidelines for living. Even highly mobile individuals may find a support system in the local church or synagogue. The church takes primary responsibility for support to enhance the spiritual dimension of health, which includes the ability to discover and articulate one's basic purpose in life; learn how to experience love, joy, peace, and fulfillment; and discover how to help oneself and others achieve full personal potential.

Faith-based communities can be a source of support for promoting healthy lifestyles. Churches represent miniature, dynamic communities that may provide social, emotional, and material support, such as child care, meals, transportation, and counseling. In addition, volunteer helpers are readily available. Churches are now participating in programs that promote healthy lifestyles and prevent obesity, such as the 2011 Robert Wood Johnson faith-based program to combat childhood obesity in diverse populations at greatest risk.

Nurses who function as parish or congregational nurses in churches support health promotion within a community setting. Parish nurses integrate concern for the spirituality of the person with holistic care within a faith-based community.

Peers as a Source of Support

Peer support systems consist of people who function informally to meet the needs of others. Many of these individuals have encountered an experience that has had a major influence in their own lives and achieved successful adjustment and growth. Because of personal insight and experiential knowledge, their advice is sought primarily in relation to resolving a problem of immediate concern with which they are familiar. Examples include the avid runner, the health-food enthusiast, or the individual who has lost a large amount of weight.

Informal support from one's peers has consistently been shown to have powerful stress-buffering and health promoting effects, which are often greater than formal support services. Support from peers is important when there is a breakdown in an individual's usual support network. The peer shares salient similarities, such as age and gender, and possesses specific concrete knowledge that is pragmatic and derived from personal experiences. Peer support can be provided through face-to-face or telephone-based sessions, self-help groups, e-mail, and online computer groups. Peer support primarily occurs through the provision of emotional, informational, or appraisal support. The more similar the peer relationships, the more likely the support will lead to understanding, empathy, and mutual help. Peer support may positively affect physical and mental health outcomes. For example, peer support from friends during adolescence has been found to influence consumption of fast foods, physical activity, and alcohol use initiation (de la Haye, Robins, Mohr, & Wilson, 2010; Mundt, 2011).

Peers must be skilled in communication, active listening, and problem solving. In addition, peers need empathy with the person's difficulties and must be willing to take a supportive role. Peer support commonly includes befriending, mediation/conflict resolution, mentoring, and counseling. Peer support systems have been developed in schools and colleges to decrease aggressive acts and social isolation, as well as to teach skills and promote health.

SELF-HELP GROUPS.   Organized support systems not directed by health professionals include voluntary service groups and self-help groups. These groups do not have an expert leader, which distinguishes them from support groups, which are led by a trained facilitator. Self-help groups are an attempt to change the behavior of members or promote adaptation to a life change such as chronic illness. They are defined by the members' expectations.

Self-help groups continue to increase in the United States. Self-help groups have been called "mutual help groups" to reflect the fact that group members give and receive advice, encouragement, and support. One therapeutic factor is the group's ability to normalize a stigmatizing condition and to take away the embarrassment of having an undesirable behavior. This is a necessary step to make cognitive, emotional, and behavioral changes.

Examples of self-help groups include Narcotics Anonymous, Alcoholics Anonymous, Mended Hearts, Compassionate Friends, and physical fitness clubs. Characteristics of self-help groups include a critical mass sufficient to form a group, a form of publicity or recruitment to attract members, and a central goal or activity that gives the group purpose and sustains the investment of its members.

The question has been raised as to why individuals use self-help groups rather than other resources, such as professional services. Two possible reasons are offered:

1. Self-help groups fulfill a need for services not being offered; and
2. Self-help groups arise because of disappointment with traditional medical models and lack of meaningful resources within the community.

Self-help groups enable group members to expand their social networks as well as receive informational, instrumental, emotional, and appraisal support. Self-help groups empower individuals by increasing self-worth, support, and affirmation. Some consider the term *self-help* misleading because members are not involved in these groups just to help themselves. Instead, they help each other, so the term *mutual-aid group* has been suggested, which implies that each person is both a helper and receiver of help. However, self-help group members prefer the term *self-help*.

The success of self-help groups in assisting individuals cope with different life experiences attests to their continuing viability as a community health resource. Self-care may be particularly effective for individuals who do not receive support from other relationships.

Virtual Communities as a Source of Support

Virtual communities or online support groups are groups of people who interact using information and communication technologies (Welbourne, Blanchard, & Wadsworth, 2013). In these online communities, individuals develop feelings of identity and belonging. Virtual communities overcome geographic distance and access to information. They are accessible for those with limited time or who do not have access to face-to-face groups. Individuals are motivated to join these groups to obtain informational as well as emotional support. In some cases, individuals prefer online support groups over offline groups when they are dissatisfied with the lack of support from their social networks or health care professionals (Chung, 2013). Virtual communities also include educational information and discussion forums. Technologies for virtual communities include online message boards, asynchronous or synchronous communication, and videoconferencing. These communities may include virtual health care delivery teams, virtual research teams, virtual disease management groups, and peer groups. Active participation in online support groups has been associated with positive outcomes and less loneliness. This is thought to be due to the development of a sense of community within the group and feelings of connectedness. The term *sense of virtual community* (SOVC) is now used to describe group members' feelings of identity and attachment with others in online groups (Welbourne, Blanchard, & Wadsworth, 2013).

Online support group messages are most helpful if they:

- Do not threaten the individual's self esteem;
- Are sensitive to the individual's feelings;
- Clearly support the individual's intentions; and
- Use explicit language in presenting messages.

The anonymity in online support groups enables members to be more selective in presenting information about themselves and allow for greater openness in sharing feelings (Chung, 2013). The downsides of online support groups include the following:

- Membership changes frequently.
- Instrumental support is not provided.
- Inaccurate or outdated information may be used.
- Problematic behavior may be promoted.

Social networking sites (SNSs) are changing the way individuals manage their relationships as well as their health care (Oh, Lauckner, Boehmer, Fewins-Bliss, & Kang, 2011). In addition to health information, many sites focus on lifestyle information and support for diet and fitness. These sites provide tools as well as support to lose weight or become physically active. For example, some websites offer food diaries to record daily calorie intake or physical activity diaries to record walking.

The Centers for Disease Control and Prevention (CDC) has developed useful guidelines and best practices for using social media and virtual worlds to communicate science-based health promotion and prevention information. In addition, guidelines for designing, implementing, and evaluating online social support groups are available in the literature. (See Weiss, Berner, Johnson, Giuse, Murphy, & Lorenzi, 2013.)

Internet technology has been shown to be acceptable across ethnically diverse groups. However, socioeconomic status continues to be a limiting factor. A 2011 report of the Pew Research Center described a new "digital divide," as minorities (Blacks and Latinos) are more challenged to gain access to new technology (see the Pew Research Center web site). Although these groups have mobile Internet access, there are limitations to mobile devices, such as completing or updating job applications. Women and young people are more likely to use social media, and older people are the least likely group to use new communication technologies. However, virtual communities may play a powerful role in meeting the informational and support needs of the elderly. Online support groups among the elderly have the potential to overcome many barriers, including mobility limitations, lack of transportation, and finances. Facebook, one of the best-known web-based social networking sites, has great appeal to young adults. However, only about one third of persons over age 65 access Facebook. Multiple sites have been developed for older adults to discuss topics such as health, difficult life transitions, and caregiver issues as older adults become more active participants.

Privacy concerns remain a challenge for social networking sites. Inappropriate access to, misuse of, and illegal disclosure of personal information can become major issues if electronic data is not protected from unauthorized users. For these reasons recommendations to protect one's personal health data have been suggested (Li, 2013). For online social support groups, individuals should share only the minimum amount of data to accomplish their purpose and learn how to protect personally identifiable information.

Advanced technologies now play an important role in the provision of social support across the life span. The rapid growth of the Internet has occurred without concurrent attention to policy, ethical, and legal issues. As nurses and other health care providers adopt these technologies they need to know the steps to address security concerns and implement strategies to evaluate the usefulness of these steps in health and health promotion.

ASSESSING SOCIAL SUPPORT SYSTEMS

It is important for both clients and health care providers to be aware of available sources of social support for individuals and families. Approaches for assessing social support networks of clients are described in Chapter 4. These approaches provide insight into existing support resources for both the client and the nurse. When assessing the adequacy of a client's support systems, it is important to be cognizant of factors that may cause the assessments to vary. Such things as one's culture, stage of life-span development, social context (school, home, work), and role context (parent, student, professional) must be considered. In addition, multiple measures are available to assess social networks, social integration, perceived and received social support, loneliness, and social isolation. Successful health promotion depends on support from friends and/or family. An assessment of an individual's support systems is essential.

SOCIAL SUPPORT AND HEALTH

The importance of social support to mental and physical health is now well established. Lower levels of support are consistently linked to higher rates of morbidity and mortality. However, the actual mechanisms linking social support to health are less well understood. Several processes have been proposed. First, social support may be directly linked to health by promoting healthy or unhealthy behaviors, supplying information, or making available tangible resources (child care, opportunities at work). Social support may foster a sense of meaning in life or be associated with more positive affective states, such as enhanced sense of self-worth and increased sense of control. Individuals may appraise events as less threatening, resulting in less physiologic arousal.

Social support may also contribute to health by buffering the effects of stress on an individual. Social support is thought to be beneficial because it decreases the negative effects of stressful experiences on one's mental and physical health. Stress promotes negative coping patterns and activates physiological systems that place a person at risk for developing mental and physical illnesses. Social support is thought to buffer the negative effects of the stress response by promoting less threatening interpretations of adverse events and effective coping strategies. Even when faced with extremely stressful events, having individuals who provide support can reduce the intensity of stress (see Uchino, Bowen, Carlisle, & Birmingham, 2013, for a review of psychological mechanisms). The physiologic mechanisms are receiving increased attention because of the role of these mechanisms on health. Social support has been associated with reduction of inflammation, a major predictor of many chronic diseases (Kiecolt-Glaser, Gouin, & Hantsoo, 2010). Studies consistently link low levels of social support and social isolation to high levels of inflammatory markers in healthy persons. These findings have been reproduced in animal models (Karelina & DeVries, 2011). Research results reinforce the positive effects of social integration and social supportive relationships and health. Nurses and other health care providers are in unique positions to assess social networks and social support and intervene to provide short-term support and to assist clients in identifying supportive relationships.

When developing social support interventions, it is important to consider the type of social support that will be targeted. Will it be emotional or informational support or an increase in social contacts? The kind of support, who will provide the support, and contextual issues all play a role. For example, interventions to increase perceived support should focus on helping persons recruit supportive others into their social network by teaching them relationship-building skills. Conditions that warrant recruitment of additional supportive network members include the following:

- The existing network is conflictual.
- The existing network reinforces unhealthy behaviors.
- The existing network does not have experiential or specialized knowledge.

If supportive network members are available, the intervention can focus on strengthening the available network to provide the needed support. Figure 9–3 provides a systematic process, known as the intervention mapping approach, for planning support interventions (Bartholomew, Parcel, Kok, Gottlieb, & Fernandez, 2011). The advantage of this approach is its focus on a needs assessment as well as theoretical intervention planning and development (Hengel, Joling, Proper, van der Molen, & Bongers, 2011)

Reviews of interventions that have been tested to improve social support have had varying long-term results. Many studies suffer from weaknesses that limit the generalizability of findings. In addition, some studies that were well designed showed no improvement in support. Although the intervention may have improved health or well-being, the client's naturally occurring social support did not change; therefore, the desired outcomes did not last when the intervention was completed. Social support is complex and includes characteristics of the person who needs or desires support (perceiver), characteristics of the person who gives the support (supporter), characteristics of the situation, and the interaction of these factors. All of these factors must be taken into consideration when designing interventions to improve social support.

Social Support and Health Behavior

Social support systems influence health behavior. It is well known that significant others function as an important lay referral system for individuals in making decisions to seek professional care for health promotion, illness prevention, or care. Concurrence by the lay

Step 1 Conduct Needs Assessment	• Establish program planning group. • Perform literature review, focus groups, interviews. • Assess socio-environmental influences. • Assess readiness for change.
Step 2 Develop Program Objectives and Outcomes	• Focus on a behavior that can be changed. • Identify behavioral determinants of behavior targeted. • Specify outcomes that will be measured. • Write measureable behavioral objectives.
Step 3 Develop Theory-Based Program Methods and Practical Application	• Generate program ideas with planning group. • Identify theoretical methods. • Choose program methods. • Design realistic application to address methods.

Step 4
Develop Program and
Materials
	• Consult potential participants and implementers.
	• Develop program outline, teaching strategies,
	  time frame.
	• Develop, tailor protocols and handouts to
	  target group.
	• Address behavioral determinants to be changed.
	• Pretest protocols and program materials.

Step 5 Develop Implementation Plan	• Identify potential participants and implementers • Select and tailor practical application methods. • Specify determinants for implementation.
Step 6 Develop Evaluation Plan	• Decide on evaluation methods. • Write process and outcome evaluation questions. • Choose evaluation time frame. • Choose evaluation measures.

FIGURE 9–3   Intervention Mapping Guide for Health Promotion Program Planning   *Source:* Adapted from http://www.interventionmapping.com/sites/default/files/im steps & tasks.png

referral system often determines the extent to which advice from health professionals is actually followed.

Social support from spouses or partners is related to health behaviors. This relationship may be due to encouragement and support of the health behavior, including giving approval and disapproval, having control over aspects of the proposed change such as food shopping and preparation; and participating in the behavior change, such as joining an exercise program. High levels of warmth, encouragement, and assistance characterize spousal and partner support. A nonsupportive family network can interfere with successful implementation of health habits by limiting the client's time and energy available for health behavior or introducing stressors that compromise healthy behaviors.

Social support and social integration have consistently been positively associated with specific health behaviors and reduced risky behaviors. In a review of social relations and health behaviors, social support was related to fruit and vegetable consumption and exercise adherence (Tay, Tan, Diener, & Gonzalez, 2013). Family ties and community-based support were most helpful in promoting physical activity. Social support, specifically greater family involvement and positive family relationships, was associated with abstinence in an alcohol abuse program. Social support and interactions with friends promote healthy behaviors through the development of social norms (Fiorillo & Sabatini, 2011). For example, exercising with a friend or playing team sports makes exercise fun. Social norms may also prevent the initiation of unhealthy behaviors, such as smoking and alcohol consumption.

Adoption and maintenance of health behaviors over time is difficult unless the behavior is supported by family members and friends. All health care providers need to help clients understand the importance of naturally occurring support and connect them with informal support systems if natural ones are not available.

Autonomy Support and Health Behaviors

Autonomy support, a concept in self-determination theory (SDT), refers to understanding and validating another's perspectives and feelings. Autonomy supportive persons offer support by respecting an individual's experiences, promoting choices, using noncontrolling language, displaying patience, acknowledging negative feelings, minimizing pressure and control, and providing relevant information (Su & Reeve, 2011). SDT operates on the belief that all persons have psychological needs of autonomy, competence, and relatedness (Ryan & Deci, 2002). Social environments that support these three basic needs are essential to health and well-being. Table 9–2 offers definitions of autonomy support used by various clinical specialties, including healthy promotion, education, and communication. The use of noncontrolling language, acknowledging perspectives and feelings, providing rationale, and nurturing motivational resources are considered the most effective components. Autonomy supportive interventions have been shown to improve eating behaviors (Leong, Madden, Gray, & Horwath, 2012); physical activity, including exercise maintenance (Hsu, Buckworth,

TABLE 9–2 Definitions of Autonomy Support

Specialty	Definition
Health Promotion	Acknowledging other's perspective, offering choices, minimizing pressure and control.
Education	Providing explanatory rationales, using noncontrolling language, showing patience for self-paced learning.
	Providing choice within limits, acknowledging other's feelings and perspectives, providing opportunities for initiative taking, providing noncontrolling feedback, avoiding controlling behaviors.
	Encouraging persons to solve their own problems, taking their perspective.
Communication	Understanding and validating the other person's frame of reference, respecting other's experiences, promoting choice through clarification of goals, emphasizing ownership and personal responsibility.

Focht, & O'Connell, 2013); and stress and coping (Weinstein & Ryan, 2011). Autonomous supportive behaviors provide an effective way to support individuals and families in implementing and maintaining health behaviors.

ENHANCING SOCIAL SUPPORT SYSTEMS

Support-enhancing strategies have three goals:

- Strengthen existing supportive relationships,
- Establish new interpersonal ties, and
- Prevent disruption of ties from evolving into mental or physical illness.

Facilitating Social Interactions

Interpersonal skills are key in developing supportive relationships with others Social skills training represents one approach to teach individuals how to develop supportive interpersonal relationships, as they learn to express positive and negative feelings honestly and communicate effectively. Training can be conducted with individuals or groups who have similar skill needs. Social skills training is based on the belief that socially competent responses can be learned. Initially, training is directed toward assessing and modifying perceptions of appropriate behavior in social situations. In addition, persons are taught to re-evaluate their thoughts about themselves in a more positive manner. Attempts are made to improve social interaction patterns using social cognitive theory concepts (modeling, role playing, performance feedback), coaching, and homework assignments. Skills taught might include initiating conversations, giving and receiving emotional and instrumental support, handling periods of silence, recognizing nonverbal methods of communication, becoming a good listener, and handling criticism and conflict. Individuals learn to identify positive and negative ways of communicating; how to use clear and accurate messages; how to differentiate between assertive, aggressive, and passive behaviors; and how to say no when necessary. More effective interpersonal communication skills enable individuals to increase social ties and foster supportive relationships.

Enhancing Coping

A lack of social ties and support may result in serious psychological and physical problems during major negative life events. Support groups for widows, children of separated or divorced parents, and parents who have lost a child, for example, can assist such persons to learn to cope effectively with these stressful life events. Effective coping skills help individuals understand emotional reactions, reduce feelings of alienation, and assist those people to move ahead into the future.

Problem-solving coping strategies are aimed at reducing stressful situations. These coping strategies enable one to identify the stressful situation, perceive it to be controllable, identify and implement a potential solution, and evaluate the outcome. Effective coping skills enable individuals to see a stressful event as a challenge or opportunity rather than a threat and to believe that a solution is possible. Effective coping enhances social support, as it functions as a resource to successfully resolve stressful life events.

Preventing Social Isolation and Loneliness

Social isolation is a state in which individuals have little or no contact with family members, friends, or neighbors and limited social participation. Loneliness is an individual's subjective feeling of social isolation due to dissatisfaction with the frequency and quality of social contacts (Saito, Kai, & Takizawa, 2012). Both social isolation and loneliness place individuals at increased risk for chronic illnesses. Preventing loneliness or social isolation is a more desirable approach than treatment of loneliness and isolation after they have occurred. Two approaches to prevention include identifying high-risk groups and implementing interventions that focus on developing social support ties. Young, unmarried, unemployed, low-income, minority persons and the elderly are particularly vulnerable to limited support and loneliness. Programs to decrease social isolation and loneliness must be congruent with the individual's wishes, and strategies should increase social interaction and reduce isolating behaviors. Programs may include transportation vehicles staffed by volunteers, respite programs for caretaker relief, religious support, and community support such as neighborhood watch groups for elders and families. Both telephone and Internet online support are additional resources to decrease isolation.

Educational approaches to prevent loss of social support and subsequent loneliness include classroom experiences for schoolchildren to help them gain skills in making friends, working cooperatively with others, and resolving differences or conflict. A body of evidence over the past 30 years has substantiated that poor social functioning in children often leads to serious personal adjustment problems in later life. Social disconnectedness and perceived isolation in older adults have been associated with increased morbidity and mortality (Steptoe, Shanker, Demakakos, & Wardle, 2013). Older adults have reduced social networks and social contacts due to death of family and friends. They must build new social relationships among people they have not previously known and create new social support systems in the face of decreasing economic resources or mobility issues. Many older persons need to learn skills to promote successful relationships, as well as skills to resolve interpersonal conflicts with people they already know. Media campaigns, such as television public service announcements about resources for formal support and the health benefits of staying connected with relatives and friends, may provide cues to initiate new relationships. Assisted living facilities may be beneficial for some elders to help them stay connected. These facilities have ready-made social networks. In addition, community programs and neighborhood activities can be designed to help persons build relationships or to reach out to others who may need emotional or instrumental support. Computer and telephone support have become viable options to provide support for the elderly.

Other general suggestions for enhancing social support include the following:

- Setting mutual goals with family members or friends to achieve common needs for support.
- Constructively resolving conflict between support network members.
- Offering assistance to individuals within one's social network to show concern and promote trust.
- Seeking counseling, if needed, to resolve marital and/or family conflict.
- Tapping nurses and other health professionals as community support resources.
- Increasing ties with online or face-to-face social groups.

Clients should be encouraged to identify specific goals to enhance personal support networks. By focusing on one or two realistic changes, clients can build effective social support systems.

CONSIDERATIONS FOR PRACTICE IN SOCIAL SUPPORT

Although evidence provides important information about social support and health, many of these findings have not been incorporated into practice. Knowledge of current evidence is necessary to be able to intervene to enhance social networks and social support. Assessment of social networks and support systems should be part of an initial assessment. Nurses should know how to obtain culturally sensitive information about support systems from diverse populations. If the social network needs to be enhanced, programs can be implemented to teach clients skills to develop or access supportive relationships. Finally, nurses should assist clients in exploring sources of support, including families, friends, neighbors, self-help, Internet and telephone support groups, and community organizations. Accessing these resources increases the potential for success in health promotion and lifestyle change.

OPPORTUNITIES FOR RESEARCH IN SOCIAL SUPPORT

The positive relationship between social networks, social support and health has consistently been documented. However, questions still need to be investigated to understand the mechanisms of social support on health outcomes. In addition, the theoretical mechanisms underlying successful interventions need further study.

1. The long-term effectiveness of interventions on sustaining health behaviors needs continued evaluation.
2. The amount or "dosage" and types of social relationships and support necessary to promote health behaviors should be explored.
3. Interventions to decrease social isolation and loneliness need further investigation across the life span.
4. The specific psychological and physiological mechanisms by which social support enhances health warrant further investigation.
5. Animal and clinical studies are needed to test the effects of social support interventions on neural pathways and immune function.
6. Measures are needed to evaluate both the short- and long-term effectiveness of online support groups.

Nurse scientists play a major role in social support research and can provide leadership for interdisciplinary teams to investigate these issues.

Summary

Social support plays an important role in the health and well-being of clients. Both the client and the social environment should be considered to facilitate holistic health promotion. The extent to which stressful events threaten health and health-promoting behaviors may well depend on the support available from primary (family) or extended (peer, community, and professional) social networks. Social support groups can help clients cope with everyday hassles and major, stressful life experiences. The design and evaluation of nursing interventions to increase social support need to include virtual environments and the new technologies available. These interventions will enhance the quality of human social transactions across the life span.

Learning Activities

1. Perform a social network review with a young adult and an elderly client, using the network components described in the chapter.
2. Design a plan, using the intervention mapping steps, to establish a self-help group for adolescents who are overweight. Incorporate both face-to-face and Internet group meetings into your plan.
3. Detail three strategies to increase your client's social support, based on the assessment you performed in the first learning activity. Take current sources as well as potential sources of support into consideration.
4. Develop four strategies to provide autonomy support for an adult who has expressed a desire to lose weight.

References

Antonucci, T. C., Ajrouch, K. J., & Janevic, M. R. (2003). The effect of social relations with children on the education-health link in men and women aged 40 and over. *Social Science & Medicine, 56*, 949–960.

Bartholomew, L. K., Parcel, C. S., Kok, G., Gottlieb, N. H., & Fernandez, M. A. (2011). *Planning health programs: An intervention mapping approach.* San Francisco: Jossey-Bass.

Berkman, L., & Syme, S. L. (1979). Social networks, host resistance, and mortality: A nine-year follow-up study of Alameda County residents. *American Journal of Epidemiology, 115*, 684–694.

Chung, J. E. (2013). Social interaction in online support groups: Preference for online social interaction over offline social interaction. *Computers in Human Behavior, 29*, 1408–1414.

Debnam, K., Holt, C. L., Clark, E. M., Roth, D. L., & Southward, P. (2012). Relationship between religious social support and general support with health behaviors in a national sample of African Americans. *Journal of Behavioral Medicine, 35*, 179–189.

de la Haye, K., Robins, G., Mohr, P., & Wilson, C. (2010). Obesity-related behaviors in adolescent friendship networks. *Social Networks, 32*, 161–167.

Fiorilla, D., & Sabatini, F. (2011). Quality and quantity: The role of social interactions in self-reported individual health. *Social Science & Medicine, 73*, 1644–1652.

Gottlieb, B. H., & Bergen, A. E. (2010). Social support concepts and measures. *Journal of Psychosomatic Research, 69*, 511–520.

Hengel, K. M., Joling, C. I., Proper, K. I., van der Molen, H. F., & Bongers, P. M. (2011). Intervention mapping as a framework for developing an intervention at the worksite for older construction workers. *American Journal of Health Promotion, 26*, e1–e9.

Hsu, Y., Buckworth, J., Focht, B. C., & O'Connell, A. A. (2013). Feasibility of a self-determination theory-based exercise intervention promoting healthy at every size with sedentary overweight women: Project CHANGE. *Psychology of Sport and Exercise, 14*, 283–292.

Karelina, K., & DeVries, A. C. (2011). Modeling social influences on human health. *Psychosomatic Medicine, 73*, 64–74.

Keene, D., Bader, M., & Ailshire, J. (2013). Length of residence and social integration: The contingent effects of neighborhood poverty. *Health & Place, 21*, 171–178.

Khatib, Y., Bhui, K., & Stansfeld, S. A. (2013). Does social support protect against depression & psychological distress? Findings from the RELACHS study of East London adolescents. *Journal of Adolescents, 36*, 393–402.

Kiecolt-Glaser, J. K., Gouin, J., & Hantsoo, L. (2010). Close relationships, inflammation, and health. *Neuroscience Biobehavioral Review, 35*, 33–38.

Kim, J. (2010). Neighborhood disadvantage and mental health: The role of neighborhood disorder and social relationships. *Social Science Research, 39*, 260–271.

Leong, S. L., Madden, C., Gray, A., & Horwath, C. (2012). Self-determined, autonomous regulation of eating behaviors is related to lower body mass index in a nationwide survey of middle-aged women. *Journal of the Academy of Nutrition and Dietetics, 112*, 1337–1346.

Li, J. (2013). Privacy policies for health social networking sites. *Journal of the American Medical Informatics Association, 20*, 704–707.

Luecken, L. L., Kraft, A., & Hagan, M. J. (2009). Negative relationships in the family-of-origin predict attenuated cortisol in emerging adults. *Hormones and Behavior, 55*, 412–417.

Mair, C., Diez Roux, A. V., & Morenoff, J. D. (2010). Neighborhood stressors and social support as predictors of depressive symptoms in the Chicago Community adult health study. *Health & Place, 16*, 811–819.

Moren-Cross, J. L., & Lin, N. (2010). Social networks and health. In R. H. Binstock, L. K. George, S. J. Cutler, J. Hendricks, & J. H. Schulz (Eds.), *Handbook of aging and the social sciences* (6th ed., pp. 111–127), Oxford: Academic Press, Elsevier.

Mundt, M. (2011). The impact of peer social networks on adolescent alcohol use initiation. *Academic Pediatrics, 11*, 414–421.

Oh, H., Lauckner, C., Boehmer, J., Fewins-Bliss, R., & Kang, L. (2013). Facebooking for health: An examination into the solicitation and effects of health-related social support on social networking sites. *Computers in Human Behavior, 29*(5), 2072–2080.

Ryan, R. M., & Deci, E. L. 2002. An overview of self-determination theory. In E. L. Deci & R. M. Ryan (Eds.), *Handbook of self-determination research* (pp. 3–33), Rochester, NY: University of Rochester Press.

Saito, T., Kai, I., & Takizawa, A. (2012). Effects of a program to prevent social isolation on loneliness, depression, and subjective well-being of older adults: A randomized trial among older migrants in Japan. *Archives of Gerontology and Geriatrics, 55*, 539–547.

Steptoe, A., Shanker, A., Demakakos, P., & Wardle, J. (2013). Social isolation, loneliness, and all-cause mortality in older men and women. *PNAS, 110*, 5797–5801.

Su, Y., & Reeve, J. (2011). A meta-analysis of the effectiveness of intervention programs designed to support autonomy. *Educational Psychology Review, 23*, 159–188.

Tay, L., Tan, K., Diener, E., & Gonzalez, E. (2013). Social relations, health behaviors, and health outcomes: A survey and synthesis. *Applied Psychology, 5*, 28–78.

Thoits, P. (2011). Mechanisms linking social ties and support to physical and mental health. *Journal of Health and Social Behavior, 52*, 146–161.

Uchino, B. N., Bowen, K., Carlisle, M., & Birmingham, W. (2012). Psychological pathways linking social support to health outcomes: A visit with the "Ghosts" of research past, present and future. *Social Science & Medicine, 74*, 949–957.

Weinstein, N., & Ryan, R. M. (2011). A self-determination theory approach to understanding stress incursion and responses. *Stress & Health, 27*, 4–17.

Weiss, J. B., Berner, E. S., Johnson, K. B., Giuse, D. A., Murphy, B. A., & Lorenzi, N. M. (2013). Recommendations for the design, implementation, and evaluation of social support in online communities, networks, and groups. *Journal of Biomedical Informatics,* http://dx.doi.org/10.1016/j.jb.2013.04.004

Welbourne, J. L., Blanchard, A. L., & Wadsworth, M. (2013). Motivations in virtual health communities and their relationship to community, connections, and stress. *Computers in Human Behavior, 29*(1), 129–139.

Wilcox, S., Parrott, A., Baruth, M., Laken, M., Condrasky, M., Saunders, R., . . . Zimmerman, L. (2013). The faith, activity, and nutrition program: A randomized controlled trial in African American churches. *American Journal of Preventive Medicine, 44*, 122–131.

Yang, Y. C., McClintock, M. K., Kozloski, M., & Li, T. (2013). Social isolation and adult mortality: The role of chronic inflammation and sex differences. *Journal of Health and Social Behavior, 54*, 183–203.

CHAPTER 10

Evaluating Health Promotion Programs

OBJECTIVES

This chapter will enable the reader to:

1. Describe the purpose of evaluation for health promotion.
2. Compare three approaches to evaluation and provide examples of each.
3. Discuss types of outcomes to consider when evaluating health promotion programs.
4. Describe the steps in program evaluation.
5. Discuss strategies that facilitate behavior change in health promotion programs.

A scientific knowledge base to guide health promotion programs and interventions is established by evaluating the results of multiple health promotion programs and interventions. Evaluation information can be used to improve health promotion programs to produce the most favorable outcomes for clients and communities. Our knowledge of the effectiveness of health promotion is based on research results and program evaluations that have been conducted and published. Nurses and other health care professionals are continually being asked about the benefits of their health promotion and risk reduction activities. This question can be answered by carefully examining the cumulative evidence produced by health promotion program evaluations.

PURPOSE OF EVALUATION

Evaluation, the process of systematically collecting and analyzing information, is undertaken to assess the value of a health promotion program or intervention. Program evaluations are considered decision oriented, whereas research evaluation involves generating scientific knowledge. Health promotion evaluations serve many purposes: to determine if program objectives were achieved, to identify strengths and weaknesses to improve the program, to compare the program with other programs, to contribute to the scientific knowledge of health promotion, to provide accountability to funding agencies, and to inform policy makers (McKenzie, Neiger, & Thackeray, 2012). Evaluations also provide information to enable health care professionals to make decisions about resource allocation, as ineffective programs can be eliminated. Health promotion evaluations enable the nurse to improve programs, to make choices between health promotion activities, and to assess if a new intervention with documented research effectiveness will translate to practice.

Questions that may be answered by a comprehensive evaluation include the following:

- Is the health promotion intervention effective in an ideal situation? (efficacy)
- Does the health promotion intervention produce the same benefits when it is translated to a practice setting? (effectiveness)
- How does the health promotion intervention work? (theory)
- What are the intended and unintended effects? (outcomes)
- How long do the effects last? (sustainability)
- What resources are needed to implement the intervention or program?
- Is the program cost-effective?
- Are the clients satisfied?
- Who will benefit most from the intervention?
- How can the program or intervention be improved?

Resources, including cost and time, pose limitations on evaluations. All stakeholders must be engaged in the evaluation process, including those who have an investment in the program as well as intended users. Credible evidence is critical to make accurate conclusions. In addition, performing an evaluation requires knowledge, skills, and administrative support. If these components are not present, the evaluation is unlikely to be performed successfully or produce useful information.

APPROACHES TO EVALUATION OF HEALTH PROMOTION PROGRAMS

Evaluation approaches provide a road map for systematically collecting, analyzing, and reporting information. Knowledge of differences in efficacy and effectiveness programs, process and outcome evaluations, and quantitative and qualitative evaluation approaches is needed to design an appropriate evaluation plan. Other approaches, such as systems analysis, goal-based evaluations, and decision-making evaluations, are not covered in this chapter.

Efficacy or Effectiveness Evaluation

Efficacy refers to changes in health outcomes of programs that are achieved under ideal circumstances. The health promotion intervention is implemented and evaluated under controlled or optimal conditions to demonstrate that the changes observed are due to the program or intervention and not to chance or other factors unrelated to the intervention. Efficacy is best demonstrated with research using randomized controlled trials.

The *effectiveness* of a program or intervention is the result it achieves in the real world, with limited resources, in entire populations or specified subgroups of a population. Effectiveness addresses the clinical usefulness of a program, as it is implemented and evaluated in a typical practice setting. Effectiveness can be demonstrated in research using randomized control trials as well as less rigidly structured methods.

Research designed to evaluate the efficacy of health promotion interventions is considered less applicable to the general population because the interventions are tested under ideal circumstances with a targeted group of clients. Efficacy studies test the usefulness of interventions. Efficacy studies are followed by effectiveness studies in which the program is applied to real-life settings for feasibility, costs, effectiveness in actual practice, and acceptance by diverse groups of clients. If the efficacy of a health promotion program or intervention has been scientifically tested, it can then be conducted and evaluated in practice settings.

Process or Outcome Evaluation

Process evaluation of a health promotion program refers to verifying the content of the program and whether it was delivered as intended, whereas *outcome* evaluations focus on the results of the program. Although the terms *formative, implementation,* and *process evaluations* are used interchangeably, some authors state that formative evaluations focus on programs that are under development, while process evaluations focus on programs that are underway. In this chapter the terms are used interchangeably. Process evaluations provide information to help improve the delivery of the program and define the needs and preferences of the targeted group or subgroups. Variations in delivery among sites and clients are identified as well as breakdowns between what was intended and what was actually delivered.

Process evaluations provide insights into what factors might hinder or facilitate achievement of program goals. Did the program fail because of a poorly conceived or designed intervention, or because of breakdowns in delivery? What contextual factors may have been operating to influence delivery of the program? Process evaluation also assesses whether the intended "dosage" of the program was delivered. *Dosage* refers to extent of participation in the program. Did the client attend all program sessions, or only half of the sessions? Dosage is important to track, as the amount of participation or exposure needs to be strong enough to produce the desired results. Ideally clients should attend all sessions. However, in the evaluation process, one may find that attending two thirds of the sessions is just as effective at promoting the desired outcomes. Process evaluations are necessary, as they offer valuable insight into the reasons for the success or failure of the intervention or program.

Outcome or summative evaluations focus on the results or changes brought about by the program, intended or unintended. The choice of outcomes to measure is determined by the program goals. If the goal is to achieve weight loss, weight should be measured prior to the program initiation and at the end of the program. If the program goal is primary prevention of cancer, clients should be followed for years to learn if and when cancer occurs. Outcome measurement enables one to evaluate if change occurred as a result of the program. In other words, was the program successful in promoting the desired change?

Outcomes may include short-term, intermediate, or long-term assessments of change. Short-term outcomes are usually measured immediately after completion of the program to assess the immediate impact of the program, whereas intermediate outcomes measure broader health and social outcomes. Long-term outcomes measure lasting or sustained effects of health promotion programs.

Quantitative or Qualitative Evaluation

The randomized controlled trial (RCT) is considered the gold standard to evaluate the intended outcomes of an intervention. Rigorously developed and precisely implemented interventions are typically evaluated with predetermined measures that can be converted to numerical (quantitative) information (data), such as questionnaires that assess changes in knowledge or health outcomes such as body weight. This information can then be analyzed statistically to evaluate the intervention effects. Although quantitative data is objective and provides evidence of the effects of the intervention, this objective information fails to account for the client's perspective.

Qualitative data represents a different perspective, as clients involved in the program are asked to provide input about the program. Information (data) may be obtained in individual or group interviews (focus groups). The recorded conversations (words) are then organized into themes or categories. This approach provides additional insight into the success or failure of the program. Qualitative approaches that include evaluation by multiple stakeholders are called *participatory evaluation* (Nitsch, Waldherr, Denk, Griebler, & Marent, 2013).

Qualitative evaluation approaches focus on the perception of the client, thus shedding light on nonhealth outcomes that may not otherwise be captured (Goebbels, Lakerveld, Ament, & Bot, 2012). Several nonhealth outcomes that have been identified with qualitative interviews include perceived self-awareness and motivation, and increased feelings of social connectedness and control over daily life. Although changing health outcomes is the ultimate goal of health promotion, nonhealth outcomes, such as empowerment, may help identify factors that lead to behavior change. Challenges in evaluating complex programs with multiple components have resulted in the use of multiple evaluation methods. Mixed methods evaluations incorporate both quantitative and qualitative data (Creswell, 2011). *Mixed methods* is an umbrella term that encompasses multiple evaluation methods. The premise of mixed methods evaluations is that no one method is adequate to evaluate a program, and multiple methods can be complementary. When using mixed methods to evaluate a program, issues to consider include how and in what sequence the methods will be implemented, and how the different types of information will be used to describe the program outcomes.

DECIDING WHICH OUTCOMES TO MEASURE

Measurement of the effectiveness of health promotion programs is necessary to determine the most relevant and cost-effective interventions. Choice of which health promotion outcomes to measure is dependent on the desired goals, the purpose and type of program, and the ability to access the information needed to measure the intended results. The challenge is to select outcomes that are comprehensive, comparable, meaningful, and accurate in reflecting the effects of the program. In addition, measurement of the outcomes must be feasible.

Nursing-Sensitive Outcomes

Although quality of care has always been a concern for nursing, quality improvement programs have focused on structure and process. The shift to effectiveness (outcomes) poses a challenge, as nurses practice in interdisciplinary teams in which health outcomes are influenced by more than one discipline. For example, in many health promotion programs nurses, nutritionists, psychologists, and exercise physiologists, may all be involved in implementing the program. The challenge is to identify and measure outcomes that are influenced by nursing actions.

Nursing-sensitive outcomes reflective of health promotion and community outcomes have been identified and published. Categories of these outcomes are summarized in Table 10–1. Biologic outcomes are the most commonly used and may include weight, skin-fold thickness, blood pressure, and blood laboratory values, such as lipid levels. Psychosocial outcomes measure patterns of behavior, communication, and relationships. Psychosocial measures may

TABLE 10–1   Categories of Nursing-Sensitive Outcomes

Category	Examples
Biologic	Blood pressure
	Weight
	Laboratory values
Psychosocial	Attitudes
	Emotions
	Moods
	Social functioning
Functional	Activities of daily living
	Mobility
	Self-care
Behavioral	Actions
	Activities
Cognitive	Knowledge
Home functioning	Family support
	Family roles
Safety	Noise-free environment
Symptom control	Smoking withdrawal
Goal attainment	Behavior change
Satisfaction	Program/service contentment
Costs	Cost effectiveness

include attitude, mood, emotions, coping, and social functioning. Functional measures include activities, mobility, and self-care outcomes. Behavioral outcomes involve the client's activities and actions, such as participation in regular physical activity. Knowledge, the cognitive level of understanding, is a common nursing-sensitive outcome because teaching is a major component of nursing practice.

Home functioning outcomes focus on the performance of the client and family in the home environment. Measures of this outcome may include family support and role function. Safety is a nursing-sensitive outcome, as nurses implement interventions to promote safe home, community, and work environments. For example, the nurse may work with clients in the community to promote a safe neighborhood environment with lighted walking paths.

Symptom control outcomes involve the management of symptoms. For example, health promotion interventions for smoking cessation may need to manage unpleasant symptoms associated with smoking withdrawal; or symptoms caused by unsuccessful health behavior change—such as depressive symptoms—may need attention.

Goal attainment outcomes refer to helping clients accomplish their health promotion goals, such as walking daily for thirty minutes or losing twenty pounds. Client satisfaction is a global measure of contentment with the services received. Measures of satisfaction or dissatisfaction with health promotion programs provide valuable information needed to make program changes.

The Nursing Outcomes Classification (NOC) is a standardized classification of patient–client outcomes developed to evaluate the effects of nursing interventions (Moorhead, Johnson, Maas, & Swanson, 2012). Seven categories have been identified: physiological health, functional health, psychosocial health, family health, health knowledge and behavior, perceived health, and community health. NOC is one of the standardized languages recognized by the American Nurses Association (ANA). Information about the NOC system is available on its website.

Health outcomes that reflect nursing's contribution to health promotion and risk reduction include lifestyle behaviors (dietary and physical activity behaviors), knowledge, attitudes, coping behaviors, biological changes (weight, blood cholesterol values, blood pressure), self-esteem, self-efficacy, and empowerment. Nursing's focus on positive lifestyle change and wellness places an emphasis on positive health-promoting behaviors.

Individual, Family, and Community Outcomes

Three categories or levels of outcomes can be measured: (1) individual or client focused, (2) family focused, and (3) community focused. These are described in Table 10–2.

Individual-focused outcomes measure the effects of health care interventions on individuals. These outcomes can be classified as biological or holistic. Biological outcomes are objective

TABLE 10–2 General Classification of Outcomes	
Category	**Types of Outcomes**
Client Focused	
Biologic	Physiologic measures
	Weight
	Body mass index
Holistic	Lifestyle change
	Functional status
	Perceptions
	Self-care
	Quality of life
Family Focused	
	Support
	Resources
Community Focused	
	Empowerment
	Participation
	Social capital
	Community health

physiologic changes in clients that reflect the effects of health promotion or risk reduction interventions. For example, a nutritional intervention may result in a change in body mass index or a normal triglyceride level.

Holistic outcomes are broad measures of behavior and health. Holistic outcomes include knowledge, lifestyle change, functional status, psychosocial functioning, perceptions, self-care, and health-related quality of life. Monitoring holistic outcomes is important in health promotion efforts, as these outcomes may be detectable before longer-term biologic effects are observed.

Family-focused outcomes have received less attention due to the challenges in measuring the contributions of family members. Family support can be assessed with published measures, as well as family cohesion and role functioning. The significant role the family plays in the development of both health-promoting and health-damaging behaviors, beginning at a very early age, is well documented. Other measurable outcomes include changes in family eating behaviors, such as a change in the frequency of shared family meals, changes in consumption of high-fat foods, or a change in leisure activity patterns, such as a change in the number of family activities that include physical activity.

Community outcomes are global measures in health promotion, as they focus on the effectiveness of the program at the community level. Community outcomes include community participation, empowerment, and changes in the community to support health promotion, such as biking paths and wellness centers. Community outcomes are measured at the neighborhood or group level. Broader measures present multiple challenges due to multiple factors that may be operating in the community to affect the program outcomes, other than the program itself.

Short-Term, Intermediate, and Long-Term Outcomes

Health promotion programs pose challenges for measuring outcomes, as the health outcomes may not been seen for many years. For this reason, different levels of outcomes have been described. An example of an outcome model for health promotion is shown in Figure 10–1. The

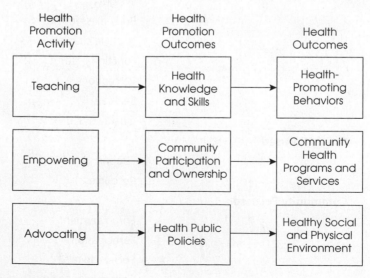

FIGURE 10–1 Outcomes for Health Promotion Activities

model differentiates health promotion (short-term) outcomes from health outcomes, which may not be evident for many months or years (Nutbeam, 1998). The model reflects outcomes associated with various types of health promotion programs.

The Centers for Disease Control and Prevention (CDC) has published a hierarchy of outcomes that also depicts levels of outcomes to measure, beginning with short-term outcomes, such as participation of the target audience (Centers for Disease Control and Prevention, 2006). The hierarchy, which is a mainstay for CDC public health program evaluations, is shown in Table 10–3. Lack of effectiveness of health promotion interventions may be due to measuring the outcomes at the wrong time. If information is collected immediately following the program, it may be too soon to capture desired changes in lifestyle behaviors. If the effects are measured many months after the program has ended, other factors may intervene

TABLE 10–3 Hierarchy of Potential Outcomes in Health Promotion

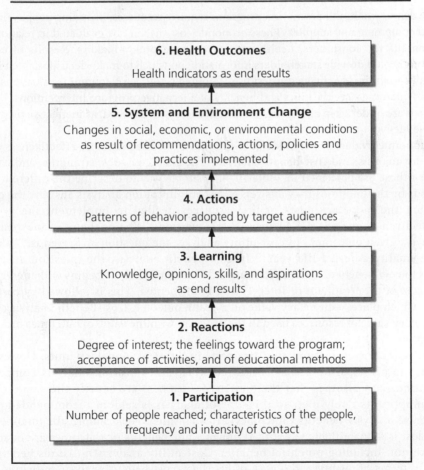

Source: Centers for Disease Control and Prevention. Office of the Director, Office of Strategy and Innovation, & National Center for Infectious Diseases, Division of Bacterial and Mycotic Diseases. *Introduction to program evaluation for public health programs: Evaluating appropriate antibiotic use programs.* Atlanta, GA: Centers for Disease Control and Prevention, 2006.

to influence the expected results. Therefore, the timing of measurement should be planned carefully to capture the anticipated effects. Measurement at multiple time points usually is necessary. Short-term outcomes are measured immediately following the program. Examples of short-term outcomes include knowledge, or a readiness to change. Intermediate outcomes are targeted at a period of time following the intervention when a change is expected to have occurred. Intermediate outcomes are measured soon enough to capture the effects before they may be due to other possible reasons. Intermediate outcomes are useful in reflecting attitude changes or attempts to change, although lifestyle change has not yet occurred. Long-term outcomes are the final or end results of health promotion programs. Long-term outcomes include such things as sustained weight loss, longevity, and improved quality of life. When measuring long-term change, it is important to monitor the potential intervening factors when interpreting the results.

Economic Outcomes

Effective delivery of health promotion programs requires resources, including people, time, facilities, and equipment and supplies. These economic costs need to be evaluated in relation to program benefits for consumers, health care payers, and policy-makers. Results of economic evaluations should provide stakeholders information on which to make decisions about investing in effective programs that make the best use of limited resources. Economic evaluations are used to quantify and measure the costs and benefits of alternative program interventions. Economic evaluations are undertaken after program effectiveness is established, as ineffective programs are not cost-effective.

Economic evaluations include cost-minimization analysis, cost-effectiveness analysis, cost-utility analysis, and cost-benefit analysis. The characteristics, strengths, and challenges of each of these are described in Table 10–4. A simple way to describe the different types of analyses is by the questions they answer. A cost-minimization analysis answers the question, "What are the monetary costs of the resources needed to implement the program?" Cost-effectiveness analysis (CEA) answers the question, "What is the most inexpensive way to achieve a given outcome?" In cost-utility analysis, the question answered is, "What is the cost per quality-adjusted life year?" In cost-benefit analysis, the question answered is, "What is the net benefit of a given alternative?" Economic analysis begins with merely reporting the cost of the treatment or intervention implemented. This is followed by cost-benefit analysis, which places a monetary value on a health outcome. Cost-benefit analysis compares the monetary value of resources used in the program with the value of outcomes produced by the program.

All economic evaluations measure costs in terms of monetary units. However, they differ in the principal outcomes measured. Cost-minimization analysis compares two interventions and assumes that the benefits (outcomes) are exactly the same. However, this assumption is rarely met, so this type of analysis is seldom recommended. In cost-effectiveness analysis, benefits (outcomes) are quantified. For example, the total number of pounds lost is a quantifiable benefit. Although some benefits or outcomes are quantifiable, many are not, including potential benefits. Cost-utility analysis measures benefits (outcomes) in terms of quality and length of life. Last, cost-benefit analysis measures benefits (outcomes) in monetary units. The issue arises when evaluators attach monetary value to such things as reduced need for health care. All types of economic analyses have potential limitations that need careful consideration when making an economic analysis. However,

TABLE 10-4 Key Characteristics of Common Economic Evaluation Methods

Type of analysis	Assessment of costs	Assessment of benefits	Characteristics	Strengths	Challenges
Cost-Benefit Analysis (CBA)	Monetary units	Monetary units	A method designed to value and compare all of the costs (C) and benefits (B) of interventions in equivalent monetary terms. It provides an absolute indicator of the "goodness" of the intervention. An intervention should be implemented only if B − C>0 or if B/C>1.	Makes it possible to compare programs that generate different types of outcomes — within the health sector and outside of it.	Difficult to assign a monetary value to the outcomes of the intervention. Ethical issues about assigning a monetary value to improvements in well-being of individuals must be resolved by evaluation team.
Cost-Effectiveness Analysis (CEA)	Monetary units	Natural health units	This method values the costs (C) in monetary terms, while benefits are expressed in natural health units or outcome of effectiveness (E). It allows comparisons among options with the same indicator of effectiveness. An intervention with a lower C/E ratio is *usually* preferable to one with a higher C/E ratio.	Comparison of health outcomes is helpful for health decision-makers. Interventions of same type competing for same resources can be compared.	Only interventions that have outcomes in the same measuring units can be compared. Limited to single dimension of effectiveness so it cannot capture the multidimensional outcomes of most health promotion programs.
Cost-Utility Analysis (CUA)	Monetary units	QALYs (Quality-adjusted life-years)	This method estimates costs in monetary terms and the benefits are expressed in QALYs (units that incorporate length of life and quality of life).	Can compare interventions with broad ranges of outcomes and from different sectors. Provides a common outcome measure so that different interventions can be compared. Can compare new programs with other programs that were evaluated with this method.	No consensus on the best method to evaluate quality of life. Many health promotion interventions have additional benefits beyond health gain. QALYs can be insensitive to small changes at the individual level even though those changes may be substantial at the population level.
Cost-Consequence Analysis (CCA)	Monetary units	Natural units (as in CEA) but not restricted to a single outcome	This is a modification of CEA. It sets out a profile of all important changes so that none may be overlooked.	It ensures that all outcomes of importance are acknowledged.	It can be difficult to determine whether an intervention is effective if some outcomes improve while others get worse.
Cost-Minimization Analysis (CMA)	Monetary units	None—outcomes are assumed to be the same	CMA just measures the relative costs of an intervention—the assumption being that outcomes are equal.	Simplest of all the forms of economic evaluation.	Rarely the case that outcomes are equivalent.

Source: Pan American Health Organization. (2007). *Guide to Economic Evaluation in Health Promotion.* Washington, DC: Pan American Health Organization.

nurses and other health care professionals need to show that health promotion is cost-effective and can save limited resources, so they should be considered when planning health promotion evaluations.

Several challenges are inherent in economic evaluations of health promotion programs. First, health promotion programs sometimes include groups that may not be representative of the general population. Second, health promotion programs and economic analyses are designed for different purposes. Economic analysis can also be time-consuming, and last, health promotion programs are often complex, while economic evaluations focus on single interventions with clearly defined outcomes. Broader outcomes of health promotion encompassed in the Ottawa Charter for Health Promotion (see Chapter 1), such as empowerment or nonhealth outcomes like self-awareness, are not easily captured, raising multiple challenges for economic evaluations.

Economic evaluations have begun to assume an important role in health care policy decisions. The approach has been standardized with principles and procedures for reporting the results. Regulatory bodies now consider cost-effectiveness part of the approval process for new medications and technologies. However, the analytic techniques are not simple and have many methodological pitfalls, so only individuals with expertise should conduct the analysis.

STEPS IN EVALUATION OF HEALTH PROMOTION PROGRAMS

Although the randomized control trial is considered the most scientifically rigorous way to evaluate health promotion interventions, alternative evaluation designs and methods are needed to shed light on the process and quality of change with complex health promotion programs in real-world settings. In community settings, traditional randomized controlled designs may not be appropriate. Control groups, for example, may not be ethical.

An alternative method for demonstrating program effectiveness is the Centers for Disease Control and Prevention's (CDC) Framework for Program Evaluation, which outlines the essential steps of program evaluation (see Figure 10–2). The comprehensive framework has become a template for program evaluation in public health because of its focus on planning, designing, implementing, and using the results of a program evaluation (CDC, 2012). Each step incorporates both planning and evaluation activities. Each step is briefly described.

ENGAGE STAKEHOLDERS.   Stakeholders include persons who have an investment in the program, including persons who implemented the program or intervention; clients who attended the program; the potential users of the results, such as community agencies; and agencies that provided resources. It is critical to engage stakeholders in the evaluation process as well as to assess their expectations. When they are not involved, the results of the evaluation may not reflect their needs and could be criticized or rejected.

DESCRIBE THE PROGRAM.   A clear description of the program includes an overview of the need for the program, the program goals, program activities, and expected measurable outcomes.

FOCUS THE EVALUATION DESIGN.   The evaluation should focus on the greatest concerns to all stakeholders. The type of evaluation design will be determined by the resources available and the time constraints of the evaluators. Any ethical and confidentiality issues need to be considered at this time. Both process and outcomes evaluations should be considered.

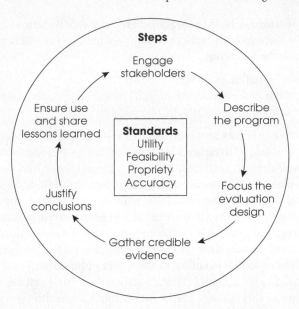

Steps

Engage stakeholders

Describe the program

Ensure use and share lessons learned

Standards
Utility
Feasibility
Propriety
Accuracy

Justify conclusions

Focus the evaluation design

Gather credible evidence

FIGURE 10–2 Framework for Program Evaluation *Source*: Centers for Disease Control and Prevention. *Framework for Program Evaluation in Public Health.* MMWR 1999; 48 (No. RR–11). Retrieved from ftp://ftp.cdc.gov/pub/Publications/mmwr/rr/rr4811.pdf

GATHER CREDIBLE EVIDENCE.   Prior to data collection, the kind of information (qualitative or quantitative) and type of data collection methods (questionnaires or interviews) need to be decided. All data should be obtained as rigorously as possible.

JUSTIFY CONCLUSIONS.   After all of the information collected is carefully analyzed, the results need to be presented as accurately as possible. The information should enable the evaluators to make recommendations for needed program changes as well as which aspects of the program were useful and effective in promoting change.

ENSURE USE AND SHARE LESSONS LEARNED.   Dissemination of the evaluation results is important and should include all stakeholders, as well as potential users of the program. In addition, the lessons learned should be used to improve the program. The information should be presented to a wider audience through written reports and publications.

The CDC website provides easy-to-use worksheets to assist with each step.

EVALUATING EVIDENCE FOR HEALTH PROMOTION PRACTICE

Current best evidence for one's practice can be obtained from many sources: a synthesis of relevant literature; international, national, and local standards of practice; cost-effectiveness analysis; clinical expertise; and client preferences. A literature search should be conducted to see if adequate information is available to evaluate the program. The literature (evidence) is critically evaluated and synthesized and then integrated into one's practice to guide health promotion decisions for clients. This process is called *evidence-based practice* or *evidence-based health promotion.* The aim of evidence-based practice is to reduce wide variations in practice, eliminate worst practices, and enhance best practices to improve quality and decrease costs. Evaluation questions to ask include the following:

- Can I trust this information (validity)?
- Will the information make an important difference in my practice (significance)?
- Can I use the information in my practice (applicability)?

Evidence-based practice involves an assessment of research-based evidence, identifying the clinical problem, conducting a literature search to find the best evidence, critically evaluating the evidence using well-defined methods, translating the evidence into one's practice, and re-evaluating the outcomes (Kelly, Morgan, Ellis, Younger, Huntley, & Swann, 2010, Melnyk, Fineout-Overholt, Stillwell, & Williamson, 2010). Table 10–5 reviews the steps to help establish evidence for a practice intervention. After an evidence-based practice change is implemented, the implementation process is monitored and expected outcomes are evaluated.

The evidence-based process does not replace clinical expertise, as the nurse must evaluate new knowledge in light of its applicability to the target population. For example, the clinical problem might be inability to promote physical activity in a rural setting and the potential of telehealth interventions in this setting. The literature about telehealth interventions to promote physical activity is reviewed to evaluate its applicability for clients in rural settings. Other considerations might include the sociocultural environment of the targeted population, prior experiences with health promotion in rural settings, and available resources. If the nurse finds that the evidence is applicable and relevant, plans are made to implement and evaluate the telehealth intervention in the new setting.

Adaptation of the program is often necessary when translating evidence-based research into practice. The program may need to be modified to accommodate the target setting or client circumstances. The setting may need to be supported throughout the implementation process. Program adaptation needs to be balanced with fidelity (agreement) to the original program, so monitoring fidelity throughout the implementation process is important (Bopp, Saunders, & Lattimore, 2013).

Current best evidence can be obtained from the Cochrane Collaboration, an organization committed to improving global health through systematic reviews of the effectiveness of health interventions. The Cochrane Collaboration's website is a valuable resource.

TABLE 10–5 Steps in Evidence-Based Practice

1. Select health prevention–health promotion area of interest.
2. Identify most effective intervention for defined area.
3. Tailor intervention to client.
4. Identify potential factors that may influence outcomes.
    Client characteristics
    Demographic factors
    Family characteristics
5. Select outcomes to measure effects of intervention.
    Short term
    Intermediate
    Long term

STRATEGIES FOR PROMOTING EFFECTIVE HEALTH PROMOTION OUTCOMES

Evaluation of results of health promotion has led to understanding program components that facilitate successful behavior change. Most research has focused on short-term change. Although knowledge about long-term maintenance of change—the last step in the change process of health promotion—is limited, several strategies have been identified.

Designing the Intervention

Theory-based, tested interventions provide greater understanding of how the intervention is expected to promote or change behavior. Theories describe the factors (concepts) that facilitate behavior change as well as suggest strategies that influence behavior change. For example, Bandura's social cognitive theory theorizes that people learn by observing and modeling others. Strategies documenting this relationship have been tested with intervention strategies such as demonstrating and modeling healthy behavior and helping the client learn skills to develop self-confidence (self-efficacy) to perform the behavior, such as cooking healthy meals. The choice of a theory or model is made by examining existing evidence and theory about behavior change. An understanding of the theoretical basis is critical to understanding what works for behavior change (Michie, 2012).

Health promotion interventions are complex and usually involve multiple components. Interventions that are complex may contain several interacting components that are difficult to change, such as weight loss and physical activity. When designing programs, the nurse first assesses whether the intervention is appropriate and feasible for the target population. If it is not, the intervention will need to be adapted to be culturally relevant or appropriate to the context. For example, a high-intensity community walking program may not be immediately appropriate for a sample of obese, older adolescents who live in a high-crime neighborhood. Feasibility questions to ask include the following: Are the facilities or other resources needed accessible in the community? Will the proposed program reach the intended audience? Will the program be acceptable to the intended audience? The program also needs to be affordable to individuals, agencies, or communities. A program that is too expensive will result in poor participation. If programs are too costly or resource intensive, community agencies will not be committed or will not offer the needed support. The program must also be manageable and compatible with existing programs in the community. Programs that are less complex and fit with existing programs have a greater chance of being successfully implemented. Evidence of the efficacy of the program should be available. If the efficacy of the intervention has not been tested, the intervention should be rigorously evaluated.

Selecting Outcomes

Program results should be evaluated with realistic, measurable outcomes. As mentioned earlier, the long-term outcomes of some health promotion programs may not be known for many years. In addition, community-level outcomes are complex and often very expensive. The outcome evaluation component needs careful planning so that outcomes reflect the purpose of the program. After a decision is made about which outcomes to assess, measures are chosen. Self-report measures, using paper-and-pencil questionnaires, are used to measure knowledge, attitudes, and self-report health behaviors. Objective measures are more precise and sensitive to change, and may include physical activity and dietary changes. Measurement of weight, for example, is a more accurate indicator of dietary change than is a self-report of eating habits. Community-level outcomes, although less well developed, also may be appropriate to measure, such as the number of new public physical activity facilities and walking paths or the number of restaurants that provide healthy choices. These broader outcomes provide information about how the program has improved the overall community, independent of behavior change of individual members. Outcomes that measure the client's perspective also should be considered. Although interviews may be time-consuming, the client's perspective may offer valuable information about the strengths and weaknesses of the program.

When long-term outcomes may not be realistic, assessment may include such things as program participation rates or client satisfaction. Although these outcomes do not measure effectiveness, they provide information about the acceptance of the intervention and its implementation. As discussed earlier, process measures are also useful to assess implementation effectiveness. Measurement of the "delivered dose," an assessment of aspects of the program that were implemented, and "received dose," the number of people who participated in the program, are useful aspects of process evaluation.

Deciding Time Frame

A realistic time frame is necessary to properly conduct the program and evaluate the results. What is realistic depends on the type, comprehensiveness, and complexity of the program and the target population. In an individual-focused intervention targeting a small group, six weeks may be a realistic period to implement and evaluate short-term results. However, five years may be needed to implement and evaluate a complex, community-based program in primary schools. The time frame should be acceptable to the target population or community as it may backfire if it is rushed or too long.

Sustaining Behavior Change

Most of the progress in health promotion has been in promoting health-behavior change; less progress has been seen in identifying strategies that sustain these changes. The current theoretical models of health behavior focus on how people decide to adopt health behaviors. Exceptions are Bandura's cognitive theory, which asserts that self-efficacy beliefs are a critical determinant of both the initiation and maintenance of behavior change, and Prochaska and DiClemente's transtheoretical model, which includes a maintenance stage. However, neither model offers detailed guidance about the process of maintenance and how it differs from initiation and adoption of behaviors. Programs that implement strategies based on change theories provide evidence for understanding the theoretical and behavioral processes that guide successful behavioral maintenance.

In health promotion programs, factors that have been shown to be associated with sustainability of weight loss include duration of the program, continuing contact or booster follow-up sessions, moderate to high levels of physical activity, ongoing self-monitoring of body weight and food intake (food and weight records), and self-efficacy. Ongoing self-monitoring has consistently been found to be effective in both eating and physical activity interventions (Akers, Cornett, Salva, Davy, & Davy, 2012; Michie, Whittington, Abraham, & McAteer, 2009). Interventions that provide ongoing support, such as regular telephone calls or mail, and ongoing self-monitoring and positive reinforcement of change, have been shown to be effective in promoting long-term (2 years) weight loss (Sherwood et al., 2013). The evidence reinforces the complexity of sustaining health-promoting behaviors and the need for continued professional support. These programs have documented changes in nutritional practices, physical activity, and weight loss for up to a year. Maintaining effective health promotion programs also is a challenge, as multiple issues influence the sustainability of a program over time. Sustainability includes helping clients maintain the health benefits achieved through the initial program, continuing the program long term, or building the capacity of the community to continue the program. Sustainability is influenced by the design of the program, implementation factors, facilitators and barriers within the targeted community setting, and factors in the broader community environment. Potential barriers include insufficient human and financial resources, lack of buy-in, reliance on volunteers, and inability to get the support of powerful persons in the community. Factors that promote sustainability include partnership formation, networking, and community capacity building (Hanson & Salmoni, 2011). Sustainability is facilitated when community capacity building has occurred and program goals have included long-term maintenance. Program sustainability is an ongoing process that is ever changing as new knowledge is gained. Building an infrastructure that integrates resources to support the program, beginning in the planning stage, is critical.

CONSIDERATIONS FOR PRACTICE IN EVALUATING HEALTH PROMOTION PROGRAMS

Health care professionals are mandated to base their practice on current research evidence as well as other factors, so it is important to understand the criteria used to evaluate the evidence. Courses that teach these skills can be offered in the clinical setting or through collaboration with local chapters of professional organizations or universities. Knowledge of the evidence-based process will enable nurses to accurately evaluate the literature and make informed decisions about the most effective programs for health promotion.

Knowledge of effective health promotion programs provides information on which to refer clients or deliver individual- or community-based interventions that have been most effective. An interdisciplinary approach has been shown to be more effective in the delivery of complex or community-based interventions.

Nurses in community settings are in pivotal positions to evaluate new models of program delivery. For example, telephone counseling and follow-up is a relatively low-cost intervention that can be effectively used to provide ongoing contact, social support, and expertise to answer questions, particularly in the elderly. Web-based health promotion interventions have shown positive effects on behavior change and are becoming a component of self-help interventions and follow-up. Program delivery using web-based technologies have a wide reach for delivery and follow-up of intensive interventions and provide tools for behavior self-monitoring. These types of interventions have special relevance for youth and individuals living in rural areas.

Maintenance continues to be a major problem in health-behavior change. Evidence supports the need for ongoing support and reinforcement for clients to maintain change. Follow-up of clients who have been successful in developing health-promoting behaviors is needed to provide ongoing support and to promote continued self-monitoring. Nurses can identify and evaluate helpful strategies through counseling and discussions with clients and their families.

OPPORTUNITIES FOR RESEARCH IN EVALUATING HEALTH PROMOTION

Evaluation of health promotion programs offers many avenues for research. First, it is evident that current theories of health promotion should be expanded or used in combination and tested, as most theories have not focused on long-term behavior change. Continuing research is needed to identify the determinants of behavior change as well as maintenance.

Second, accurate and sensitive measures of behavior change are needed to evaluate community outcomes. Self-report measures of behavior change should be developed that are reliable and valid and sensitive to both short-term and long-term change. Measures of behavior change that are easy to administer are needed to assess change in family behaviors and communities. Outcome measures also need to be standardized across studies of health behaviors, such as physical activity, to enable researchers and practitioners to compare findings.

Research to promote long-term maintenance has been limited. Studies are needed to answer such questions as these: "What factors promote successful maintenance of healthy behaviors?" "What factors contribute to preventing or promoting relapse?" "What are the greatest challenges encountered in maintenance?" Factors associated with maintenance of behaviors long term as well as factors that predict success in diverse populations across the life span also are avenues for investigation. Theory-driven research to evaluate interventions that promote long-term maintenance also is needed.

Summary

Evaluation of health promotion programs sheds light on what is most effective to promote wellness and behavior change as well as what does not work. Evaluation facilitates the development of a knowledge base on which to make decisions about programs that are most effective for behavior change. The evaluation process is complex, time-consuming, and requires advanced knowledge. However, learning to evaluate programs provides valuable information about the usefulness of individual- and community-based interventions.

Learning Activities

1. Select a health promotion intervention of interest, such as physical activity in the elderly, and, using the steps in Table 10–5, evaluate the literature and establish the evidence on which to base your planned intervention.

2. Develop an evaluation plan for a health education program to teach adolescents proper nutrition.
   a. What would you consider in designing the program?
   b. What factors will you need to consider when assessing the feasibility of the program for your population?
   c. Develop a process evaluation plan, describing how you will evaluate the dosage of the intervention received by the participants.
   d. Describe your outcome evaluation plan. Which outcomes will be appropriate to measure, and how will you measure them? Consider both short-term and intermediate outcomes.
   e. Describe the time frame you will use to evaluate the results of the program and the rationale for choosing the particular time points.
   f. What factors do you need to consider in promoting sustainability of the program?

References

Akers, J. D., Cornett, R. D., Salva, J. S., Davy, K. P., & Davy, B. M. (2012). Daily self-monitoring of body weight, step count, fruit/vegetable intake, and water consumption: A feasible and effective long-term weight loss maintenance approach. *Journal of the Academy of Nutrition and Dietetics, 112*, 685–692.

Bopp, M., Saunders, R. P., & Lattimore, D. (2013). The tug-of-war: Fidelity versus adaptation throughout the health promotion program life cycle. *Journal of Primary Prevention, 34*(3), 193–207.

Centers for Disease Control and Prevention (CDC). (2006). *Introduction to program planning for public health programs: Evaluating appropriate antibiotic use programs.* Atlanta, GA: Centers for Disease Control and Prevention.

Centers for Disease Control and Prevention (CDC). (2012). *Overview of the framework for program evaluation.* Accessed June 19, 2012 at http://www.cdc.gov/eval/framework/index.htm

Creswell, J. W. (2011). *Designing and conducting mixed methods research.* Thousand Oaks, CA: Sage Publications.

Goebbels, A. F., Lakerveld, J., Ament, A. J., & Bot, S. D. (2012). Exploring non-health outcomes of health promotion: The perspective of participants in a lifestyle behavior change intervention. *Health Policy, 106*, 177–186.

Hanson, H. M., & Salmoni, A. W. (2011). Stakeholders' perceptions of programme sustainability: Findings from a community-based fall prevention programme. *Public Health, 125*, 525–532.

Kelly, M., Morgan, A., Ellis, S., Younger, T., Huntley, J., & Swann, C. (2010). Evidence based public health: A review of the experience of the National Institute of Health and Clinical Excellence (NICE) of developing public health guidance in England. *Social Science & Medicine, 71*, 1056–1062.

McKenzie, J. F., Neiger, B. L., & Thackeray, R. (2012) *Planning, implementing, and evaluating health promotion programs* (6th ed.). San Francisco, CA: Pearson—Benjamin Cummings.

Melnyk, B., Fineout-Overhold, E., Stillwell, S. B., & Williamson, K. M. (2010). The seven steps of evidence-based practice. *American Journal of Nursing, 110*, 51–53.

Michie, S. (2012). Theories and techniques of behavior change: Developing a cumulative science of behavior change. *Health Psychology Review, 6*, 1–6.

Michie, S., Whittington, C., Abraham, C., & McAteer, J. (2009). Effective techniques in health eating and physical activity interventions: A meta-regression. *Health Psychology, 28*, 690–701.

Moorhead, S., Johnson, M., Maas, M. L., & Swanson, E. (2012). *Nursing Outcomes Classification (NOC)* (5th ed.). St. Louis, MO: Elsevier Mosby.

Nitsch, M., Waldherr, K., Denk, E., Griebler, U., & Marent, B. (2013). Participation by different stakeholders in participatory evaluation of health promotion: A literature review. *Evaluation and Program Planning, 40*, 42–54.

Nutbeam, D. (1998). Evaluating health promotion—progress, problems, and solutions. *Health Promotion International, 13*, 27–44.

Sherwood, N. E., Crain, A. L., Martinson, B. C., Anderson, C. P., Hayes, M. G., Anderson . . . Jeffery, R. W. (2013). Enhancing long-term weight loss maintenance: 2 year results from the Keep It Off randomized controlled trial. *Preventive Medicine, 56*, 171–177.

CHAPTER 11

Self-Care for Health Promotion Across the Life Span

OBJECTIVES

This chapter will enable the reader to:

1. Differentiate between self-care and self-management.

2. Contrast the focus of self-care in children and adolescents with young, middle-aged, and older adults.

3. Discuss the steps in the self-care empowerment process to promote health.

4. Describe the role of the Internet in self-care to promote health.

Professional nurses play a major role in enhancing clients' capacity for self-care throughout the life span. Nurses have long recognized the right of individuals and families to be informed and active participants in their care. Broad-based efforts to activate the general public for self-care must be a priority for all health professionals and community leaders. Activation of consumers to "take charge" of their health is based on the assumptions that consumers are willing to do the following:

1. Be actively involved in solving their health problems
2. Make rational, informed decisions about their health and health care
3. Develop competencies and skills that foster health and adaptation amid changing life circumstances
4. Strive for greater mastery over environmental conditions that influence health
5. Promote public policy to build healthy communities
6. Advocate for financing plans that pay for self-care education for all people

Individuals, families, and communities should be empowered for health promotion. Advances will be achieved when all groups work in concert to make health promotion a social movement that influences the quality and cost of health.

SELF-CARE OR SELF-MANAGEMENT

Self-care is a universal requirement for sustaining and enhancing life and health. Self-care directed toward health promotion can be defined as deliberate activities initiated or performed by an individual, family, or community to achieve, maintain, or promote maximum health (Orem, 2001; Richard & Shea, 2011). Care of self and others to maximize health includes actions to minimize threats to personal health, self-nurturance, self-improvement, and continued personal growth. Self-care approaches embody the notion of empowerment and autonomy. Active involvement in self-care is widely acknowledged as an important strategy for achieving national health goals. The government initiative, *Healthy People 2020*, emphasizes the importance of prevention and health promotion (see the *Healthy People 2020* website). Self-care is the basis for implementing health promotion and prevention strategies.

Self-care is considered a basic form of primary care. Engaging in self-care means taking responsibility for one's health and well-being. Self-care includes eating a healthy diet, being physically active, getting adequate rest, and avoiding harmful substances and environments, as well as other behaviors to enhance well-being. Characteristics of self-care include the following:

- It is situation and culture specific.
- It is influenced by one's social and physical environments.
- It involves the capacity to make choices and act.
- It is influenced by knowledge, skills, values, motivation, and self-efficacy.
- It focuses on aspects of health under individual control.
- It occurs independent of health care professionals.

Self-care and *self-management* are used interchangeably. However, they are not the same. *Self-management* is an individual's ability to detect and manage symptoms, treatments, physical and psychosocial consequences, and lifestyle changes associated with living with a chronic illness (Jones, MacGillivary, Kroll, Zahoor, & Connaghan, 2011). In self-management, an individual participates in activities to manage the illness, such as adjusting medication, eating special foods, or taking direct action, such as making a doctor's appointment. Clients and families assume responsibilities that previously were carried out by health professionals.

Self-care refers to individual responsibility to promote one's health and well-being, whereas self-management *focuses* on managing an illness. Self-management may be considered *shared care*, as health care professionals and clients work together to manage health conditions. In *dependent care*, individuals completely rely on health professionals with little opportunity for self-care. Self-care to promote health across the life span continues to gain significance as consumers become empowered and decrease their dependence on traditional medical care.

Consumer or patient activation, a concept that is similar to both self-management and self-care, refers to an individual's capability and willingness to manage his or her health and health care (Hibbard & Mahoney, 2010). Clients who score high on patient activation are more likely to engage in self-care behaviors as well as self-management behaviors. Activation is measured with the Patient Activation Measure (PAM), a scale that assesses self-reported knowledge, skills, and confidence necessary to be an activated consumer in both health promotion and health care decisions (Fowles, Terry, Xi, Hibbard, Bloom, & Harvey, 2009; Hibbard, Mahoney, Stockard, & Tusler, 2005). The authors of the scale have validated four stages in the activation process.

Stage 1: Clients believe that an active role in managing their health is important.

Stage 2: Clients have the confidence and knowledge to take action to manage or promote their health.

Stage 3: Clients take action.

Stage 4: Clients maintain the new behaviors and have confidence they can continue them under stressful situations.

Supportive social environments are precursors to activation, as individuals in supportive, less stressful environments report higher levels of activation and are engaged in more health-promoting behaviors (Hibbard & Mahoney, 2010). Ongoing research is beginning to shed light on how educational strategies can be tailored to each stage of activation, similar to tailoring strategies using Prochaska's stages of change. In addition, the role of gaining self-confidence and experiencing success in promoting effective self-care and self-management reinforces the value of focusing on self-efficacy described in Bandura's theory.

SELF-CARE AND HEALTH LITERACY

Self-care for health promotion requires that clients have the knowledge and competencies needed to maintain and enhance health independent of the medical system (Whitehead, 2011). An individual's ability to obtain, process, and understand information is essential to being able to make appropriate decisions for self-care. As described in detail in Chapter 12, limited literacy skills have been associated with less knowledge and skills, negative health behaviors, and less access to screening and preventive health services (Ferguson & Pawlak, 2011; Institute of Medicine, 2013).

The client's reading and comprehension levels should be assessed prior to conducting health education to promote self-care. Health literacy screening questions can be asked using available measures in the literature. (See Chapter 12 for strategies to increase health literacy.) Health information should be written in a language and at a level the client and all family members can understand. Interventions to promote understanding include the following:

- Simple, oral communication using lay terms
- Plain, culturally appropriate language materials
- Pictorial illustrations and models
- Audiovisual aids
- Group educational sessions
- Tailored individual sessions

Health literacy is an empowerment strategy that enables individuals and families to take responsibility for their health, as it allows individuals to gain control over the personal, social, and environmental determinants of their health. Health literacy skills enable clients and families to participate fully in health promotion activities and practice self-care behaviors to promote wellness.

Health policy-makers and health professionals must be sensitive to the extent to which problems of literacy and poverty present barriers to health education and self-care. Competent, literacy-appropriate self-care must also be economically feasible for individuals and families living in poverty. This requires coordination of public, private, and volunteer services to provide coherent self-care education and options for all age groups who are trying to change unhealthy behaviors.

OREM'S THEORY OF SELF-CARE

Dorothy Orem, a pioneer in nursing theory, began publishing about the concept of self-care in 1959 (Taylor, 2011). The theory continues to be tested and expanded and is reviewed briefly here, as it has relevance for self-care in health promotion.

In Orem's Self-Care Nursing Model, three types of self-care requisites are described: (1) universal, (2) developmental, and (3) health deviation requirements (Orem, 1995, 2001; Orem & Taylor, 2011). Universal self-care requirements include sufficient air, water, food, elimination, a balance between activity and rest, a balance between isolation and social interaction, protection from hazards, and protection of human functioning and development. Developmental self-care requirements fall into two categories:

1. Maintaining conditions that support life processes and promote progress toward higher levels of human structure and maturation, and
2. Providing care either to prevent the occurrence of deleterious effects of conditions that can affect human development or to lessen or overcome these effects.

Three concepts are central to the model: self-care, self-care agency, and basic conditioning factors (Orem, 2001). Orem's definition of self-care is similar to the one provided earlier in the chapter. *Self-care agency* refers to the complex capabilities needed to perform self-care, such as one's knowledge and skills. Self-care agency includes foundational capabilities such as memory, self-concept, and self-awareness; and power capabilities specific to self-care actions, such as motivation and decision making. *Basic conditioning factors*, which include age, developmental state, life experiences, sociocultural background, resources, and health state, are factors that influence an individual's self-care and self-care agency. Self-care activities are learned in everyday life. To promote health, nurses should focus on conditioning factors as well as health deviation requirements, such as knowledge and skill needs.

In Orem's model, individuals perform self-care to meet needs and demands consistent with their age, maturation, experience, resources, and sociocultural background. In her model, three systems are described within professional practice: a compensatory system, a partially compensatory system, and an educative-developmental system. In the *compensatory system*, total care is provided for the client. This can be considered self-management support or dependent care and is most common in acute-care settings, such as hospitals during acute illness episodes. The *partially compensatory system* of care is implemented when there can be shared responsibility for care (shared care). Care during rehabilitation from illness is partially compensatory. In contrast, the *educative-developmental system* gives the client primary responsibility for personal health, with the nurse functioning as a consultant or collaborative partner. The educative-developmental system is compatible with self-care in health promotion. Orem's model of self-care has been criticized because it is based on the assumption that individuals are able to exert control over their environments in the pursuit of health. However, many individuals and families do not have control over their physical and social environments, two components that influence health and health behaviors. Therefore, it is important to evaluate the client's context when applying the model to environments in which the ability to change factors may be limited.

According to Orem's theory, nurses, as self-care agents, design and produce systems of care (Banfield, 2011). Systems of care include health-promoting systems. Educative-developmental strategies for self-care in health-promoting systems include promoting physical activity and physical fitness; healthy eating; stress management; risk reduction; maintenance of social support systems; avoidance of high-risk and violent behaviors; and environmental modifications in homes, schools, work sites, and communities to reduce barriers to health. Education, counseling, and environmental interventions are a shared responsibility of federal government, state, and local governments, policy-makers, health care providers, community leaders, and individuals.

SELF-CARE TO PROMOTE HEALTH THROUGHOUT THE LIFE SPAN

Self-Care for Children and Adolescents

Children represent the potential for a healthy society. This population faces multiple challenges, as the assumption that school-aged children are healthy is no longer valid. The prevalence of obesity in industrialized societies continues to increase, and childhood obesity is a global epidemic with far-reaching consequences for the health of our nations (Ogden, Carroll, Kit, & Flegal, 2012). Childhood is a critical period for the adoption of healthy behaviors and a health-promoting lifestyle. Behaviors are developed and learned based on developmental level, social and physical environment, and family and personal experiences. Thus, health promotion efforts need to begin before unhealthy behavior patterns are established, as these early learned behaviors will continue into adulthood.

During childhood social and cognitive skills for autonomous decision making and health behaviors are developed. Health behaviors can be linked to family structure and support, family functioning and stress, and level of parental authority, as well as socioeconomic variables (Pelicand, Fournier, Le Rhum, & Aujoulat, 2013). The family environment plays a significant role in self-care for health promotion through positive, stable childhood experiences. A supportive family shapes the child's behavior through the use of rewards and punishment in behavior choices. Family role modeling of self-care behaviors facilitates the development of healthy behaviors such as physical activity. Socioeconomic status also plays a significant role in health behaviors, as increased socioeconomic status enables the family to provide resources, such as a safe neighborhood, a more affluent school system, nutritional food choices, and access to physical activity programs.

Parents exert influence over their child's health-promoting behaviors by serving as role models. For example, in families where one or two parents smoke, the risk of the child becoming a future smoker is increased. Programs that target parents as well as children can reduce high-risk behaviors such as tobacco use, sedentary habits, and unhealthy food choices. Parents can become positive role models by being actively involved in school-based programs with their children whenever possible to promote physical activity and healthy eating. Although it may be difficult to involve parents due to work and other commitments, flexible options for their inclusion should be available, as the success of these programs warrants the effort.

The family also influences eating patterns. Dietary patterns, such as regular breakfast eating, that are established in childhood and adolescence continue into adulthood. Eating breakfast regularly has been shown to have multiple positive effects. However, breakfast is the most frequently skipped meal in young people. Parental breakfast eating and living in a two-parent family have been shown to be associated with adolescent breakfast consumption (Pearson, Biddle, & Gorely, 2009). Adolescents in nontraditional families (single parent, step-parent, no parent) are more likely to display unhealthy eating behaviors such as skipping breakfast and lunch, eating fewer vegetables, and eating more fast foods than adolescents in traditional (two-parent) households (Stewart & Menning, 2009). Parents can role model positive behaviors, such as ordering healthy choices at fast-food restaurants.

Schools are critical resources for implementing health promoting programs. Traditionally, schools concentrated on the role of peer pressure in the adoption of self-care behaviors, rather than focusing on health in the curriculum. However, efforts have been expanded, based on research showing that targeted education can make a difference in adoption of healthy behaviors. Schools can reach many children and adolescents; have available personnel, such as teachers and school nurses, who can implement health promotion programs; have an organizational structure and facilities to incorporate healthy behaviors; and are capable of interacting with families and communities. Successful school programs teach self-care skills for healthy behaviors and include the family in programs to promote healthy living.

Strategies to reduce time in sedentary activities should be implemented in the home as well as in the school setting. For example, computer and television use time can be limited daily. Instead, family outdoor activities should be planned and fostered. Physical activities can be planned for recess times, and the physical activity time can be extended in schools. At both the family and community levels, physical activity programs are needed in neighborhoods that involve participation by peers as well as family members. Walking instead of riding should be rewarded, and parents should be encouraged to take regular walks with their children. Communities can map safe walking areas if school tracks are not available in the neighborhood. The walking school bus program for elementary children implemented in several states to promote walking to school is an example of a strategy to promote physical activity in children (Sayers, LeMaster, Thomas, Petroski, & Ge, 2012).

Adolescence is a critical period of physical, cognitive, emotional, and social development in a dynamic and uncertain period between childhood and adulthood. Developmentally, it is a time characterized by change and transitions. The primary biological transition is puberty. Cognitively, adolescents begin to think more abstractly. However, as children, they lack the ability to apply their cognitive skills to solving problems in stressful situations. The mismatch between biological and social maturity has implications for behavioral choices under stress, such as being pressured by peers to drink alcohol or experiment with illegal drugs. Socially, the family remains an important source of support. Parents can play a positive role in providing emotional support and encouragement and promoting healthy peer interactions, as peers also serve as a source of support and important role models. Beginning in the 1990s, health care professionals began to view adolescents as a resource to be developed instead of a problem to be managed. This has led to moving beyond a single focus on reducing adolescent risks, such as avoiding drugs, to also fostering resiliency or protective factors, such as family and peer support, to promote positive behaviors (Viner et al., 2012). Protective (positive supportive) factors counteract the effects of potential risks and are safeguards that increase an adolescent's ability to resist stressful life events. Developmental domains have been identified that can be targeted for positive self-care behaviors (Kia-Keating, Dowdy, Morgan, & Noam, 2011). Developmental areas include social, emotional, behavioral, cognitive, educational, and structural and can be described as either a risk or protective factor. Targeting the protective factors of these areas will promote positive qualities, including self-efficacy, optimism, self-determination, prosocial behavior, and positive identity for positive youth development (Hoyt, Chase-Lansdale, McDade, & Adam, 2012). See Table 11–1.

Adolescents are considered a high-risk group for engaging in risky and health-damaging behaviors, such as cigarette smoking, alcohol use, illicit drug use, early sexual activity, and physical aggression. Parental factors, including open communication, consistent monitoring and

TABLE 11–1   **Risk and Protection Behaviors in Development Areas of Adolescence and Their Relationship to Self-Care Outcomes**

Area of Development	Positive Elements of Youth Development Programs	Risk Behaviors	Protection Behaviors	Examples of Self-Care Outcomes
Social	Social support, sense of belonging	Alienation	Sense of belonging	Motivated to practice positive self-care behaviors
Emotional	Self-efficacy, resilience	Helplessness	Self-efficacy	Develops effective self-care strategies
Behavioral	Sharing and helping activities	Antisocial behaviors	Sharing behaviors	Participates in healthy self-care activities with family and peers
Cognitive	Perspective-building	Hopelessness	Hope	Practices goal-directed self-care behaviors
Educational	Competence-building	Disengagement	Engagement	Actively involved in regular healthy self-care activities
Structural	Structure and safety	Unsupervised	Monitored	Achieves health promotion self-care goals

control, and positive support, help to reduce these risks. The social environment of adolescents has an important influence on development of health-damaging or health-promoting behaviors. Connectedness to family and school is protective against developing health-compromising behaviors. Being connected to others promotes positive well-being, which has been associated with fewer risk behaviors and better perceived health during young adulthood (Hoyt, Chase-Lansdale, McDade, & Adam, 2012). Stronger connection in family and community contexts during adolescence also has been associated with greater civic engagement as young adults, including a greater likelihood of voting, participation in community volunteer services, and involvement in social groups (Duke, Skay, Pettingell, & Borowsky, 2009). The importance of parental factors reinforces the need for adolescent health-promotion programs with a parent component. Although these programs may vary in the amount of parental involvement, evidence continues to show that strengthening parent–adolescent relationships promotes healthy adolescent self-care behaviors.

Children and youth who have dropped out of school or are homeless need special attention in developing self-care behaviors for health promotion. Homeless youth do not benefit from family ties and depend on peers for support. Education sessions may have to take place in parks, food kitchens, or homeless shelters. Children of one-parent families as well as "latchkey youth" of two working parents also may require special attention. Special sensitivity to the lack of resources for daily living, lack of parental influence and supervision, and low levels of motivation because of life conditions is critical for promoting a healthy lifestyle.

Today, children enter puberty at an earlier age and take on adult roles at a later age than they did in the past, resulting in a longer time spent in adolescence, despite the traditional age of 18 years signifying adulthood (Sawyer, Bearinger, Blakemore, Dick, Ezeh, & Patton, 2012). The rapid developmental changes that occur for children and adolescents and the emerging behavioral patterns that will carry into adulthood make the preschool and school-age years a critical time to enhance skills for health-promoting behaviors. Many groups and persons influence the lifestyle behaviors of children and adolescents, including family members, peers, religious groups, popular entertainers, athletes, teachers, and other adults. Peer groups play a critical role in molding lifestyles for school-aged children, particularly adolescents. When peers reinforce the active health consumer role, peer pressure becomes a positive force. Parents serve as powerful role models of health and health-related behaviors. Approaches to enhance the health-promoting behaviors of children and adolescents should focus on families, peer groups, and the communities in which they live. The multiple approach is critical because values, attitudes, beliefs, and behaviors of families, peers, and the community context influence children's and adolescent's lifestyles.

Self-Care for Young and Middle-Aged Adults

Contextual factors that shape the health of young adults include a prolonged transition to adult roles and responsibilities and the weakening of the family support safety net. Young adults pursue multiple pathways, such as college, military service, employment, parenthood, and marriage. Each path has its unique set of role expectations and potential barriers to health. Many health problems peak during this period, including homicide, motor vehicle injuries, substance abuse, and sexually transmitted infections. University students frequently engage in unhealthy behaviors, including poor diet, little physical activity, alcohol consumption, and smoking. Although parental involvement diminishes during the transition to adulthood, evidence indicates that parental, community, and institutional support is needed to address the health behaviors of this group.

Young and middle-aged adulthood is the time in the life cycle when many young people are intensely involved in careers and child rearing. The momentum of everyday life and demands of dependent others may leave little time for focusing on health in the absence of an illness crisis. Strengthening support within the family for self-care is particularly important at this time. Young adults need to learn to accept responsibility for modeling and teaching children competent self-care by increasing their family self-care knowledge and skills and learning how and when to access health care resources for the family. Adult learners bring many assets to self-care education, including life experiences, self-direction, problem- or interest-centered (as opposed to subject-centered) specific learning needs, and interest in immediate rather than delayed application. Self-care education for adults should include the following strategies:

1. Provide time to express feelings.
2. Express a supportive attitude.
3. Reinforce client's self-esteem.
4. Provide access to health information.
5. Teach self-care skills that can be applied immediately.
6. Present alternative views on health issues.
7. Offer views about complementary self-care therapies.
8. Provide timely feedback and reinforcement.
9. Offer flexible learning pathways.

Adults who are aware of their own needs for self-care may be more effective in reducing the stress inherent in multiple roles, including family and work responsibilities. Systematically planning health-promotion activities into daily routines at work or with family members can both enhance health in a busy lifestyle and model healthy lifestyles to family members. For example, physical activities in place of watching television can be planned prior to dinner; or, if feasible, children can walk to school rather than be driven. Adequate attention to self-care during the young and middle-aged years promotes optimal productivity and life satisfaction and lays the groundwork for a healthy and productive retirement and old age.

Activities of everyday life shape and influence the health of family members. Family practices either promote or hinder the development of good health habits and well-being in children. Life transitions and traditional caregiving roles by women promote physical inactivity or lack of attention to their own self-care needs. Nurses should implement interventions that take into consideration family roles and demands, employment status, educational levels, cultural traditions, and available resources to promote self-care for healthy behaviors for partners and their children.

Self-Care for Older Adults

Older adults are the fastest growing population group in the United States. Research indicates that chronic health problems associated with old age can be prevented or postponed and controlled, and early death can be reduced with health behaviors such as not smoking, regular physical activity, and good nutrition (Ford, Bergman, Li, & Capewell, 2012). Physically active older adults maintain health functioning longer than do sedentary adults and report higher levels of subjective well-being (Garatachea et al., 2009). Exercise can enhance the self-esteem of older adults and, in some cases, decrease depression and anxiety. Physical inactivity is greater in older adults and continues to be associated with poor health outcomes (Seguin et al., 2013). Sedentary activities, such as television viewing or computer time, should be limited. Neighborhood environments that support walking need to be facilitated, including short walking paths, safe pedestrian areas, and parks. Psychological barriers such as loneliness and depression are common in the elderly (Bekhet & Zauszniewski, 2012). Health barriers may include limited mobility or vision and hearing difficulties. Regular participation in physical activity has the potential to reduce the burden of chronic diseases and disability and improve quality of life in this group.

Self-care for older adults focuses on maximizing independence, vigor, and life satisfaction. The ability for self-care is high for many older adults, and most function well. Personal autonomy, the ability to make self-directed choices, is important in older adults. The older person should be a partner in the self-care educational process rather than a passive recipient. Information should promote informed decision making and independence. Self-care education must also take into account the physical, sensory, mobility, and psychosocial changes that accompany aging as well as feelings of isolation, dissatisfaction, and helplessness. Personality and coping styles do not seem to change significantly with age. Thus, persons who develop positive coping skills early in life are able to meet social demands in later years, find meaning in life, and direct energy to appropriate self-care activities. Older individuals who have been characterized as information seekers have more effective health-promoting behaviors. Other patterns linked with health-promoting behaviors include positive perceptions of one's health and aging, education, social integration, involvement in groups and organizations, and contact with family members (Lyyra, Leskinen, Jylhä, & Heikkinen, 2009; Meléndez, Tomás, Oliver, & Navarro, 2009).

Retirement is a significant life event that presents major financial, social, and emotional challenges for the older population (Wang & Shi, 2013). The challenges are likely to be magnified, as the length of time an individual will live following retirement continues to increase. Employment is a fundamental role central to an individual's identity, so retirees may feel they have lost an important role if it is not replaced with new activities. Appropriate self-care in the form of anticipatory planning in the preretirement phase is associated with successful adaptation. Self-care actions that have been shown to facilitate healthy retirement include the following:

1. Plan ahead to ensure adequate income.
2. Develop friends not associated with work.
3. Decrease time at work in the last years before retirement by taking longer vacations, working shorter days, or working part-time.
4. Develop routines, including adequate physical activity, to replace the structure of the workday.
5. Rely on other people and groups in addition to spouse or partner to fill leisure time.
6. Develop leisure time activities before retirement that are realistic in energy and financial cost.
7. Engage in volunteer work in the community.
8. Assess living arrangements, and if relocation is necessary, take time to develop new social networks.

Although retirement is considered a positive life transition, a growing number of retired adults need to continue to work part-time. In addition, many Americans, age 60 and older, are delaying retirement, and the number of women over age 65 in the workforce is increasing faster than that of men (Burtless, 2012). For this group, self-care strategies to promote healthy lifestyles need to consider financial resources as well as limited leisure time. Retired adults often have more time available to pursue personal wellness than do younger adults. They should be challenged to use the time productively and counseled about resources available within the community to facilitate healthy behaviors.

The fastest growing segment of the population in the United States is the group aged 85 and older. Less than one fourth of persons in this age group live in nursing homes, so these individuals need safe, health-promoting communities as well as support services to assist them in continuing activities that focus on quality versus quantity of life. With adequate support from families, friends, and health professionals and access to resources, older adults are able to remain in their own homes throughout their old age.

Older adults are at risk for consuming inadequate diets and decreasing functional capacity due to decreased mobility. Physical inactivity may be due to lack of opportunities to participate in activities as well as lack of encouragement. Homebound community-dwelling elderly should be encouraged to go outdoors on a regular basis to maintain functional capacity (Seguin et al., 2013). Community-based interventions in senior centers are ideal places to promote physical activity and healthy eating behaviors. Physical activity programs that include chair exercises or chair yoga and promotion of walking improve physical function. Self-care ability in older adults has been associated with being physically active, not being at risk for undernutrition, and good mental health, so focusing on these health behaviors is critical in older adults (Sundsli, Soderhamn, Espnes, & Soderhamn, 2012). Health and well-being in old age depend on freedom from disease, adequate functional status, and sufficient social and environmental supports. Promotion of self-care activities to maintain and improve functional status includes strategies for safe mobility and prevention of falls, and activities that promote social functioning and social integration. All evidence to date indicates that the elderly can become physically fit. However, it is much easier to remain physically active if self-care behaviors are developed earlier in life.

Self-care for health promotion in older women needs attention because of different experiences of aging and old age in women. Women live longer than men and are more likely to live their later years alone with substantially lower incomes, more vulnerability to poverty, and more chronic health conditions than are men in the same age group. However, mortality in women has started to increase at a greater rate than that of men in some parts of the United States. Factors that have been identified for this increase include smoking, educational level, and area of the country in which a woman resides (Kindig & Cheng, 2013). Women are also more likely to have no or inadequate insurance coverage, resulting in barriers to health care. Unsafe environments and living alone are negative influences on the performance of health behaviors. Personal, social, and environmental barriers need to be addressed that prevent elderly women from being able to participate in healthy behaviors, such as fear of leaving the security of their home, lack of transportation, and inadequate financial resources. The socioeconomic conditions of the older person's residence also affect the person's participation in leisure-time physical activity. Low-cost interventions such as walking groups can be implemented in communities. Interventions that take into account the social context in which women live their lives, as well as their perceptions of their health and well-being must be incorporated into all health promotion activities.

THE ROLE OF *HEALTHY PEOPLE 2020* IN PROMOTING SELF-CARE

Healthy People 2020's ten-year agenda was introduced in 2010 to continue the national objective for improving the health of all Americans (see the Healthy People 2020 web site). Self-care is implicit in one of the four overarching goals, which is to promote quality of life, healthy development, and healthy behaviors across all life stages. In addition, new information is provided for early and middle childhood, adolescent health, and older adults. For both early and middle childhood and adolescents, the critical role of being connected to a parent or positive adult caregiver is explicit in the objectives. In addition, health education in schools is articulated in an objective as well as supportive and safe environment. The goal for older adults is to increase health, function, and quality of life, reinforcing the need to implement self-care strategies in this group. Increasing physical activity, a self-care behavior that is important for preventing mental and physical decline, is an objective for this group. Another relevant topic describes the role of community-based programs in the promotion of health, including programs that focus on injury and violence prevention, tobacco use, nutrition and obesity prevention, and physical activity. Health promotion activities can be developed and implemented in community sites, including schools, by nurses in collaboration with other health professionals, using existing facilities and resources. The user-friendly *Healthy People 2020* website has vast resources available to use in implementing these objectives.

THE PROCESS OF EMPOWERING FOR SELF-CARE

Empowerment is a process through which individuals gain mastery over their lives. The aim of health empowerment is to enable clients to take proactive actions to promote their health. Health empowerment has an intrapersonal dimension, or self-reliance through individual choice, as well as an interpersonal dimension. The interpersonal dimension may incorporate professionals or the community. Empowerment is embedded in health promotion, as both are based on the assumption that individuals have the capacity to bring about changes in their personal behaviors as well as their communities (Holmstrom & Roing, 2010). Characteristics of empowerment to promote health include the following:

- A helping process
- A partnership in which both individuals and health care professionals are valued
- Client decision making using resources, opportunities, and authority
- Freedom to make choices and accept responsibility

Empowered persons actively participate to promote self-care, are well-informed about the need to engage in healthy behaviors, are actively involved in decisions related to their health, and are committed to their health (Johnson, 2011). In the nurse–client relationship, empowerment is a process of communication and education in which knowledge, values, and power are shared. When individuals are empowered, they have the self-efficacy, knowledge, and competence to take proactive actions to reach their health promotion goals. Empowerment emphasizes rights and abilities rather than deficits and needs of individuals and communities. Characteristics of an empowering relationship include the following:

- Continuity
- Client-centered
- Relatedness
- Autonomy

In empowered relationships, health professionals are not in control; they are facilitators. Client choice, mutual decision making, nonjudgmental responses, and experiential learning are part of empowerment-based interventions. Self-care results when clients determine their own goals and the strategies to reach these goals.

The process of empowering health education for self-care is multidimensional and complex. The client brings a unique personality and learning style, established social interaction patterns, numerous group affiliations, cultural norms and values, proximal and distal environmental influences, and a level of readiness to adopt self-care behaviors. The nurse also brings innate personality characteristics, values, attitudes, and social circumstances that affect the nature of the interaction. Critical elements need to be considered in the empowering health education process. These include the following:

- Enabling the client to express concerns
- Promoting a partnership
- Providing information to facilitate client decision making
- Supporting autonomy
- Acknowledging cultural norms

The self-care education process as an empowering collaborative endeavor between client and nurse is depicted in Figure 11–1. The interaction for self-care education brings the professional expertise of nurses and other health care professionals together with the knowledge and goals of the client. Mutual assessment of health care competencies, strengths, and needs by the client and nurse will enable the client to prioritize the learning activities, set the pace of learning, establish long- and short-term goals, and identify any interpersonal and environmental support needed for learning. Barriers to learning and implementing self-care behaviors are identified by the client and directly addressed. Failure to identify and decrease barriers can result in frustration and a lack of progress toward self-care goals. For example, barriers to obesity reduction might include low

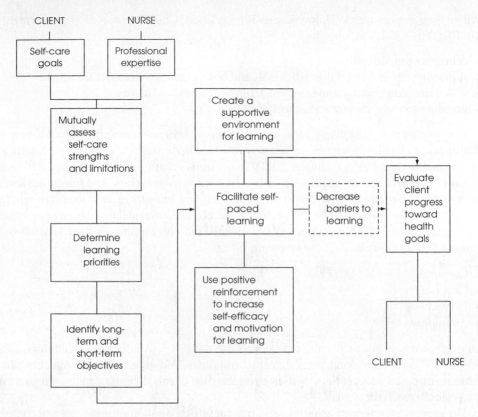

FIGURE 11–1   The Self-Care Education Process

socioeconomic status, time constraints, intimate saboteurs, and attitudes and beliefs. Lack of attention to these barriers results in a sense of failure, low self-efficacy, and low self-esteem.

Mutually Assess Self-Care Competencies and Needs

The client often comes to the encounter with certain self-care goals in mind. Competencies related to these goals can be assessed through informal discussion health-knowledge checklists (Table 11–2), or structured tests of knowledge in specific content areas. Informal discussions are recommended for low-literacy clients or individuals who are uncomfortable with paper-and-pencil tasks. Observation of actual behavior can also provide useful insights, if this is possible.

The activated client is motivated to seek health information that will assist in self-care. Apathy, lack of interest, and inattention should alert the nurse to a lack of motivation or low activation. Reasons for lack of interest should be explored so that strategies can be designed to increase motivation and activation for self-care.

Determine Learning Priorities

Deciding where to begin is often a dilemma when the client needs information about many health topics and behaviors. The empowerment process enables clients to make decisions about what they want to know and what is important to them. Sometimes their priority may not be the

TABLE 11–2 Health-Knowledge Checklist for Physical Activity

In the list below, check the behaviors that you are comfortable performing without assistance from others.

_____ Counting your pulse at the wrist for 1 minute

_____ Setting and reading your pedometer

_____ Selecting appropriate shoes and clothing for walking or jogging activities

_____ Planning a regular schedule of physical activity to meet your personal needs

_____ Indicating your ideal weight range for your height

_____ Calculating your maximal heart rate during exercise

_____ Planning time for physical activity that is convenient and realistic

_____ Selecting warm-up exercises that you can do before brisk walking, bicycling, or jogging

_____ Performing cool-down exercises after vigorous activity

_____ Participating in a physical activity such as walking at least five times a week for 30 minutes

_____ Maintaining a record of your physical activity progress weekly for three months

_____ Knowing what to drink and eat before and after physical activities such as walking

_____ Avoiding injuries during physical activity

area of greatest threat to personal health. For example, a client may smoke but be more interested in starting to exercise than quitting smoking. Although the nurse may believe that smoking constitutes a more serious threat than does a sedentary lifestyle, it is important that client choice be honored. If an exercise program is implemented, the client may develop a heightened awareness of the negative impact of smoking on lung capacity and physical endurance. At a later point, the client may exhibit readiness to discuss approaches to smoking cessation based on symptoms during exercise.

Identify Short- and Long-Term Objectives

Mutual identification of both short- and long-term objectives is important in self-care education. Long-term objectives guide large segments of learning. Short-term objectives identify the specific content or activities that must be progressively mastered to meet long-term objectives. The objectives should be realistic, not so easy as to result in boredom, and not so difficult as to cause discouragement. An example of a Goal and Objectives Identification Form is presented in Table 11–3. The form enables the client to check each objective as it is attained and maintain awareness of the desired behavioral and health outcomes. Both the nurse and the client should retain a copy for continuing reference and update.

Facilitate Self-Paced Learning

The pace at which clients learn depends on personal motivation, self-confidence, perseverance, skills, and learning styles. The pace of learning may also vary with age, health status, and educational level. Self-pacing is important to enable the client to be self-directed and maintain control over the learning process. The pace at which the client meets each short-term objective will vary, and expectations of both the client and the health professional should be adjusted accordingly. The important factor is not how rapidly knowledge or skill is attained but the extent of mastery.

TABLE 11–3 Goal and Objectives Identification Form	
Health Goal: Increased Physical Activity	
Long-Term Objective: To walk briskly for 30 minutes five times a week	
Related Short-Term Learning Objectives	**Objectives Attained**
1. Demonstrate how to check my pulse by counting beats for 10 seconds and multiplying by six.	
2. Read my pedometer steps and record after walking.	
3. State heart rate that I should achieve during walking.	
4. Demonstrate two warm-up exercises to use before walking.	
5. Demonstrate two cool-down exercises to use after walking.	
6. Plan a weekly schedule for walking.	
7. Map out three different routes to take when walking.	

The nurse must be realistic about teaching and learning and accept both good and bad days in clients of all ages. Sometimes the nurse and client will be elated with the results, sometimes discouraged. When efforts are less rewarding than anticipated, the pace of learning as well as the short-term objectives should be reviewed carefully and renegotiated. Focusing on resources rather than deficits and praising small steps are important to maintain motivation. Expanding the time frame for learning may also facilitate success. This is especially true for young children and adolescents, who have less experience in the learning process than adults have.

Use Autonomy Support to Increase Competence and Motivation for Learning

Persons are more likely to develop internal motivation to change or implement new behaviors when they feel supported and feelings of being pressured to change by others are minimized (Niemiec & Ryan, 2009). In education for self-care, the client, nurse, and family play important roles in supporting the client's autonomy. The nurse should be attuned to small steps in client progress and use positive support such as praise and compliments frequently to enhance feelings of success in developing competence in self-care. Specific information about the proposed change needs to be provided without pressure. Skills should be practiced, and immediate feedback is needed to correct errors in performance. When feedback is intermingled with autonomy support, it is helpful and nonthreatening and enhances intrinsic motivation. Immediate and consistent positive autonomy support facilitates learning and results in client satisfaction. After learning has occurred, intermittent support strengthens the behavior, making it more resistant to extinction. Autonomy supportive strategies include the following (see Deci & Ryan, 2012 for a discussion of autonomy support and self-determination theory):

- Use neutral language when offering a clear rationale for the new behavior, avoiding terms like "should" or "must."
- Provide a menu of options instead of only one way, if possible.

- Promote a sense of ownership of the change.
- Acknowledge the client's feelings and perspective.
- Focus on strengths, not weaknesses.
- Handle lack of progress or relapses positively and constructively.
- Remain neutral and avoid telling clients what they should do. Help them see what they are doing.
- Avoid criticism and judgment.
- Avoid pressuring language.

Family support without pressure or criticism is critical to successful behavior change. Family members should also learn to serve as sources of support for one another in developing health behaviors. For example, achievement of a specific goal may be rewarded by the family spending time together in a favorite activity. By providing mutual support, a sense of healthy interdependence rather than crippling dependence is created within the family.

Actual performance of new behaviors that lead to success is a powerful strategy to strengthen self-efficacy, as successfully performing the new behaviors promotes self-confidence to continue the behavior. Other sources of self-efficacy (e.g., modeling, observational learning, and verbal persuasion) can be learned during the educational sessions. (See the discussion of Bandura's model in Chapter 2 to review these concepts.)

Clients should learn to practice self-reward or self-support in the health education process. Self-reward of one's own efforts and achievements is important because much of the time support and reinforcement for self-care cannot be given by others. Rewards can be tailored to personal preferences. Use of foods or negative behaviors should be discouraged. Instead, such things as an outing with family or friends or a small purchase of a favorite item can be rewarding. Clients should learn to use self-praise and self-compliments. Learning to use internal self-reward in an appropriate manner permits the client to be less dependent on the availability of tangible objects to facilitate the learning process.

Create a Supportive Environment for Learning

The health-education environment for self-care is important for successful educational efforts. Classrooms should be warm, comfortable, and informal. Tables, chairs, and sofas should be placed in a conversational setting. Pictures and textured materials should be used to create a supportive and nonthreatening climate. Visual aids such as flip charts or bulletin boards should be at a comfortable height to use while seated in a chair. If very young children are present during the sessions, an area with toys and books may need to be provided for their use. This will minimize distraction of the parents. If children are old enough to be included in the sessions, they should be actively involved. Often, use of bright colors and interesting figures or designs on flip charts will amuse children and maintain their interest. Children can play an important role in reinforcing learning or in reminding parents and other family members to engage in the recommended behaviors.

To the extent possible, materials available in the home should be used in teaching. If a client is expected to use a booklet on low-cholesterol foods to prepare meals at home, the booklet should be the basis for instruction. If the client is learning relaxation techniques, audiotapes or videos for practice must be usable in the client's home. They should be demonstrated in the classroom and questions answered about their use. Well-illustrated materials should be supplied liberally to the client to take home to provide reinforcement of knowledge and skills gained during health-education sessions. Pictures are especially important for clients with low health literacy.

The minimum time span needed for most health instruction is 15 to 30 minutes. Either individual or small-group teaching methods may be used. Groups should be kept small (four to six individuals) to facilitate interaction and attention to the specific needs of group members. A combination of group and individual instruction often is helpful. A combined approach allows for efficient use of professional time yet meets the unique educative-developmental needs of clients.

Decrease Barriers to Learning

Barriers to learning can result from various sources: personal values, beliefs, and attitudes; lack of motivation; poor self-concept; and inadequate cognitive or psychomotor skills, to name a few. These barriers present major challenges for behavior change. For this reason, if the client is not making progress, personal and environmental factors should be explored. In addition, family barriers should be assessed and reduced or eliminated to the extent possible.

Strategies to manage obstacles to healthy behavior should be an integral part of the health-education plan. In this way, problems are addressed systematically, and progress in decreasing barriers can be periodically assessed. The client may be unaware of what is inhibiting progress or reluctant to share information. A climate of trust facilitates effective communication and enables the client to discuss perceived and real obstacles to learning and performance.

Evaluate Progress Toward Health Goals

Evaluation is a collaborative process by which the nurse and client judge the extent to which short- and long-term objectives and goals have been attained. Evaluation involves direct or indirect assessment of behavior change. Although the target behaviors may be observed during limited clinic or home visits, it must be kept in mind that this may not reflect actual behaviors. Self-report behavior change also is limited, as clients may not be completely honest, or they may ascribe a "halo effect" to themselves, seeing their performance as more frequent or more intensive than it actually is.

A combination of methods should be used to evaluate progress. These may include checklists of objectives, client daily records, laboratory results, paper-and-pencil tests, verbal questioning, and direct observation. The primary purpose of evaluation is to provide an accurate picture of the progress that clients have made in attaining their health goals. The desired outcome from self-care education is knowledge and skills to enhance self-care behaviors and promote a healthy lifestyle.

Other Considerations in Self-Care Empowerment

Each client's desire for change must be assessed. Some individuals do not want to be responsible for their own self-care but instead wish to function in a highly dependent role. Their desire for self-care competence may have been frustrated by prior health care experiences, which may have made them feel dependent and helpless. Before initiating a health education program, it is critical to assess the extent to which clients desire to assume responsibility for their own health when they are given the opportunity to gain the knowledge and skills to do so.

Culture, gender, and age also need to be taken into account when implementing the empowering health education process. In some cultures, it is inappropriate to question authority. Also, in some cultures women are unable to participate in a collaborative health care relationship.

In addition, older generations may view questioning authority figures as disrespectful. The nurse will need to identify cultural norms and plan self-care education within the client's frame of reference. Although these norms may limit the empowerment process, the process can be introduced through shared decision making and a supportive, nonthreatening environment.

Clients' conceptualization of health also will play a role in the type of content to share in self-care health promotion education. When health is defined as maintaining stability or avoiding overt illness, prevention behaviors such as immunization, self-examination for signs of cancer, and periodic multiphasic screening may be the priority. When health is defined as self-actualization or well-being, emphasis may be placed on physical activity, relaxation techniques, healthy eating, and other health-promoting behaviors.

THE ROLE OF THE INTERNET IN SELF-CARE EDUCATION

Health care costs and the shortage of qualified health professionals to deliver effective health promotion programs reinforce the importance of empowering individuals and families to take responsibility for their health and well-being. Internet and mobile device technology offer viable, effective, lower-cost options for delivering health information and self-care interventions to large segments of the population. Internet technology is now an essential part of everyday life. Millions of people today are seeking health information and finding self-help groups of people who want to learn from each other. Internet virtual communities fulfill the need for affiliation, information, and support. The potential of the Internet as a platform for self-empowerment through development of feelings of competence and control is beginning to be realized. Extensive information that traditionally was not available is now accessible on almost any topic. The information can be accessed at any time in almost any geographic location. This has important implications for persons living in rural or inaccessible areas, who are homebound, and who work. The quality of health information available is highly variable, indicating that clients need to learn to evaluate the information.

The Internet is still inaccessible to many who do not have adequate financial resources or lack computer or health literacy skills. The "digital divide" refers to the gap in computer and Internet access between groups based on income, age, and education. Emerging issues that will have to be addressed by this technology include the possibility of diminished involvement in face-to-face interactions with family members and friends, as well as weakening attachments to one's local environment with greater access to remote people and places. Privacy and confidentiality of information remains a major challenge as well.

A layperson usually leads self-help groups that meet online. These virtual electronic networks enable persons with similar health interests to converse and pose questions, provide mutual information and support, and minimize feelings of isolation. Nurses should share knowledge of effective programs and Internet sites that will strengthen their clients' role in their self-care.

Advantages of online self-help groups have been identified (see Chapter 9). These groups are convenient to access, and there is increased access of diverse members, including people in rural or remote areas. They provide access to peers with similar interests and issues, and the fear or embarrassment of public speaking is removed. In addition, lasting relationships may be formed. Disadvantages include misunderstanding that may result from text-based relationships; few controls to prevent erroneous information; absence of rules and guidelines; and ethical issues related to identity, deception, privacy, and confidentiality.

Mass education available through advanced technology is changing the way the public obtains health information and relates to health professionals. Young persons perceive the Internet as a primary source of information, not an adjunct to traditional informational modes.

Nurses should work to ensure that the information revolution is used to empower individuals and communities and is accessible to those who do not currently benefit because of poverty or ther social, environmental, and cultural conditions. In addition, health care professionals must monitor the content and quality of the sites they recommend. Last, formal evaluation of participants' health outcomes and satisfaction with information must be conducted. Formal evaluations will provide evidence of the effectiveness of this application to health promotion. Virtual communities may empower clients; however, the evidence is not yet sufficient.

Mobile technology also is gaining recognition as a platform for delivering personal health and disease management information (Mattila, Korhonen, Salminen, Ahtinen, Koskinen, & Sarelia, 2010). This technology is available 24 hours a day, and it is taken almost everywhere. Wellness Diary (WD), a personal application for wellness management, was introduced in 2010 to support self-observation and feedback. Health-related behavior, such as weight, physical activity, and alcohol consumption, is recorded, and feedback is automatically provided in graphic form. While users have found it easy to use and helpful in wellness management, shortcomings have been identified. These include the need to make it more engaging and motivating. However, the simplicity and mobility of this type of application is rapidly increasing, as design factors are being modified to support behavior change.

CONSIDERATIONS FOR PRACTICE IN SELF-CARE

The nurse's role as collaborator, facilitator, resource, and teacher has become more important than ever, as clients are asked to assume more responsibility for their health. Empowerment for self-care should be considered a priority of all health care professionals. Development of health-promoting behaviors at a young age and maintenance of these behaviors throughout the life span is critical. A multidisciplinary team approach is needed to implement health promotion programs in families, schools, work sites, and in community locations that are easily accessible. These programs should target the individual, the family, and social and environmental factors in the community that facilitate or inhibit adoption of self-care behaviors. Strategies that strengthen parental communication and support should be implemented to promote adoption of healthy behaviors in children and adolescents. The nurse can also work with school systems to include instruction for healthy nutrition and regular physical education. Opportunities should be created for after-school sports and other activities. Partnerships with community organizations are needed for children and adolescents as well as the elderly. Self-care education is complex. However, use of new technologies, such as the Internet and mobile devices, and active involvement of individuals and their family members in the educational process can help ensure the adoption of healthy behaviors.

OPPORTUNITIES FOR RESEARCH IN SELF-CARE

Although self-care has been practiced for centuries, it did not become the focus of research for health professionals until the 1980s. The theoretical work by Orem (2001) was the initial driving force in nursing for empirical work on the various dimensions of self-care and related nursing care systems. Opportunities for research in self-care include the following:

1. Develop and test new models of self-care that account for sociocultural and environmental antecedents across the life span.
2. Develop interventions to test the effects of self-care practices for preschool children.

3. Conduct longitudinal studies to describe the long-term health care outcomes of self-care behaviors in preschool children, adolescents, and young adults.
4. Develop and test health literacy intervention to increase self-care behaviors in low-income groups.
5. Test culturally appropriate interventions to enhance self-care empowerment among diverse individuals and families.
6. Conduct intervention studies to increase self-care health behaviors in community-dwelling older persons.

Summary

Empowerment for self-care emphasizes the competencies of clients for self-direction and self-responsibility in promoting and managing their health. Environmental constraints that impair self-care must be addressed and resolved to optimize client success. Education to empower and support autonomy enables clients to achieve their health goals. As a major resource, the nurse can enhance the client's success in becoming empowered by acquiring the needed knowledge and skills. Technology can play an important role in promoting wellness for individuals across the life span. Further research on self-care within the context of health promotion will provide important information for facilitating optimum self-care across the age continuum.

Learning Activities

1. Plan a preschool-based program that has parent involvement to decrease television or other screen time by children.
2. Develop a program to increase physical activity in community-dwelling, rural older persons, identifying and addressing potential barriers.
3. Design a program for healthy eating for adolescents using the steps in the empowerment education process to implement the program. Describe how you plan to evaluate the program's effectiveness.

References

Banfield, B. E. (2011). Nursing agency: The link between practical nursing science and nursing practice. *Nursing Science Quarterly, 24*, 42–47.

Bekhet, A. K., & Zauszniewski, J. A. (2012). Mental health of elders in retirement communities: Is loneliness a key factor? *Archives of Psychiatric Nursing, 3*, 214–224.

Burtless, G. (2012). Who is delaying retirement? Analyzing the increase in employment of older ages. In G. Burtless and H. J. Aaron (Eds.), *Closing the deficit: How much can later retirement help?* (pp. 11–35). Washington, DC: The Brookings Institution.

Deci, E. L., & Ryan, R. M. (2012). Motivation, personality, and development within embedded social contexts: An overview of self-determination theory. In R. M. Ryan (Ed.), *The Oxford handbook of human motivation* (pp. 85–110). New York, NY: Oxford University Press.

Duke, N. N., Skay, C. L., Pettingell, S. L., & Borowsky, I. W. (2009). From adolescent connections to social capital: Predictors of civic engagement in young adulthood. *Journal of Adolescent Health, 44*, 161–168.

Ferguson, L. A., & Pawlak, R. (2011). Health literacy: The road to improved health outcomes. *The Journal for Nurse Practitioners, 7,* 123–129.

Ford, E. S., Bergman, M. M., Li, C., & Capewell, S. (2012). Healthy lifestyle behaviors and all-cause mortality among adults living in the United States. *Preventive Medicine, 55,* 23–27.

Fowles, J. B., Terry, P., Xi, M., Hibbard, J., Bloom, T., & Harvey, L. (2009). Measuring self-management of patients' and employees' health: Further validation of the Patient Activation Measure (PAM) based on its relation to employee characteristics. *Patient Education and Counseling, 77,* 116–122.

Garatachea, N. M., Molinero, O., Martínez-García, R., Jiménez-Jiménez, R., González-Gallego, & Márquez, S. (2009). Feelings of well being in elderly people: Relationship to physical activity and physical function. *Archives of Gerontology and Geriatrics, 48*(3), 306–312.

Hibbard, J. H., & Mahoney, E. (2010). Toward a theory of patient and consumer activation. *Patient Education and Counseling, 78,* 377–381.

Hibbard, J. H., Mahoney, E. R., Stockard, J., & Tusler, M. (2005, December). Development and testing of a short form of the patient activation measure. *Health Services Research, 40*(6), 1918–1930.

Holmstrom, I., & Roing, M. (2010). The relation between patient-centeredness and patient empowerment: A discussion of the concepts. *Patient Education and Counseling, 79,* 167–172.

Hoyt, L. T., Chase-Lansdale, P. L., McDade, T. W., & Adam, E. K. (2012). Positive youth, healthy adults: Does positive well-being in adolescence predict better perceived health and fewer risky behaviors in young adulthood? *Journal of Adolescent Health, 50,* 66–73.

Institute of Medicine. (2013). *Health literacy: Improving health, improving systems, and health policy around the world: Workshop summary.* Washington, DC: The National Academies Press.

Johnson, M. O. (2011). The shifting landscape of health care: Toward a model of health care empowerment. *American Journal of Public Health, 101,* 265–270.

Jones, M. C., MacGillivary, S., Kroll, T., Zahoor, A. R., & Connaghan, J. (2011). A thematic analysis of the conceptualization of self-care, self-management and self-management support in the long-term conditions management literature. *Journal of Nursing and Healthcare in Chronic Illness, 3,* 174–185.

Kia-Keating, M., Dowdy, E., Morgan, M. L., & Noam, G. G. (2011). Protecting and promoting: An integrated conceptual model for healthy develop-ment in adolescents. *Journal of Adolescent Health, 48,* 220–228.

Kindig, D. A., & Cheng, E. R. (2013). Even as mortality fell in most US counties, female mortality nonetheless rose in 42.8 percent of counties from 1992–2006. *Health Affairs, 32,* 451–458.

Lyyra, T.-M., Leskinen, E., Jylhä, M., & Heikkinen, E. (2009). Self-rated health and mortality in older men and women: A time-dependent covariate analysis. *Archives of Gerontology and Geriatrics, 48*(1), 14–18.

Matilla, E., Korhonen, I, Salminen, J. H., Ahtinen, A., Koskinen, E., & Sarelia, A. (2010). Empowering citizens for well-being and chronic disease management with Wellness Diary. *Transactions on Information Technology in Biomedicine, 14,* 456–463.

Meléndez, J. C., Tomás, J. M., Oliver, A., & Navarro, E. (2009). Psychological and physical dimensions explaining life satisfaction among the elderly: A structural model examination. *Archives of Gerontology and Geriatrics, 48*(3), 291–295.

Niemiec, C. P., & Ryan, R. M. (2009). Autonomy, competence, and relatedness in the classroom: Applying self-determination theory to educational practice. *Theory and Research in Education, 7,* 133–139.

Ogden, C. L., Carroll, M. D., Kit, B. K., & Flegal, K. M. (2012) Prevalence of obesity and trends in body mass index among US children and adolescents, 1999–2010. *JAMA, 307,* 483–490.

Orem, D. E. (1995). *Nursing: Concepts of practice* (5th ed.). St Louis, MO: Mosby.

Orem, D. E. (2001). *Nursing: Concepts of practice* (6th ed.). New York, NY: Mosby.

Orem, D. E., & Taylor, S. G. (2011). Reflecting on nursing practice science: The nature, the structure, and the foundation of nursing sciences. *Nursing Science Quarterly, 24,* 35–41.

Pearson, N., Biddle, S. J. H., & Gorely, T. (2009, February). Family correlates of breakfast consumption among children and adolescents: A systematic review. *Appetite, 52*(1), 1–7.

Pelicand, J., Fournier, C., Le Rhum, A., & Aujoulat, I. (2013). Self-care support in pediatrics patients with type 1 diabetes: Bridging the gap between patient education and health promotion: A review. *Health Expectations,* doi: 10.1111/hex12041

Richard, A. A., & Shea, K. (2011). Delineation of self-care and associated concepts. *Journal of Nursing Scholarship,* doi:10.1111/j.1547-5069.2011.01404.x

Sawyer, S. M., Bearinger, L. H., Blakemore, S., Dick, B., Ezeh, A. C., & Patton, G. C. (2012). Adolescence: a foundation for future health. *Lancet, 379,* 1730–1640.

Sayers, S. P., LeMaster, J. W., Thomas, I. M., Petroski, G. F., & Ge, B. (2012). A walking school bus program. Impact on physical activity in elementary children in Columbia, Missouri. *American Journal of Preventive Medicine, 43*(5S4), S384–S389.

Seguin, R., LaMonte, M., Tinker, L., Lin, J., Woods, N., Michael, Y. L., . . . LaCroix, A. (2013). Sedentary behavior and physical function decline in older women: Findings from the Women's Health Initiative. *Journal of Aging Research,* doi: 10.1155/2012/271589

Stewart, S. D., & Menning, C. I. (2009). Family structure, father involvement, and adolescent eating patterns. *Journal of Adolescent Health, 45,* 193–201.

Sundsli, K., Soderhamn, U., Espnes, G. A., & Soderhamn, O. (2012). Ability for self-care in urban living older people in southern Norway. *Journal of Multidisciplinary Healthcare, 5,* 85–95.

Taylor, S. G. (2011). Dorothea Orem's legacy. *Nursing Science Quarterly, 24,* 5–6.

Viner, R. M., Ozer, E. M., Denny, S., Marmot, M., Resnick, M., Fatusi, A., & Curric, C. (2012). Adolescence and the social determinants of health. *Lancet, 379,* 1641–1652.

Wang, M., & Shi, J. (2013) Psychological research on retirement. *Annual Review of Psychology, 65,* 1, 1–25.

Whitehead, D. (2011). Before the cradle and beyond the grave: A lifespan/setting-based framework for health promotion. *Journal of Clinical Nursing, 20,* 2183–2194.

CHAPTER 12

Health Promotion in Vulnerable Populations

OBJECTIVES

This chapter will enable the reader to:

1. Discuss the social and economic determinants of health and their role in health disparities.
2. Describe the concept of equity in health.
3. Discuss approaches to address health inequities in diverse populations.
4. Examine strategies to promote health literacy.
5. Describe the continuum of interpersonal skills necessary for cultural competence.
6. Review strategies that facilitate culturally competent communication in vulnerable populations.
7. Describe approaches to ensure culturally competent health promotion programs.

Vulnerable populations are diverse groups of individuals who are at greatest risk for poor physical, psychological, and/or social health outcomes. Vulnerable populations are more likely to develop health problems, usually experience worse health outcomes, and have fewer resources to improve their conditions. Various terms have been used to describe vulnerable populations, including underserved populations, special populations, medically disadvantaged, poverty-stricken populations, and American underclasses. Vulnerable groups include persons who experience discrimination, stigma, intolerance, and subordination, and those who are politically marginalized, disenfranchised, and often denied their human rights. Vulnerable populations may include people of color, the poor, non-English-speaking persons, recent immigrants and refugees, homeless persons, mentally ill and disabled persons, gay men and lesbians, and substance abusers.

The values, attitudes, culture, and life circumstances of individuals who are poor, socially marginal, or culturally different from traditional mainstream society, and the communities in which they reside, must all be considered when planning health promotion and prevention activities. Taking into account the factors that reflect the health determinants of vulnerable populations is key to promoting positive health behaviors.

In spite of improvements in health and spending more money on medical care than any other nation, the United States ranks near the bottom on key indicators of health, and health disparities continue to persist, based on an individual's racial/ethnic background and socioeconomic (income and education) characteristics (Braverman, Egerter, & Mockenhaupt, 2011). Blacks, Hispanics and other racial/ethnic minorities are more likely to be socioeconomically disadvantaged, a more likely explanation for health differences by race and ethnicity. Health disparities are the differences in the incidence, prevalence, mortality, and burden of diseases and other adverse health conditions that exist among groups who are defined by certain characteristics. Health disparities disproportionately affect individuals who are members of the racial, ethnic minority, underserved, and other vulnerable groups mentioned previously, as well as persons who live in geographic (rural) areas where they are socially and physically isolated. Elimination of disparities to improve the health of all groups is an overarching goal of *Healthy People 2020*, and determinants of health and health disparities are included as outcome measures of the national health objectives. (See the *Healthy People 2020* website for details.) Although the major causes of health disparities need the input of society and government, development of empowering health promotion programs tailored for diverse individuals and communities is a major responsibility of nurses and other health care professionals.

DETERMINANTS OF HEALTH DISPARITIES AND HEALTH INEQUITIES

Social determinants of health are the structural and economic conditions in which people are born, live, work, and age (World Health Organization, 2013). These conditions are also responsible for health inequities and are shaped locally, nationally, and globally by economic distribution, social policies, and politics. In other words, money, power, and resources are responsible for the major inequities in health. *Health inequities* are avoidable *inequalities* in health between groups of persons that arise from social and economic conditions which increase their risks for illness and access to health promoting and preventive services. *Health equity*—the absence of disparities in health across populations, genders, and geographic areas—can be achieved by empowering individuals and communities to challenge and change the distribution of social resources and advocate for social policies for equal access for all.

Inequities in health are well documented and are considered to be the result of complex interactions among multiple factors:

- Biological variations
- Health care access
- Personal health behaviors
- Social and economic resources
- Culture

One way to view health disparities is by examining the range of risk factors that increase the potential for inequalities (Table 12–1). The risk factors include personal health behaviors, population characteristics, health care characteristics, the social and physical environments, and the types of diseases that are disproportionately diagnosed in vulnerable groups (Koh, Oppenheimer, Massin-Short, Emmons, Geller, & Viswanath, 2010).

TABLE 12–1   Range of Potential Risk Factors for Health Disparities

Potential Risk Factor	Examples
Personal Health Behaviors	Tobacco use, illicit drug use, personal hygiene, dietary habits, physical inactivity, unsafe sexual practices.
Population Characteristics	Race, ethnicity, immigration status, education, social position, occupation, employment, income, age, sexual orientation, health literacy.
Health Care Characteristics	Insurance, access to health care services, access to prevention and screening services, regular physician, medication affordability.
Residential Physical Environment	Housing density, housing quality, traffic density, air pollutants, hazardous wastes, drinking water quality, urban or rural, zoning policies, proximity to health care services, and proximity to quality food.
Social Residential Environment	Civic engagement, crime rate, isolation, neighborhood cohesion, neighborhood social capital.
Diseases	Obesity, hypertension, cardiovascular diseases, diabetes, mental illness, HIV/AIDS, cancer, respiratory illnesses, foodborne and waterborne illnesses.

The most important social determinants of health inequities are considered to be structural influences, or factors that generate and reinforce social stratification and social class divisions in a society and define one's socioeconomic position (Solar & Irwin, 2010). Socioeconomic position provides access to power, prestige, and resources and is based on a person's income, education, and occupation. Other important structural determinants include gender, social class, and race/ethnicity. These determinants are shown in the model in Figure 12–1 that describes the social determinants of health. This model was first drafted at the World Health Organization (WHO) Commission on Social Determinants of Health Meeting in 2005 (Solar & Irwin, 2010). The model depicts how governance structures or the sociopolitical context influences one's socioeconomic position through the distribution of resources. Socioeconomic position shapes intermediate health determinants. Intermediary determinants that are determined by socioeconomic position include the following:

- Material characteristics: neighborhood, housing, physical working conditions, buying potential
- Behavioral factors: nutrition, physical activity, tobacco use, alcohol use
- Psychosocial factors: stressful living conditions and relationships, social supports, coping resources

Intermediary determinants are reflective of an individual's place in the social hierarchy, which results in differential exposure and vulnerability to health-compromising conditions (Solar & Irwin, 2010). All of these factors determine one's health status and well-being.

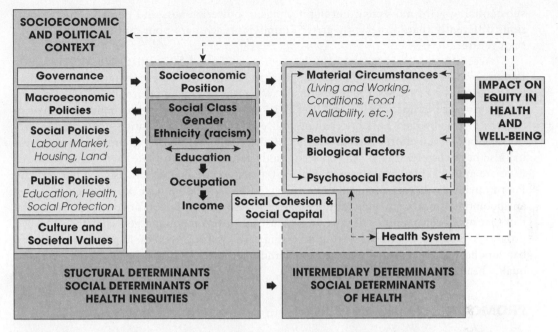

FIGURE 12–1 WHO Framework Describing Structural Determinants of Health   *Source:* Solar, O., & Irwin, A. (2010). A conceptual framework for action on the social determinants of health. Social Determinants of Health Discussion Paper 2 (Policy and Practice). Accessed at http://www.who.int/sdhconference/resources/ConceptualframeworkforactiononSDH_eng.pdf

Socioeconomic Determinants

The key components of socioeconomic position depicted have been substantiated to be the root of health inequities, measured at the population level (Solar & Irwin, 2010). Low economic status is the most consistent predictor of life expectancy, morbidity and mortality, and health status (Braverman, Cubbin, Egerter, Williams, & Pamuk, 2010). Although there is great diversity among minority populations, overall, minorities have substantially lower incomes and educational levels than do whites. Income is a powerful variable that explains health status. Low income and education result in economic hardship, such as the inability to meet one's living expenses, while higher incomes and educational levels facilitate access to care, better housing in safer neighborhoods, increased opportunities for healthy food purchases, and access to club memberships and health-promotion programs. In addition, low-status occupations expose individuals to physical health hazards. Educational attainment also is lower in minority groups. High-risk behaviors have been correlated with lower educational levels. More-highly educated persons are also more likely to obtain health-related information at understandable levels.

A socioeconomic gradient exists for almost every health indicator for every racial and ethnic group (Braverman, Egerter, & Mockenhaupt, 2011). The effects of low socioeconomic status are long lasting. Low socioeconomic status in childhood has been associated with poorer health in adulthood. The cumulative wear and tear of the adverse experiences of living in poverty, with its multiple challenges, results in chronic illnesses. Families who have been poor over several generations and suffer ongoing discrimination and frustration without substantial upward movement develop feelings of powerlessness and perceive their conditions differently than do recently arrived immigrants who are poor, but are hopeful about their future.

Access to care can be measured by the proportion of a population that has health insurance. Because of their socioeconomic situation, racial and ethnic minorities are much more likely to be underinsured or to lack health insurance. When they do have insurance, it is likely to be public insurance, primarily Medicaid. Health insurance contributes to the amount and type of health services obtained. Lack of health insurance has important implications for health promotion and prevention efforts, such as screening and access to wellness programs. Insurance status has also been correlated with self-reported health status. Those who rate their health as fair or poor are more likely to be uninsured than are those who rate their health as good or excellent. Poor individuals also experience greater barriers in accessing care, have more difficulty getting an appointment, and wait longer during health care visits. These factors are compounded by the fact that many communities of poverty mistrust the government and government-controlled programs. Socioeconomic barriers to accessing care exist for vulnerable populations. These barriers have been repeatedly documented and need to be addressed to improve access to quality health care.

PROMOTING EQUITY IN HEALTH

Achieving equity in health means that everyone has the opportunity to attain their full health potential, and no one is disadvantaged because of social, demographic, or geographic differences. Health disparities can be eliminated through the promotion of health equity, which minimizes avoidable differences between groups of people who have diverse levels of underlying social advantage (Braverman, Kumanyika, Fielding, LaVeist, Borrell, Manderscheld, & Troutman, 2011). The early literature on health disparities focused on racial/ethnic differences in health and "closing the gap"; however, "achieving health equity" is now more commonly discussed. Equity in health places emphasis on the multiple influences on individual and population health and draws attention to the many challenges that must be addressed. Promotion of health equity moves health promotion to a political activity, as it moves from the individual level to a broader focus on strategies to also change the distribution of social and economic resources (Raphael, 2011a).

Health equity can be achieved only through interventions that address the multiple health determinants:

- Social: networks, connections, institutional links
- Economic: money, time, prestige
- Sociocultural: skills, education, knowledge, language, religion, family background
- Political: power, distribution of resources

A study of the economic value of improving the health of less-educated American adults if they were to experience mortality rates and health status similar to those of adults with a college education was commissioned by the Robert Wood Johnson Foundation in 2007 (Schoeni, Dow, Miller, & Pamuk, 2011). In spite of limitations, results showed an annual economic value of $1.2 trillion. The economic burden of health disparities over a three-year period was estimated to be $1.24 trillion. Although these analyses do not uncover the causal pathway of education on health or account for costs in eliminating disparities, the results from these and other studies document the important role of socioeconomic characteristics in health.

Multilevel Interventions

Successful outcomes result from multilevel interventions and programs that are directed to individuals, communities, and social policies. Multilevel interventions address several factors to effect change in individuals and their socioeconomic context. Multilevel interventions go beyond individual-focused strategies to structural and socioeconomic influences to promote change (Trickett & Beehler, 2013). Multilevel interventions have been called *fourth-generation health disparities research* (Thomas, Quinn, Butler, Fryer, & Garcia, 2011). These types of interventions incorporate both qualitative and quantitative methods to implement programs and evaluate outcomes. They are complex, pose many challenges, and require input from multiple sources, such as interdisciplinary health care teams, community organizations, and local and state governments.

Community Empowerment

At the community level, empowerment is a key strategy for reducing health inequities. (See Chapter 11 for a discussion of individual empowerment and Chapter 14 for more discussion on community empowerment.) Community empowerment is a social action process that enables individuals, communities, and organizations to gain control over their lives within their social and political context to promote equity (Wiggins, 2011). It involves a shift in power between individuals and other social groups. Local community organizations empower individuals by working together to build trust and improve neighborhood programs. They also work with community members to advocate for new programs and resources for their neighborhoods. For example, they may work together to advocate for after-school programs for youth, parks for leisure activities for families, or increased law enforcement presence; or they may work to bring affordable health screening services to the neighborhood for those without transportation. Community agencies can advocate for local school board participation. In addition, they can empower community members to take an active role in promoting healthy and safe schools and neighborhoods.

Empowered communities believe in their capacity to change inequities and use that capacity to bring about change. Empowered community members feel a sense of community, which increases a sense of caring and support for each other and facilitates participation in change, such as working to obtain affordable housing, public transportation, safe walking places, and access to healthy foods. Empowered communities work with external powers to address community needs. For example, they may lobby and engage in policy decisions that impact the health of their communities. The ultimate goal of community empowerment is to create relationships and policies to promote health equity (Wiggins, 2011).

Focusing on working conditions, household and neighborhood hazards, and availability of community resources such as healthy foods and physical activity areas brings attention to environmental factors that can be changed within communities and work sites. Empowered community members can organize walking groups, community lectures, and health fairs. Community members need to be able to participate in decisions that influence their health and the health of the community. Empowerment means having a political voice to garner resources to change the community.

Community-based organizations (CBOs) are logical places to begin to bring about community change, as these organizations are enmeshed in the life of the community (Griffith et al., 2010). They are organizational sites where community members meet to socialize or address their concerns. CBOs are places where individuals can learn skills that empower them to address community issues. Leaders of CBOs can represent and advocate for the community. Empowering CBOs enables members to establish new projects and programs, as well as use their collective power to advocate for policy changes. Empowered CBOs are able to build community capacity, as they know the strengths, weaknesses, and availability or lack of resources within their community.

Community-based Participatory Research

Community-based participatory research (CBPR) is a method that integrates research with social action (Masuda, Poland, & Baxter, 2010). It is an effective way to build community capacity, as the method functions to transform power structures to create knowledge and promote actions for social change through community engagement. CBPR has been successfully implemented to expose power inequities in disadvantaged communities. This strategy enables community voices to be heard. Wallerstein and Duran (2010) have identified barriers to implementing CBPR and strategies to address these barriers.

Policy Advocacy

The socioeconomic and structural gradients in this country and their relationship to differences in health mandate that policies be created to address the social determinants of health inequities (Braverman, Cubbin, Egerter, Williams, & Pamuk, 2010). Canada, England, and Australia are considered leaders in implementing health-promoting public policies through legislation, fiscal measures, taxation, and organizational change (Raphael, 2011b).

Public policies influence the prerequisites of health in three key areas: early childhood development, employment, and income (Raphael, 2011a). Public policies to address these key areas have all been associated with lower rates of poverty and income inequities, Notably, the United States has the second lowest percentage of gross domestic product expenditures allocated in the form of public expenditures and the highest poverty rates in families and children among 21 selected countries (Raphael, 2011a). These rankings point to the need for policy to shift from a focus on individual health risk behaviors to the redistribution of economic resources to promote a healthy society for all.

Nurses and all other health professionals need to become knowledgeable about the political economy of health and public policy analysis to be able to advocate for health policies that promote healthy communities and equitable socioeconomic conditions. In community settings, nurses may become spokespersons for the poor in order for their voices to be heard. At the individual level, strategies to alleviate poverty include helping families obtain available benefits, providing information about available services and how to access them, targeting those in greatest need, teaching skills, and partnering individuals with community agencies to provide additional supports (Cohen & Reutter, 2007). At the community level, empowerment strategies promote community dialogue between community members, CBOs, and persons in positions to influence policies. Nurses can also work with their professional associations to place the elimination of health inequities on their agendas for action. Membership in organizations that promote agendas to reduce health inequities is another avenue for action. Political competence can be developed through courses and dialogues with knowledgeable others. Working in collaboration with all stakeholders enables nurses to raise awareness of health inequities, advocate for change, and take action, such as lobbying to promote change.

Primary Care

Primary care offers an effective mechanism for achieving health equity, as interventions are directed at individuals versus diseases. Primary care was established as a framework for health in the 1960s with the World Health Organization Declaration of Alma-Ata. It includes first contact and continuous, coordinated, decentralized care to address health promotion and disease prevention. Primary care is complex and requires community engagement and respect for individual and family viewpoints. It is an efficient, rational way to provide care for all people.

Investments in a primary care infrastructure have been shown to impact health equity. Primary care services in community health centers can reach socially disadvantaged, racial/ethnic minorities and isolated groups. Nurses are leading primary health care interdisciplinary teams and conducting community-based initiatives to promote community participation in health, provide health care and education, and advocate for communities. Primary care continues to increase in value with the passage of the Affordable Care Act, and nurses play a major role in promoting behavior change as primary care providers.

HEALTH LITERACY AND VULNERABLE POPULATIONS

Vulnerable populations are adversely affected by low health literacy, which has been associated with worse health status, poorer health knowledge and comprehension, increased hospitalizations and use of medical services, and decreased participation in preventive activities, such as mammogram screening and influenza immunizations (Berkman, Sheridan, Donahue, Halpen, & Crotty, 2011). In the United States, a third of the population is estimated to have limited health literacy skills. Vulnerable populations that are disproportionally affected include minorities, the elderly, individuals with less than a high school education, those who spoke another language prior to starting school, persons who do not speak English, and persons living in poverty. The importance of health literacy to understanding one's health care and having adequate knowledge to promote healthy self-care led the U.S. Department of Health and Human Services (USDHHS) to publish a national action plan to address health literacy issues (USDHHS, 2010). This document has brought national attention to the problem of health literacy and has been important in the development of strategies and programs to decrease health literacy. Health literacy is an empowerment tool, as persons with higher health literacy are able to access and analyze information to make better health care decisions, which results in positive health outcomes.

Medical Health Literacy or Health Literacy

Health literacy is considered to be a constellation of skills an individual needs to function effectively in the health care environment and act appropriately on health information. Multiple definitions of health literacy exist in the literature. (For a review see Sorensen, Van den Broucke, Fullam, Doyle, Pelikan, Slonska, & Brand, 2012.) A commonly cited definition of health literacy in this country is the Institute of Medicine (IOM) one, which describes health literacy as an individual's capacity to obtain, process, and understand basic information and services needed to make appropriate health care decisions (IOM, 2004). This definition was adopted by the Centers for Disease Control and Prevention (CDC). Other common descriptions of health literacy include medical health literacy, clinical health literacy, or functional health literacy, as health literacy refers to the skills needed to function in the health care system. These skills include basic reading and writing (*print literacy*), using quantitative information (*numeracy*), and speaking and listening effectively (*oral literacy*). Medical health literacy enables persons to read and understand health information such as specific instructions or prescriptions and consents, to make appointments, to complete medical forms, and to self-manage chronic conditions.

The World Health Organization adopted a broader definition, as it defines health literacy as the cognitive and social skills that determine the motivation and ability of an individual to gain access to, understand, and use information in ways that promote and maintain good health (Kumareson, 2013). This broader definition includes persons who are not in the health care system and indicates that individuals must have the knowledge, skills, and self-confidence needed to take action to improve their personal health as well as the health of the communities in which they reside. Within this definition, three typologies of health literacy have been identified:

- Functional: basic reading and writing skills to understand and use information
- Interactive: cognitive skills to interact with health care professionals, interpret and apply information
- Critical: cognitive skills to analyze information to be able to exert control over one's health

Clients with low health literacy need specific skills to manage their health effectively, including reading, writing, and numeracy skills, as well as the following (Frisch, Camerini, Diviani, & Schulz, 2012):

- When to seek health information or care
- Where to seek health information
- Verbal communication skills
- Assertiveness skills
- Skills to process and retain information
- Skills to apply information

Health literacy involves an individual's cognitive, emotional, and social skills outside the control of the health care system (Peerson & Saunders, 2009). Health literacy involves the ability to access information and use it in one's everyday life. Medical health literacy is more limited, as it focuses on the ability to read, understand, and carry out health care instructions. Vulnerable groups need to be taught health literacy skills to become empowered to navigate the health care system as well as participate in preventive and health-promoting behaviors.

Strategies to Promote Health Literacy

Addressing the literacy needs of vulnerable populations is a basic component of designing health promotion programs and interventions. Numerous resources for developing literacy and culturally appropriate messages are available on federal websites. In addition, the federal plain language guidelines are available online. These guidelines were written to support the Plain Writing Law of 2010 that mandates plain language usage in all public documents, presentations, and electronic communications. Plain language is a strategy for making information easier to understand. The key elements include the following:

- Presenting the most important information first
- Breaking complex information into small, understandable chunks

- Using simple language and defining technical terms
- Using the active voice

ORAL MESSAGES. Strategies for delivering clear messages incorporate plain language principles. Some of the major strategies to keep in mind are listed in Table 12–2. Messages need to reflect the age, language, literacy level, and cultural diversity of the target individual or group. Messages must be relevant to the key beliefs, attitudes, and values of the group, using familiar and acceptable language and images. Messages may need to be presented multiple times using narratives and visual illustrations to capture attention and reinforce content. Tailored cultural messages that use the client's personal information are more effective than standard communication. In addition, communication channels that are familiar to the client and are easily assessable are more effective.

CULTURALLY TAILORED MESSAGES. Culture influences how individuals understand and respond to information. For low-literacy, culturally diverse populations, only terms that the individual or groups are comfortable with should be used. Do not assume that all minority groups are alike. Consider the subpopulation and geographic location. Mexican Americans in the Southwest, for example, may respond differently from Puerto Rican Americans in the Northeast. Differences also exist within the same culture or ethnic group, depending on the age, gender, class, or religious practices. Collaboration with organizations in the participant's community enables the nurse to learn local beliefs and attitudes. If an interpreter is needed to convey information, someone from the same community who has experience in translating and knows the local language should be chosen instead of relatives or minors.

TABLE 12–2 Health Literacy Teaching Strategies

- Begin with warm greeting and welcoming attitude.
- Focus on specifically what needs to be done or known.
- Use plain, non-technical language and avoid jargon.
- Use terms and analogies that are familiar.
- Cover most important points first.
- Stick to one idea at a time.
- Clearly state what needs to be done.
- Repeat key points.
- Use pictures, illustration or demonstrate with models.
- Use teach-back method.
- Highlight the positive.
- Avoid long lists.
- Limit use of statistics and general terms.
- Invite and encourage questions.
- Avoid questions with yes/no responses.

Source: Dewalt, D. A., Callahan, L. F., Hask, V. H., Broucksou, K. A., Hink, A., & Brach, C. *Health Literacy Universal Precautions Toolkit*, AHRQ publication No. 10-0046-EF, Rockville, MD: Agency for Healthcare Research and Quality, April, 2010.

TEACH-BACK METHOD.   The "teach-back" technique is an effective method to assess and verify an individual's understanding of information provided during an interaction. This method goes beyond asking clients if they understand. Instead, they are asked to state or demonstrate how they will use the information. For example, after a demonstration that shows how to wear a pedometer and reset the steps, the client is asked to do the procedure. If it is not performed correctly, the information is clarified or another approach is implemented to teach the information. The client should practice until the skill is mastered, or the instructions are understood. It is important not to rush, and to remain patient and provide positive feedback with each step of the procedure or activity being demonstrated. Statements such as "Do you understand?" or "Do you have any questions?" are replaced with statements such as "Show me how you will do it when you get home" or "Tell me so I know you understand." This method has been shown to be an effective tool for pharmacists to verify understanding of medications (Watermeyer & Penn, 2009).

WRITTEN MESSAGES.   Written information should be attractive and easy to read. (See the federal government's plain language website.) Strategies for effective written messages include the following:

- Write specifically for your target audience.
- Use positive words and "must" when stating a requirement instead of "shall."
- Use a large font.
- Avoid using fancy script and all capital letters.
- Use headings and bullets and leave large amounts of white space between sections.
- Write short sentences.
- Avoid jargon, legal, or technical language.
- Present numerical information in tables.

Nonprint materials also can be used to communicate information. For example, videos are helpful for demonstrating procedures such as how to wear a pedometer. Pictures can supplement written or verbal information.

INTERNET MESSAGES.   Persons with limited health literacy are less likely to use the Internet and online health information, although this information may lower literacy demands through the use of audio, video, and graphic information (Sarkar, Karter, Liu, Adler, Nguyen, López, & Schillinger, 2010). As mentioned in an earlier chapter, this disparity is referred to as the "digital divide." Limited Internet use is thought to be due to absent or limited computer access, lack of computer training, and lack of skills or family support for skill building. These issues can be addressed with hands-on training and design features that facilitate navigation of the Internet. Other strategies include the following:

- Engage users with interactive content using plain language.
- Incorporate audio and video features and organize information to minimize searching and scrolling.
- Provide simple search options.
- Apply user-centered design principles.
- Conduct usability testing.

Usability is a measure of the user's experience and satisfaction in interacting with a webpage. Usability questions to ask might include the following:

- How fast can the participant learn to use the website?
- How fast can the participant accomplish tasks?
- Can the participant remember how to access the site the next time she or he visits?
- How often does the participant make mistakes?
- How well does the participant like the site?

Persons with limited literacy skills need opportunities to learn the skills needed to obtain online health information. They also need access to computers in public places within the community, such as public libraries.

Health Literacy Training for Health Professionals

Health literacy is a key component of effective communication between individuals and health professions. In order for health literacy to become an effective component of all health promotion activities, nurses and other health professionals need to understand and apply health literacy principles and strategies in their communication and in the design of written health information and websites. However, a gap exists between professional awareness of low health literacy and effective communication practices to address low health literacy (Coleman, 2011). Health literacy is not being adequately addressed in many nursing and health professional schools and continuing education programs.

An assessment is the first step to identify health literacy training needs. This should be following by training, which can be incorporated into orientation programs, didactic courses, and ongoing staff meetings. Health literacy skills can also be added to position descriptions in the work environment. One successful strategy that has been implemented with students is an interdisciplinary international program that combines service learning with cultural immersion (Smit & Tremethick, 2013). These programs provide opportunities for students to learn how to work with diverse cultures by practicing in diverse cultural settings.

At the national level, the United States Department of Health and Human Services (USDHHS) Office of Disease Prevention has responded to the need for information for health care organizations and professionals with a website that provides information and resources to learn about health literacy and how to implement health literacy strategies in practice. In addition, videos are available that show interviews with individuals to illustrate health literacy issues. PowerPoint presentations also can be downloaded to teach health literacy skills. The Centers for Disease Control (CDC) has an online course to teach health professionals and students about health literacy. Resources available on the CDC website can be used in workshops or small groups, or they can be reviewed individually.

The National Action Plan to Improve Health Literacy (USDHHS, 2010) is a framework for organizations to use to identify priorities, strategies, and activities for health literacy. The plan reinforces the critical role of health care professionals in improving health literacy and suggests learning strategies, which include participation in ongoing training and education in health literacy. Organizational assessments should be conducted with follow-up training and development, as well as implementation of policies to promote health literacy.

HEALTH CARE PROFESSIONALS AND CULTURAL COMPETENCE

Expertise in cultural competence and sensitivity to differences among cultures is a needed skill, considering the diversity of vulnerable populations and the number of interacting factors operating to create health disparities. *Cultural competence* is defined as appropriate and effective communication that requires one to be willing to listen and learn from members of diverse populations. It also includes the provision of information and services in appropriate languages, at appropriate comprehension and literacy levels, and in the context of the individual's health beliefs and practices. In culturally competent health promotion programs, the beliefs, interpersonal style, attitudes, and behaviors of individuals and families are respected and incorporated into all program activities. Culturally competent nurses continually adapt their practice to be consistent with the culture of their clients. Culturally competent health professionals are aware of their own cultural values and beliefs and recognize how these influence their attitudes and behaviors toward another group.

Continuum of Cultural Competence

Cultural–linguistic competence has been described by various authors, using a continuum of interpersonal behaviors. Bushy's (1999) classic continuum, which addresses individuals, ranges from *ethnocentrism* at one end to *enculturation* at the other end of the spectrum. *Ethnocentrism* refers to assumptions or beliefs that one's own way of behaving or believing is most preferable and correct and the standard by which all cultural groups will be judged. This view devalues the beliefs of other cultural groups or treats them with suspicion or hostility. *Cultural awareness*, the next stage on the continuum, refers to an appreciation of and sensitivity to another person's values, beliefs, and practices. Next, *cultural knowledge* refers to gaining understanding of and insight into different cultures. The continuum progresses to *cultural change* and then *cultural competence*, the level at which health care providers are aware, sensitive, and knowledgeable about another's culture and have the skills to conduct culturally competent health promotion activities. *Enculturation*, the final anchoring point, refers to fully internalizing the values of the other culture. Enculturation is evident when the nurse develops culturally sensitive health promotion programs in collaboration with individuals in the cultural group and incorporates members of the culture to deliver and evaluate the intervention.

A similar cultural competence continuum is used for health care organizations and systems in which services and care are delivered. It ranges from *cultural destructiveness* to *cultural proficiency* (Cross, 2011). The two continua are shown in Figure 12–2. *Cultural destructiveness*, the most negative anchoring point, represents attitudes, beliefs, and behaviors that are damaging to the culture and individuals within the culture. *Cultural incapacity* refers to cultural bias due to the lack of capacity to assist vulnerable individuals and communities. Agencies that are characterized by this dimension have patronizing and paternalistic attitudes, low expectations for minority groups, and may implicitly practice segregation and paternalistic attitudes. *Cultural blindness* occurs in uninformed organizations that may have the right intentions and may profess cultural equality and a philosophy of being unbiased. However, the system espouses the belief that the dominant culture should be universal and encourages assimilation, ignoring the other culture's strengths. *Cultural precompetence* refers to being aware of limitations in cross-cultural communication and relationships and having a desire to provide fair and equitable services. Although intentions are good, the system lacks the knowledge needed to implement culturally competent programs and services. These agencies may

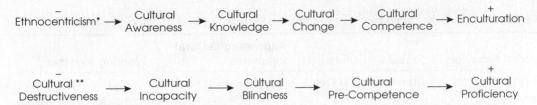

FIGURE 12–2 Two Continua of Cultural Competence *Sources:* *Bushy, A. (1999). Resiliency and social support. In J. G. Sebastian & A. Bushy (Eds.), *Special Populations in the Community: Advances in Reducing Health Disparities.* Gaithersburg, MD: Aspen Publications, Inc. **Cross, T. L., (2008). *Cultural Competence Continuum.* Accessed at http://pbsnetwork,org/up_content/uploads/2011/04/Cultural-Competence-Continuum, Accessed September 3, 2013.

pay attention to culture differences and begin to try to adapt practices that take cultural differences into account. *Cultural competency* is evident when diversity is valued and differences are respected and accepted. Systems develop awareness of cultural practices as self-assessments are implemented. *Advanced cultural competence* or *cultural proficiency,* the final anchoring point, occurs when individuals and systems are committed to culturally competent practice and hold cultural diversity in high esteem. System personnel have the knowledge and skills to implement culturally sensitive principles, and policies and practices reflect culture competence.

Developing cultural competence is not a linear process. Progress depends on attitudes, life experiences, exposures to other cultures, and receptivity to learning about new cultures. Progress also depends on institutional policies and practices. Acquisition of cultural competence skills is an ongoing process to ensure delivery of health promotion interventions that are appropriate, acceptable, and meaningful for persons of diverse backgrounds. Diversity is embedded in cultural competence, but it is just one component. Accepting and understanding differences in customs and patterns of thinking are ways in which diversity is valued.

These continua offer a mechanism for assessment of individuals and systems to facilitate designing training courses and workshops that are tailored to the level of cultural competence. Cultural competency programs have three essential components: awareness, knowledge, and skills (Hong, Garcia, & Soriano, 2013). First, awareness of one's own cultural beliefs, values, and biases is the focus. Second, cultural knowledge and life experiences of the other's culture as well as cross-cultural communication are taught. The third component incorporates the development of skills. These skills, including verbal and nonverbal communication skills, need to be practiced under supervision, using role-playing or other teaching strategies, such as videotaping, practice interviews, and client encounters.

Strategies for Culturally Competent Communication

Culturally competent communication skills build trust relationships with diverse clients. Trust is necessary to obtain valid information to develop interventions or manage issues of concern. The culturally competent communication model emphasizes verbal and nonverbal skills, recognition of potential cultural differences, incorporation of cultural knowledge, and negotiation and collaboration (Teal & Street, 2009; see Table 12–3). *Verbal skills* should reflect respect and empathy, nonjudgmental concern and interest, reflections, and follow-up questions. *Nonverbal behaviors* should also reflect respect, concern, and interest in the client's well-being. Skills include

TABLE 12–3 Culturally Competent Communication Techniques and Illustration of Their Use

Nonverbal Behaviors	Verbal Behaviors	Addressing Cultural Influences	Working Together
Be on time; don't rush. Be attentive; – Do not interrupt. – Indicate interest with body language. – Do not write notes during encounter. – Respect preferences for physical space. – Make eye contact but do not stare. Limit gestures. Show nonjudgmental expressions.	Communicate in client's preferred language. Address with client's last name unless asked to do otherwise. Indicate interest in client. ("Tell me about yourself.") ("How are you feeling?") Use nonjudgmental language such as "how," "what," etc. Reflect client's observed emotions. ("How are you feeling about your weight?") ("You seem sad, tired, frustrated.") Reflect what the client states about the problem. "Sounds like you think …") Summarize. Ask for feedback. ("Did I get that right?") ("What else do you want to talk about?") Invite questions about proposed behavior change plan. ("Do you understand or have questions?") ("Stop me if you're not sure what I'm saying.")	Assess causes of negative perceptions. Include others present in the discussion. Explore changes in client's life. Assess education and knowledge levels. Assess social factors that can influence ability for self-care (SES, family, living arrangement, stressors, literacy, language). Ask client's preferences for information and decision making. Ask for client's understanding of proposed plan. Acknowledge client's perspective. Invite questions ("Do you understand?" "Do you have questions?") Observe body language, facial expression that may indicate discomfort with plan. Use plain language consistent with client's education, knowledge, and health literacy level.	Assess client's priorities. Assess client's acceptance of the proposed plan. ("How do you feel about this plan?") Assess client's confidence in carrying out plan. ("Do you think you can do this?") ("What things or persons can help you?") Assess concerns and expectations. ("What worries you most about this plan?") Assess client's reluctance to commit to the change. ("You seem hesitant about making the change. Let's talk about your concerns.") Include family in making the plan. ("What else do you need to know that we haven't talked about?")

active listening and focusing on the client. *Recognizing cultural differences* entails monitoring potential cultural misunderstanding to prevent crossing cultural boundaries. Observing the client's reactions, asking for the client's perceptions, and exploring client preferences and understanding are useful strategies. Differences are acknowledged, and information and priorities are based on client input and preferences. Communication skills for *negotiation and collaboration* require awareness and adaptability to come to a shared understanding and agreed-upon priorities. Shared decision making is vital, as the client is a partner in a culturally competent communication model. Advanced communication skills and cultural awareness enable the nurse to avoid stereotyping clients and ignoring cultural issues. If the nurse is working with a translator, an additional layer of complexity is added. Translators must be both content and contextual experts who are using the client's local language. Translators should be immersed in the same native language and community as the client, if possible, and understand the dialect and context in which the words are being used.

In summary, health professionals must challenge their own practices and cultural values and develop effective culturally competent communication skills to avoid reinforcing stereotypes to be able to successfully manage client encounters.

Considerations in Designing Culturally Competent Programs

Assessment of characteristics of vulnerable populations that may affect successful health promotion is the first step to achieving goals established in partnership. These factors include demographic, cultural, and health care system variables.

Because language is an obvious demographic difference among diverse groups, knowledge of the language spoken is a key feature in the delivery of programs. Inability to communicate in the dominant language creates barriers in accessing programs and health care. It may also result in errors and/or inappropriate care. Even in some English-speaking minority clients, communication may be problematic, as clients may not fully understand the information and may avoid further verbal communication to get their questions answered. The National Institutes of Health Office of Minority Health's national standards for culturally and linguistically appropriate services (CLAS) address the need to offer language assistance services, including interpreters, and to offer verbal and written notices of clients' rights in their preferred language. These standards can be accessed at their website.

Geographic location is another major factor to consider, as the physical environment plays a significant role in promoting healthy behaviors. Poor urban neighborhoods are associated with areas that are unsafe. Research on "walkability" indicates that attractive, aesthetically pleasing settings are more conducive to physical activity. Fear due to drug sales or violence may be a major factor in limiting outside activities. Poor neighborhoods have fewer services available, such as clinics or community centers and public transportation. In addition, limited grocery stores result in higher prices paid for fresh fruits and vegetables that may be scarce and of lesser quality.

Cultural factors that may affect the success of health education also should be identified. Social customs and norms—including touching, shaking hands, eye contact, and smiling—may have different connotations. Religious or spiritual practices also need to be considered. For example, prayer and chanting, dancing rituals, and purification ceremonies are important in the Native American culture to reestablish harmony in one's physical, mental, and spiritual life. The cultural, religious, or spiritual framework must be respected in the health promotion encounter.

Communication, body language, and word meanings vary across cultures. In low-literacy groups, abstract concepts may not be understood, so traditional written communication is not appropriate. Health promotion programs are more successful when they are delivered in the language of the participants. Persons who represent the target culture and speak the same language should be involved in developing and implementing the intervention. In addition, culturally specific newspapers and radio and television stations can be targeted to deliver health messages in the appropriate language.

Family relationships and the concept of family also differ across cultures. In some cultural groups, the family is an extension of the individual. It is also common for the family to include more than the immediate relatives. Traditionally, the needs of the family have had priority over the needs of the individual in some cultures, such as Asians and Hispanics. In these groups, support from family members is more important than external support, so family members should be intimately involved to support the individual and participate in the interventions and programs. Family-oriented approaches, using family and extended family networks, are more likely to be successful in behavior change in African American and Hispanic cultures. In cultures in which the woman's role is subordinate, the value of the behavior change of the woman for the entire family needs to be emphasized. Family networks may also include church relationships, as they offer social support and communication networks. In these cultures, the church is an effective place to implement health-promotion programs. Educational strategies should capitalize on the powerful effects of family networks to promote behavior change.

Time orientation refers to how the perception of time varies among cultures. A present orientation is common in vulnerable populations, as the focus is on surviving in the present, so the future may have less meaning. Vulnerable persons with a present orientation have more difficulty changing behaviors, as current, day-to-day needs take priority. Knowledge of an individual or culture's dominant time orientation as well as values related to "clock" time helps to eliminate misunderstandings, such as missed appointments or tardiness.

Health care system factors also are important to assess prior to health promotion efforts. Vulnerable populations have problems accessing care and participating in health-promoting programs due to costs, distance, transportation, and language. Missed appointments or program sessions may not mean that the individual is not interested. Transportation or child care may not be available, or bilingual support may be inadequate. Program acceptance depends on multiple factors, including lack of trust, prior interactions with health care providers, and a failure to incorporate the client's cultural values. Culturally sensitive approaches enhance access and acceptance of health interventions. Focus group or individual interviews in the target community may reveal missed culturally relevant information on which to base interventions. Community priorities and availability of community resources also should be identified. Churches or other sites within the community should be used whenever possible to facilitate easy access as well as offer a familiar environment. The Office of Minority Health Resources Center's standards for culturally and linguistically appropriate health care services are relevant for the delivery of health promotion programs. These are summarized in Table 12–4.

Strategies for Culturally Competent Interventions

Strategies to make health promotion programs and materials more culturally appropriate are available. These strategies can be classified into six categories: (1) peripheral, (2) evidential, (3) linguistic, (4) constituent involving, (5) sociocultural, and (6) cultural tailoring.

TABLE 12–4   Recommended Standards for Culturally Appropriate Health Promotion Programs

1. Acquire the attitudes, behaviors, knowledge and skills needed to work respectfully and effectively with individuals in a culturally diverse environment.
2. Use formal mechanisms to involve communities in the design and implementation of health promotion programs.
3. Develop strategies to recruit and retain culturally competent staff who are qualified to address the health promotion needs of the racial and ethnic communities.
4. Provide ongoing education and training in culturally and linguistically competent program delivery.
5. Provide all participants with limited English proficiency programs conducted in their primary language.
6. Translate and make available signage and commonly used written educational material.
7. Ensure that the participants' birthplace, religion, cultural dietary patterns, and self-identified race-ethnicity are documented.
8. Undertake assessments of cultural competence, integrating measures of satisfaction, quality and outcomes of health promotion programs.

Source: Reprinted from *Public Health Reports*, 115, D. Chin, "Culturally Competent Health Care," 25–33, Copyright 2000, with permission from Royal Institute of Public Health.

Peripheral strategies involve packaging programs or materials to reflect the target culture. Colors, images, pictures, or titles are used to reflect the social and cultural world of the targeted group. Thus, the information is viewed as familiar and comfortable. Materials that are matched to one's culture also help establish credibility and create interest, increasing acceptance and receptivity of the information.

Evidential strategies are those used to present information in a way that increases the perceived relevance of the topic for the specific cultural group. For example, provision of information on the prevalence of diabetes has been used to raise awareness to promote lifestyle change in high-risk groups. The message becomes more meaningful when it is perceived to be directly applicable to those receiving the message.

When materials and programs are provided in the cultural group's dominant language, *linguistic* strategies are applied. Strategies, such as translating materials or delivering the program in the target culture's native language, are essential. Guidelines are available for translating information from one language to another.

Constituent-involving strategies are implemented to capitalize on the experiences of those within the target population. For example, using peers or lay helpers, as well as professional members of the target population, facilitates culturally competent teaching. Lay health advisors serve as role models and advocate for community members. They have been used extensively in the Hispanic/Latino community to eliminate health disparities.

Sociocultural strategies build on the group's values and beliefs. Implementing sociocultural strategies facilitates the cultural meaningfulness of the material or programs. For example, interventions to change dietary behaviors for African Americans may be more successful when the beauty salon or barber shop is used, as these places have meaning and familiarity. Programs that are culturally meaningful and delivered in familiar locations have been shown to be more effective to change behavior in vulnerable populations.

Cultural tailoring strategies are any combination of change strategies intended to reach an individual based on characteristics unique to that person. Targeted strategies differ from tailored strategies; the group is the focus when targeted strategies are used. Both targeted and tailoring strategies are important. When individual differences are small, the group can be the major target. When unique individual differences are evident, cultural tailoring strategies that focus on the individual are needed.

In summary, multiple strategies facilitate the development and implementation of culturally appropriate interventions. Effective communication is a core concept. Using interpreters, bilingual staff, and lay health advisors; integrating the cultural values of the family and community; culturally tailoring health information; and attending to health literacy issues are key strategies to promote health in vulnerable groups.

CONSIDERATIONS FOR PRACTICE IN VULNERABLE POPULATIONS

Nurses have multiple opportunities and challenges with vulnerable populations because of the diversity, poverty, and other socioeconomic factors that increase their risks for diseases and chronic illness. When working with diverse populations, nurses first examine their own attitudes and values and how these may either facilitate or impede culturally appropriate client encounters. A commitment to becoming culturally competent is necessary to effectively promote healthy behaviors with vulnerable groups. Culturally competent communication skills and knowledge are necessary to design culturally and literacy appropriate programs. These skills can be learned through courses and practice. Factors such as potential language difficulties, educational level, poverty, unsafe housing or neighborhoods, and different cultural beliefs are challenges that need to be confronted to change lifestyles. Collaborative partnerships with other health care professionals and organizations within the community are critical. The significant role of public policy in reducing health inequities stresses the need for nurses to learn policy analysis and advocacy to represent the voices of vulnerable groups and lobby for policies and changes that promote health equity for all.

OPPORTUNITIES FOR RESEARCH IN VULNERABLE POPULATIONS

Although evidence documents the adverse health outcomes caused by health disparities, research to eliminate disparities and promote health equity is limited due to the multiple determinants and the complex, multilevel interventions needed. Multiple methodologies, including community-based participatory research, and many stakeholders are needed to support multilevel interventions that target sociocultural, behavioral, and environmental systems. The effects on health outcomes of changing policies that increase socioeconomic status and access to quality services and care need rigorous investigation. Appropriate health literacy interventions that target subpopulations such as children and adolescents, the elderly, and rural residents should be designed and tested, as these subgroups have received less attention.

Interdisciplinary research teams are crucial in research to address the complex social determinants of health inequities. Community interventions that partner with stakeholders should be implemented to evaluate changes that target living conditions within the community. Health policy research also is a priority, and the effects of policy in achieving health equity must be evaluated.

Vulnerable groups traditionally have been underrepresented in research for many reasons, including unsuccessful recruitment and retention strategies, lack of culturally sensitive interventions and measures, literacy levels, and lack of trust. Recruitment of communities for interventions that evaluate large-scale changes, such as improved living conditions, is an even bigger challenge. However, research is needed to evaluate large-scale change in order to influence policy.

Summary

Although great progress has been made in the health of the American people due to basic improvements—such as safe drinking water, sanitation, the availability of nutritious food, and advances in medical care—evidence shows that, in addition to these improvements, structural factors that define a person's social class and socioeconomic position in society are powerful predictors of health status. At all levels of income, health and illness follow a social gradient, with lower socioeconomic levels associated with poorer health. Vulnerable populations have diverse threats to health that require attention from clinicians, researchers, and policy-makers. Although the contributing factors are multiple and complex, many components are amenable to change. Nurses, as primary care providers, are well positioned to take a leadership role in designing and implementing culturally competent health promotion programs to promote health equity for diverse populations.

Learning Activities

1. Develop a plan describing the steps you would take to become culturally competent in a culture different from your own.
2. Design a program to promote physical activity in low-income Mexican American families using health literacy strategies discussed in the chapter.
3. Describe strategies you would use to address environmental barriers to promoting physical activity, such as unsafe places to walk, that the families in Learning Activity 2 might face.
4. Identify an issue in a poverty-stricken community, such as unsafe housing. Describe how you would advocate at local and state levels to promote change that targets resources to provide safe housing for the community.
5. Using the guidelines found in the Making Health Literacy Real Toolkit (see the CDC website), conduct a health literacy assessment on an organization, such as the county health department. Identify potential barriers and strategies to overcome in improving health literacy in the organization.

References

Berkman, N. D., Sheridan, S. L., Donahue, K. E., Halpen, D. J., & Crotty, K. (2011). Low health literacy and health outcomes: An updated systematic review. *Annals of Internal Medicine, 155*, 97–107.

Braverman, P., Cubbin, C., Egerter, S., Williams, D., & Pamuk, E. (2010). Socioeconomic disparities in health in the United States. What the patterns tell us. *American Journal of Public Health, 100*, S186–S196.

Braverman, P. A., Egerter, S. A., & Mockenhaupt, R. E. (2011). Broadening the focus. The need to address the social determinants of health. *American Journal of Preventive Medicine, 40*, S4–S18.

Braverman, P. A., Kumanyika, S., Fielding, J., LaVeist, T., Borrell, L. N., Manderscheld, R., & Troutman, A. (2011). Health disparities and health equity: The issue of social justice. *American Journal of Public Health, 101*, S149–S55.

Bushy, A. (1999). Resiliency and social support. In J. G. Sebastian & A. Bushy (Eds.), *Special populations in the community: Advances in reducing health disparities.* Gaithersburg, MD: Aspen Publications, Inc.

Cohen, B. E., & Reutter, L. (2007). Development of the role of public health nurses in addressing child family poverty: A framework for action. *Journal of Advanced Nursing, 60*, 96–107.

Coleman, C. (2011). Teaching healthcare professionals about health literature: A review of the literature. *Nursing Outlook, 59*, 70–78.

Cross, T. L. (2011). Cultural Competence Continuum. Accessed 9/03/2013 at http://pbsnetwork.org/up_content/uploads/2011/04/Cultural-Competence-Continuum.

Frisch, A., Camerini, L., Diviani, N., & Schulz, P. J. (2012). Defining and measuring health literacy: How can we profit from other literacy domains? *Health Promotion International, 27*, 117–126.

Griffith, D. M., Allen, J. O., DeLoney, E. H., Robinson, K., Lewis, E. Y., Campbell, B., . . . Reischl, T. (2010). Community-based organizational capacity building as a strategy to reduce racial health disparities. *Journal of Primary Prevention, 31*, 31–39.

Hong, G. K., Garcia, M., & Soriano, M. (2013). Responding to the challenge: Preparing mental health professionals for the changing US demographics. *Handbook of Multicultural Mental Health.* doi: http://dx.doi.org/10.1016/B978-0-394420-7.00030-8

Institute of Medicine. (2004). *Brief report: Health literacy: A prescription to end confusion.* Washington, DC: National Academies Press.

Koh, H. K., Oppenheimer, S. C., Massin-Short, S. B., Emmons, K. M., Geller, A. C., & Viswanath, K. (2010). Translating research evidence into practice to reduce health disparities: A social determinants approach. *American Journal of Public Health, 100*, S72–S80.

Kumareson, J. (2013). Health literacy perspectives. In Institute of Medicine Report on *Health literacy: Improving health, health systems, and health policy around the world: Workshop summary* (pp. 9–13). Washington, DC: The National Academies Press.

Masuda, J. R., Poland, B., & Baxter, J. (2010). Reaching for environmental justice: Canadian experiences for a comprehensive research, policy, and advocacy agenda in health promotion. *Health Promotion International, 25*, 453–461.

Peerson, A., & Saunders, M. (2009). Health literacy revisited: What do we mean and why does it matter? *Health Promotion International, 24*, 285–296.

Raphael, D. (2011a). The political economy of health promotion: Part 1, national commitments to provision of the prerequisites of health. *Health Promotion International, 28*, 95–111.

Raphael, D. (2011b). The political economy of health promotion: Part 2, national provision of the prerequisites of health. *Health Promotion International, 28*, 112–132.

Sarkar, U., Karter, A. J., Liu, J. Y., Adler, N. E., Nguyen, R., López, A., & Schillinger, D. (2010). The literary divide: Health literacy and the use of an Internet-based patient portal in an integrated health system—results from the Diabetes Study of Northern California (DISTANCE). *Journal of Health Communication, 15*(Suppl 2), 183–196.

Schoeni, R. F., Dow, W. H., Miller, W. D., & Pamuk, E. R. (2011). The economic value of improving the health of disadvantaged Americans. *American Journal of Preventive Medicine, 40*(1S1S), S67–S72.

Smit, E. M., & Tremethick, M. J. (2013). Development of an international interdisciplinary course: A strategy to promote cultural competence and collaboration. *Nurse Education in Practice, 13*, 132–136.

Solar, O., & Irwin, A. (2010) *A conceptual framework for action on the social determinants of health.* Social Determinants of Health Discussion Paper 2. Geneva, Switzerland: World Health Organization Press.

Sorensen, K., Van den Broucke, S., Fullam, J., Doyle, G., Pelikan, J., Slonska, Z., & Brand, H. (2012). Health literacy and public health: A systematic review and integration of definitions and models. *BMC Public Health, 12*, 1–13.

Teal, C. R., & Street, R. L. (2009). Critical elements of culturally competent communication in the medical encounter: A review and model. *Social Science & Medicine, 68*, 533–543.

Thomas, S. B., Quinn, S. C., Butler, J., Fryer, C. S., & Garcia, M. A. (2011). Toward a fourth generation of disparities research to achieve health equity. *Annual Review of Public Health, 32*, 399–416.

Trickett, E. J., & Beehler, S. (2013). The ecology of multilevel interventions to reduce social inequities in health. *American Behavioral Scientist, 57*, 1278–1246.

U.S. Department of Health and Human Services, Office of Disease Prevention and Health Promotion. (2010). *National Action Plan to Improve Health Literacy.* Washington, DC. Accessed at http://cdc.gov/healthliteracy/planact/index.htm

Wallerstein, N., & Duran, B. (2010). Community-based participatory research contributions to intervention research: The intersection of science and practice to improve health equity. *American Journal of Public Health, 100*(Suppl 1), S40–S46.

Watermeyer, J., & Penn, C. (2009). "Tell me so I know you understand": Pharmacists' verification of patients' comprehension of antiretroviral dosage instructions in a cross-cultural context. *Patient Education and Counseling, 75,* 205–213.

Wiggins, N. (2011). Popular education for health promotion and community empowerment: A review of the literature. *Health Promotion International, 27,* 356–371.

World Health Organization. (2013). *Social determinants of health.* Accessed at http://www.who.int/social_determinants/sdh_definition/ed/index.html

CHAPTER 13

Health Promotion in Community Settings

OBJECTIVES

This chapter will enable the reader to:

1. Describe the difference between promoting the health of individuals and promoting the health of the family.

2. Describe the health-promoting school concept.

3. Discuss four advantages of the workplace as a setting for health promotion programs.

4. Discuss the impact of behavioral economics on health promotion in the workplace.

5. Justify the rationale for nursing-managed health centers to increase their emphasis on health promotion.

6. List the factors that facilitate successful community-based health promotion programs.

7. Discuss the domains of expertise needed to develop community partnerships.

HEALTH PROMOTION TO IMPROVE THE HEALTH OF POPULATIONS

Health promotion to improve the health of populations has increased in value worldwide. People of all ages can benefit from gender and culturally sensitive health-promoting care and services delivered at sites where they spend their time: home, school, work, and the community at large. However, the many demands on public/private sector resources have led to a reluctance to fund health promotion programs. With the implementation of the Affordable Health Care Act in January 2014, selected screenings and health promotion activities are mandated and will have a positive impact on coverage of health promotion activities by most insurance carriers. Demonstrated cost-effectiveness of health promotion programs is also making an impact on the delivery of health promotion programs in schools, worksites, and the community at large.

This chapter presents an overview of community health promotion settings including home, school, workplace, and the community at large and the key roles they play in developing healthy behaviors. Also discussed are the keys to fostering healthy lifestyles within diverse communities: (1) partnerships to foster health promotion services in the community, (2) partnerships in research and education, and (3) multi-agency collaboration.

Health Promotion in Families

Families provide the context in which most health values, attitudes, and health-related behaviors are learned. Factors that influence values, attitudes, and behaviors include the following:

1. Family structure
2. Employment patterns
3. Gender and age differences
4. Stage of parenting
5. Family dynamics
6. Communication patterns
7. Power relations
8. Decision-making processes (Wright & Leahey, 2012)

Just as individuals are responsible for their own health decisions, so families must assume similar responsibilities for the health decisions of the family as a unit. The essential role of the family is to build human capital by investing in the health, education, values, and skills of its members so they may have productive roles in society. The family is the *major* unit responsible for socialization of children, and thus it is an ideal target for health promotion and prevention planning efforts (Ziebarth, Healy-Haney, Gnadt, Cronin, Jones, & Viscuso, 2012).

Approaches to the family generally focus on either family *structure* or family *functioning*. The *structural* approach defines how family members operate by their relationship to each other, such as a parent or sibling. Family *functioning* describes what families do together to meet their needs within a context of mutual responsibility.

Variant family forms are common in today's society. Family units may be traditional two-parent families, one-parent families (often mother-only families, although the number of father-only families is growing), blended families (parts of two preexisting families), extended families (nuclear plus a relative, often older), augmented families (additional members, not blood relations), married same-sex adults, and unmarried adults (blood and nonblood relations). The nurse, working with families, must be sensitive to both the commonalities and differences across varying family forms. Understanding the milieu for the promotion of health in nontraditional families is essential to successful family health-promotion planning. By focusing on the responses to the questions in Table 13–1, the nurse is able to assist the family in developing a health promotion plan that includes critical information about family values, beliefs, and lifestyle.

Families demonstrate a spectrum of abilities, insights, and strengths and exert three types of influences:

1. Cultural/attitudinal, such as church attendance or school engagement
2. Social/interpersonal, including social support, such as family activities
3. Intrapersonal, such as self-esteem, coping, and depression

TABLE 13–1	**Questions to Generate Information about Family Values, Beliefs, and Lifestyles**

1. How does the family define *health*?
2. What health-promoting behaviors does the family engage in regularly?
3. What health-promoting behaviors are particularly enjoyable to family members?
4. Do all family members engage in these behaviors, or are patterns of participation highly variable in the family?
5. Is there consistency between stated family health values and their health actions?
6. What are the explicit or implicit health goals of the family?
7. What factors are operating to prevent health-promoting behaviors?
8. What resources are available to facilitate health-promoting behaviors?

The family is a pivotal unit to *decrease* risky behaviors and *increase* healthy behaviors among its members. Family-centered collaborative negotiations are effective in facilitating behavior change. A collaborative partnership, rather than a prescriptive one, engages parents, supports parent–child relationships, and enhances motivation to change health behavior. The challenge for the nurse is to assist the family unit in identifying relevant health goals, planning for positive lifestyle changes, and capitalizing on family members' strengths to achieve desired health outcomes. The nurse can make families aware of technology-delivered and community programs to assist them in meeting their goals.

Health Promotion in Schools

The majority of the nation's children attend private or public preschool, kindergarten, elementary, or secondary schools. Therefore, schools are excellent settings for programs to increase health-promoting behaviors among children and adolescents before certain behavior patterns solidify. School health programs over the last four decades have been successful in building health-enhancing environments.

The earliest programs to target health promotion in schools focused on providing information about potential health threats and risks of certain behaviors. The second phase of program development included the influence of teachers, parents, and peers. Teachers and school health personnel not only set the normative expectations for healthy behaviors, but also serve as role models for health-enhancing lifestyles. Positive peer influences foster *health-promoting* rather than *health-damaging behaviors* and have a significant impact on their peers' behavior. Interested and involved parents also play important roles in creating healthy school environments and modeling healthy lifestyles that are crucial to the success of school-based health promotion programs.

The assumption in both phases was that *individuals determine their lifestyle.* Individual-level theories such as social cognitive theory (see Chapter 2, Individual Models to Promote Health Behaviors) provided the framework, and most school-based interventions focused on specific topics—such as physical activity, smoking cessation, or dietary behaviors. These programs usually provided health education within the confines of the school curriculum. National Health Education Standards, shown in Table 13–2, provide schools the framework to meet the goal of enabling students to acquire the knowledge and skills needed to promote personal, family, and community health. Education is an important determinant of health-promoting behaviors, and it is an accepted fact that healthy children learn better.

TABLE 13–2	National Health Education Standards
Standard 1	Students will comprehend concepts related to health promotion and disease prevention to enhance health.
Standard 2	Students will analyze the influence of family, peers, culture, media, technology, and other factors on health behaviors.
Standard 3	Students will demonstrate the ability to access valid information, products, and services to enhance health.
Standard 4	Students will demonstrate the ability to use interpersonal communication skills to enhance health and avoid or reduce health risks.
Standard 5	Students will demonstrate the ability to use decision-making skills to enhance health.
Standard 6	Students will demonstrate the ability to use goal-setting skills to enhance health.
Standard 7	Students will demonstrate the ability to practice health-enhancing behaviors and avoid or reduce health risks.
Standard 8	Students will demonstrate the ability to advocate for personal, family, and community health.

Source: CDC National Health Education Standards-SHER-Adolescent and School Health. Accessed at http://www.cdc.gov/healthyyouth/sher/standards

HEALTH-PROMOTING SCHOOLS.   More recently, the social-ecological model (Bronfenbrenner, 1979) has been used to understand the interrelated effects of the individual and her or his social and physical environments. By using this model to create health-promoting programs, one has a better understanding of the relationship between the student, his family, school, community, and the society and culture at large (Figure 13–1). These programs not only build resilience, but also assist children in improving health knowledge and developing healthy behaviors, such as better food choices and regular exercise habits (Keshavars, Nutbeam, Rowling, & Khavarpour, 2010). This approach results in holistic health promotion programming that is likely to sustain health-promoting behaviors over time.

The World Health Organization (WHO) Health Promoting Schools Framework defines a *health-promoting school* as one where the policies, infrastructure, procedures, and activities promote the health and well-being of its students, faculty, staff, and the community (WHO, 1996). The *health-promoting school concept* combines traditional classroom education with actions that improve the social and physical environments with input from the home and community (Keshavars, Nutbeam, Rowling, & Khavarpour, 2010).

Competence, confidence, character, connection, and caring are key attributes of positive youth development. Programs that focus on developing these attributes assist children and adolescents in developing into healthy, productive adults. *Effective* programs take into account both individuality and social context and have a vision of positive development; a focus on participation in *all* facets of the program, including design, conduct, and evaluation; and are conducted in accessible, safe settings. In addition, they recognize the interrelated challenges facing children and adolescents so they integrate support services, provide training to adult leaders, emphasize life skills development, incorporate program evaluation, and pay attention to group diversity (Keshavars, Nutbeam, Rowling, & Khavarpour, 2010).

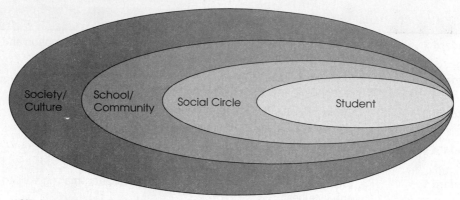

Student: The first level identifies the biological and personal history factors such as age and education

Social Circle: Student's peers, family members, and others who influence one's behavior and experiences

School/Community: Settings that influence the student and where social relationships form

Society/culture: Broad societal factors such as health, economic, and educational policies, and social and cultural norms that influence the student's environment

FIGURE 13–1   Social-Ecological Model   *Source:* Adapted from the Centers for Disease Control and Prevention. http://www.cdc.gov/violenceprevention/overview/social-ecologicalmodel.html

HEALTH-PROMOTING INTERVENTIONS.   Youth development programs based on the best current evidence improve quality, lead to more reliable results, and give direction to resource allocation in schools (Inman, van Bakergem, LaRosa, & Garr, 2011). Examples of evidence-based study outcomes follow.

1. **The Gatehouse Project** targeted three aspects of the school social context: security, communication, and participation (Patton, Bond, Bulter, & Glover, 2003). School-wide strategies include (1) mentoring programs, (2) promotion of positive classroom climates, and (3) introduction of a curriculum to promote social and emotional skills, and have resulted in substantial positive changes in the behaviors of children in the intervention schools, including a reduction in health risk behaviors. The findings document the value of including both the individual and the social contexts of the school, where young people spend more than a third of their waking hours.

2. **The Adolescent Health and Social Environments Program (AHSEP)** grew out of The Gatehouse Project and focused on building capacity in schools that are most often the adolescents' key social environment. This research demonstrated that system-level changes in schools reduced adolescents' health risk behaviors (Centre for Adolescent Health, 2013).

3. **The Child and Adolescent Trial for Cardiovascular Health** was one of the largest school-based health education studies conducted in the United States (McCullum-Gomez, Barroso, Hoelscher, Ward, & Kelder, 2006). The study design included a curriculum component augmented by a family component, a physical activity component, a school food service component, and a program to promote smoke-free school policies. An evaluation five years after the intervention showed that these environmental changes supported healthy behaviors.

However, compliance was less than desired. The researchers concluded that *staff training* is a significant factor in achieving institutionalization of these programs.

4. **"Action Schools! BC,"** designed to promote cardiovascular health in elementary school children, found that children in the intervention group had a 20 percent greater fitness level and 5.7 percent lower blood pressure than children in the control group. When school and after-school settings incorporate physical activity into their programs, both physical activity and other health behaviors improve (Beets, Beighle, & Huberty, 2009; Reed, Warburton, MacDonald, Naylor, & McKay, 2008).

5. **Physical Activity Intervention for Girls.** A two-year study involving 36 schools in six geographically diverse areas of the United States targeted schools and communities to increase opportunities, support, and incentives to increase physical activity in middle-school girls. In the third year of the program, community leaders requested measurement of the effectiveness of a staff-directed intervention versus school- and community leader–directed interventions. Physical activity level of the girls slightly improved in the community leader–directed intervention compared to the staff-directed intervention. Physical fitness or percent body fat did not differ in the two groups (Webber, Catellier, Lythe, Murray, Pratt, Young, et al., 2008). Continued study is essential to determine how best to get school-age girls to increase their level of physical activity.

Health-promoting behaviors acquired in childhood are more likely to persist as an integral part of one's lifestyle than are health behaviors acquired later in the adult years. Development of healthy behaviors in school-aged children and adolescents is critical to increasing the prevalence of healthy lifestyles in the total population.

Health Promotion in the Workplace

The workplace and the health of the workers within it are inextricably linked. The structure and nature of work, as well as the profile of the worker in the United States, have evolved over time. In 2013 the workforce has become older, more racially and ethnically diverse, with proportionally more women in the workforce. The primary jobs now are (1) *knowledge work*, requiring a relatively high level of education or technical training, and (2) *service* jobs.

CHANGES IN WORK AND WORKPLACES.   Changes in work and workplaces have many implications for health. Figure 13–2 addresses how work shapes the health of workers and their families.

Average American adults spend about half their waking hours at work. When they have untreated health problems, they do not perform as effectively as they can, or as well as their employers would like. Poor employee health results in absenteeism, accidents, and high health care and related cost. In 2011, American businesses lost more than 153 billion dollars due to lost productivity from absenteeism. For example, workers who are above normal weight, or have at least one chronic health problem, take an extra 450 million sick days compared with healthy workers.

A relatively new field in workplace health is *presenteeism*. Presenteeism is being present at work, but limited in some aspect of the job due to a health problem, so that there is a decrease in overall performance (Cancellere, Cassidy, Ammendolia, & Cote, 2011). Presenteeism likely contributes to lost revenue and needs further study to determine its role in the formula that determines lost productivity. Figure 13–3 shows work-based strategies to improve health.

Work sites offer access to large numbers of adults and serve as a vehicle for delivering interventions at multiple levels, including individual, interpersonal, environmental, and organizational. Work site programs have the potential to (1) increase healthy behaviors, (2) increase productivity,

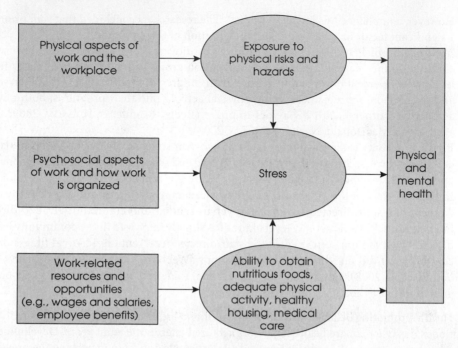

FIGURE 13–2   How Work Shapes Health for Workers and Their Families   *Source:* Robert Wood Johnson Foundation Commission to Build a Healthier America. Issue Brief 4: Work Matters for Health, December 2008. Accessed at http://www.commissiononhealth.org/PDF/0e8ca13d-6fb8-451d-bac8-7d15343aacff/Issue%20Brief%204%20Dec%2008%20-%20Work%20and%20Health.pdf

(3) decrease absenteeism, (4) decrease use of expensive medical care, and (5) lower disability claims. These outcomes ultimately result in a more productive and globally competitive workforce.

Workplace programs have access to employees over an extended period and therefore have the opportunity to modify policies and promote environmental change to enhance employees' healthy behaviors. Also significant is the potential to modify social norms and increase interpersonal support for coworkers who are motivated to change.

Work site programs range from annual events, such as health fairs, to software programs, to ongoing comprehensive programs. Some programs are available only to employees of a certain level, or the work site may subsidize membership at an independently operated facility. Programs typically include on-site exercise capabilities as well as opportunities to improve diet, stop smoking, control substance abuse, relieve stress (see Chapter 8, Stress Management and Health Promotion), and control obesity (see Chapter 7, Nutrition and Health Promotion).

A multifaceted on-site program is likely to attract and retain a broader spectrum of workers, is more cost-effective, and is more likely to have successful long-term results—if it addresses risk reduction counseling, modifies workplace policies, and makes changes in the physical work environment. For example, *smoke-free* workplaces made a major contribution to the decline in cigarette smoking in the United States. Policy changes also resulted in a decrease in exposure of nonsmokers to environmental tobacco smoke at the work site.

Offering a variety of health-promotion programs at the work site and using different approaches can increase the appeal of the program to employees of varying cultural backgrounds and ages. In addition, work site programs can create a cultural milieu that supports

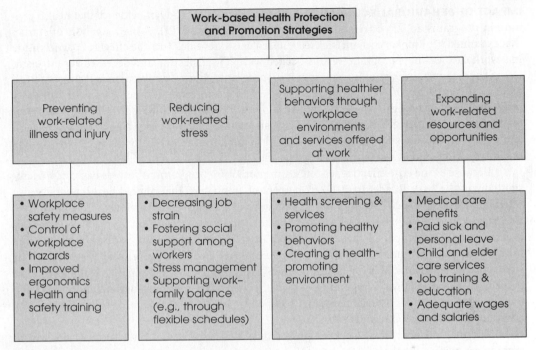

FIGURE 13–3 Work-Based Strategies to Improve Health *Source:* Robert Wood Johnson Foundation Commission to Build a Healthier America. Issue Brief 4: Work Matters for Health, December 2008. Accessed at http://www.commissiononhealth.org/PDF/0e8ca13d-6fb8-451d-bac8-7d15343aacff/ Issue%20Brief%204%20Dec%2008%20-%20Work%20and%20Health.pdf

health-promoting behaviors. Change in the workplace culture is important to achieve broad-based support for health-promotion programs.

Examples of changes at the work site include the following:

1. Availability of culturally sensitive health materials
2. Healthier foods in cafeterias and vending machines
3. Discounted rates at fitness centers for employees and families
4. Periodic health screenings
5. On-site health fairs
6. Computer application health programs

Programs are more likely to succeed when they not only address multiple risk factors for change, but also integrate families and neighborhoods. Including families in health promotion programs is of interest, as many employers pay much of the health care costs for family members as well as the primary employee. Smokers are more likely to have spouses who smoke, and individuals with physically active spouses are more likely to be active themselves. Their children also are likely to be more active.

Local school staffs, including teachers and school nurses that seek to participate in work site programs, can ensure consistency and integration of health promotion concepts across both schools and work sites. This effort, if expanded, could give rise to "seamless" health promotion programming in communities, which would accelerate behavior change efforts across the life span.

IMPACT OF BEHAVIORAL ECONOMICS.   There is a growing body of evidence that health promotion programs are effective and cost-effective (Chapman, 2013). A meta-analysis of studies that examined health plan cost and sick leave absenteeism revealed that the effects of participation in a workplace wellness program were associated with job satisfaction and deceased absenteeism.

The financial impact of health promotion programs showed a return on investment (ROI) of $3.27 for medical cost savings and $2.73 for absenteeism reduction per $1 invested in these programs. These findings provide significant support for the adoption of health promotion programs (Baicker, Cutler, & Song, 2010). Most organizations recognize the value of these programs and appear not to question whether they should offer programs, but to ask about the design, implementation, and evaluation of such programs.

Because of the cost-effectiveness of health promotion programs, offerings have grown substantially in the past decade. In 2011, 67 percent of companies that offered health benefits also offered at least one health promotion program such as physical examinations, screenings, exercise programs, or vaccinations. Although worksite programs are prevalent in major corporations (Chapman, 2013), companies that employ fewer than 50 people have not made a strong showing in offering health promotion programs to their employees. Cost is the primary reason given by small companies for *not* offering health promotion programs (Witt, Olsen, & Ablah, 2013). The overall goal is for employers, large and small, to offer health promotion programs and activities to their employees through on-site programs, technology-based applications, or collaboration with other businesses and community agencies.

The major *weakness* of worksite programs is that they attract only 10 to 64 percent of employees, with a median of 33 percent participation (Robroek, van Lenthe, Empeten, & Burdorf, 2009). Because the primary motivator for most employees' participation in workplace health promotion programs is concern for their health, many workers may hesitate to identify health problems that are not evident, as they may fear loss of their job and/or privacy. Workers need assurance that sharing their health problems will not lead to punitive outcomes. Other barriers to participation include time commitment, use of off-site facilities and programs, and lack of interest.

Participation is the whole point of worksite health programs. "Nudging" employees with the right incentives can lead to significant improvement in participation. The study of behavioral economics underlies the buy-in decisions in other industries, but has been used only recently in health care. Cognitive, emotional, social, cultural, and psychological factors influence whether one participates in programs, and employing strategies that use these concepts can boost or "nudge" employees to participate (Saravis, 2013).

For example, some companies are trying new and innovative strategies to encourage exercise while at work. The nature of many work settings involves sitting for long periods, and sedentary behavior is associated with adverse health markers. To reduce prolonged sitting, employees are using treadmill desks, stand-up desks, or other moving workstations, as well as large exercise balls in place of chairs. Others are using prompting software on their work computer to remind them to stand up every 30 minutes to decrease uninterrupted sedentary periods (Evans, Fawole, Sheriff, Dall, Grant, & Ryan, 2012). These efforts respond to individual employee interests and motivation, demonstrate the company's concern for their employees' health, and promote a health-promoting worksite.

BEST PRACTICES TO INCREASE PROGRAM PARTICIPATION.   Some of the most effective practices to increase participation in worksite health programs include (1) management support,

(2) employee involvement in program planning, (3) incentives/rewards, (4) marketing and communication activities, and (5) workplace policy and environmental changes (Ryan, 2011). The use of incentives to encourage or "nudge" employees to participation in worksite health programs is receiving significant attention. There are three strategies to boost participation:

1. *Encourage commitment:* Partner with spouse or coworker to meet a shared goal such as increased physical activity.
2. *Inspire action:* Build intrinsic motivation by discovering what's important to employees and helping them achieve their goals.
3. *Include a retention or incentive item:* Offer rewards and recognition for achieving goals.

(Saravis, 2013; The Incentive Research Foundation Resource Center, 2011)

Examples of successful worksite programs are the following:

- A study of 3,272 employees of a Midwestern company randomly sent one of three reminder mailings encouraging them to get a flu shot at an on-site health clinic. The Control group received the times and locations of clinics. Treatment group A received that information plus a mailing with a suggestion to write down the day they planned to get the flu shot. Treatment group B received the same information as the Control group and Treatment group A, and a mailing that prompted them to write down the time and day. The overall vaccination rate for the Control group was 33.1 percent. The Treatment A group participation rate was 34.6 percent, while the Treatment B group had a 37.3 percent participation rate. "Nudges" appear to move people from good intentions into actual behavior (Milkman, Beshears, Choi, Laibson, & Madrian, 2011).
- Walk@Work: An automated web-based intervention to increase walking in university employees not achieving 10,000 daily steps demonstrated its effectiveness in reducing cost and the investment of time required to manage a successful walking program. Across the sample, step counts increased significantly, the group that was least active at baseline had the greatest increase in steps. Overall, participants in the study increased their workday walking by 25 percent (Gilson et al., 2013).

Worksite health promotion programs will continue to expand in the future as research demonstrates that healthy lifestyles help control health care costs and improve the work environment. Programs that include physical, mental (stress reduction), and social health increase the overall effectiveness of the company as well as the health and life quality of employees. Exciting possibilities exist for integrating health promotion programs into a coordinated effort through technology-based applications and on-site delivery.

It is in these efforts that nurses can have a significant impact. While employers are responsible for ensuring that workplace demands are reasonable, expectations are clear, and goals are set and achievable, employees are responsible for achieving their own work–life balance. Being aware of the work environment, the nurse can encourage the integration of health promotion concepts such as assertiveness, openness to learning, adequate rest, nutritious food, exercise, and humor into the work setting (Budin, Brewer, Chao, & Koyner, 2013). Through active participation and conscience awareness, the nurse can serve as a role model for peers and colleagues and can be a leader in making positive changes in the workplace. With a commitment to teamwork, camaraderie, and a "no tolerance" stance for BHHV (bullying, harassment, and horizontal violence; Versey, Demarco, Gaffney, & Budin, 2010), the nurse can make the workplace one in which everyone can thrive.

THE COMMUNITY AS A SETTING FOR HEALTH PROMOTION

Community *organizing* and community *building* are central to changing the health behavior of communities (Minkler, 2012). Community-based health promotion and prevention programs encompass a range of activities, such as (1) health education, (2) risk-reduction intervention programs, (3) environmental awareness and improvement programs, and (4) initiatives to change laws or regulatory policies to be supportive of health.

Skills and values needed in the community are not necessarily the same as those that have been effective in the traditional health care system. The success of nurses and other health care professionals who work in communities is influenced by four basic values:

1. Health care professionals respect the wisdom of the community.
2. Health care professionals share health information in an understandable form.
3. Health care professionals use their capacities, skills, contacts, and resources to empower the community.
4. Health care professionals focus on capacities, not needs and deficiencies (Minkler, 2012).

Community activation, a health promotion strategy, includes (1) organized efforts to increase community awareness and consensus about health problems, (2) coordinated health promotion partnerships to plan environmental change, (3) allocation of resources across organizations within the community, and (4) the promotion of citizen involvement in these processes. Community activation matches programs to actual community needs as identified by those who reside in the community. The community is a "living" organism with interactive webs among organizations, neighborhoods, families, and friends. The challenge of community activation is to involve community members in all aspects of planning to achieve the goals they have defined.

Four principles facilitate community capacity building and ownership of the project:

1. Community members are equal partners.
2. Intervention and evaluation are essential components.
3. Community demands influence organizational and program flexibility.
4. The program is a learning project for everyone involved. (Hacker, Tendulkar, Rideout, Bhuiya, Trinh-Shervrin, Savage, et al., 2012)

A successful community project requires that participants not only have ongoing knowledge of the community but also view the community as a true partner. Community programs are dynamic processes as defined through an ongoing negotiation process among all members. A community partnership, based on honesty and respect, requires time, people, and resources.

Community-based health promotion programs offer an excellent approach to reach impoverished communities that have limited resources. A community-based intervention to improve low-income parents' interaction with their children showed that improved parenting skills contributed to the children's participation in daily family functions and strengthened the family and community (Powell & Peet, 2008).

Another example of a community-based family study is an 8-week intervention for 47 Hispanic families that promoted the importance of physical activity and awareness of healthy food choices. The program, selected, translated, and adapted for the Hispanic community, was successful in increasing knowledge and attitudes of participants and had an impact on the community as well. Improved access to parks and schools allowed families to participate together in physical activities (Ziebarth, Healy-Haney, Gnadt, Cronin, Jones, Jensen, & Viscuso, 2012).

Health promotion services—provided where people live, work, worship, and play—are likely to be more successful than those offered *outside* the community. For example, offering nutrition services in churches and mammography screening in malls brings valuable services to people in real-life settings. The synergy of bringing community strengths and resources together, and the empowerment that results from early successes, warrant continued attention to designing and planning community-wide innovative and culturally sensitive health promotion programs. Integrating evidence-based clinical knowledge and community strategies improves the health of the entire community.

CREATING HEALTH PARTNERSHIPS

A major strategy to optimize the health of communities is health partnerships across settings. Partnerships promote continuity of care in health promotion and prevention and synergistic use of resources to achieve optimal effectiveness and efficiency. Partnerships may consist of any combination of worksites, schools, nursing centers, nonprofit organizations, community organizations, health agencies, or universities all working together to improve the health of an entire community.

A *community health partnership* is defined as a relationship between collaborating parties (people and organizations), committed to work together to achieve a common purpose (Jenerette, Funk, Ruff, Grey, Adderley-Kelly, & McCorkle, 2008). Community health partnerships recognize the value of community members, corporate leaders, and health care providers all working together to create health care systems that are user-friendly, accessible, and culturally sensitive. Partnerships optimize the combined resources of all partners to achieve mutual goals. These goals include helping to empower individuals and families to manage their own health; improve the health of people in socially, racially, and culturally diverse communities; and eliminate health disparities.

In successful community health partnerships, respect for the community's right to identify problems and potential solutions to those problems is clearly established and communicated. Initially, the following questions frame the community's norms for participation:

1. Is current community problem-solving an individual or collective effort?
2. How in touch are citizens with each other?
3. What are the units of interaction (e.g., neighborhoods, townships, housing complexes)?
4. Does crime or other factors deter citizens from interacting?

Some communities have established structures to address health concerns. To learn how partnerships might be shaped in any given community, carefully review current patterns of citizen involvement and existing relationships among community organizations and organizations known for activating community involvement (churches, recreation centers, and service clubs). For some communities, flexible coalitions are the appropriate organizing framework to address community health needs, whereas for others, a leadership board or council balances the power of key community activists.

An important goal of community partnerships for health promotion is *empowerment*. Community empowerment is a social-action process in which individuals and groups act to gain mastery over their lives by changing their social and political environment (Minkler, 2012). Members of such a partnership create conditions that empower their joint efforts. Community partnerships for health promotion have the potential to bring about institutional and policy changes that affect many people. The commitment of partnerships to the broader goals of positive social, structural, and individual change is essential to improving the overall health of communities.

Building partnerships requires substantial time and effort. Putting collaborative partnerships into practice is complex and represents a challenge for all the stakeholders involved in the partnership. It is important for the stakeholders to both acknowledge their diverse interests in the early stages of the partnership and implement strategies to address any cultural gaps that exist.

Partnership principles include the following:

1. Find the right mix of ownership and control among partners.
2. Recognize the assets of all partners.
3. Develop relationships based on mutual trust and respect.
4. Acknowledge and honor different partner agendas.
5. Acknowledge the difference between community input and active community involvement.
6. Resolve ethnic, cultural, and ideological differences between and among partners. (Centers for Disease Control and Prevention, 2011)

A shared vision among partners creates a common *identity* and a *shared* purpose. A *vision* is an image of what partners see as outcomes of their collaboration. A shared vision facilitates a shared mission that identifies the primary reasons for existence of the partnership. An example of a mission statement is as follows:

> To assist individuals and families in the community in adopting healthy lifestyles and to assist the community in developing culturally sensitive, cost-effective health promotion and prevention services.

The potential for fostering healthier lives for citizens of all ages lies in the power of partnerships that are multidisciplinary and reach beyond the bounds of traditional medicine. Partnerships enable members to appropriately plan, implement, and evaluate community-based health promotion interventions. For example, the community must be a major player in meeting the health needs of adolescents and young adults who are disconnected from traditional education and work settings. This may be accomplished by integrating health promotion activities into all youth employment and training programs in the community (Tandon, Marshall, Templeman, & Sonenstein, 2008).

Basic concepts in the community approach to health promotion collaboration are (1) self-determination, (2) shared decision making, (3) bottom-up planning, (4) community problem solving, and (5) cultural relevance. The philosophy underlying this approach is that health promotion is likely to be more successful when the community at risk identifies its own health concerns, develops its own intervention programs, forms a board to make policy decisions, and identifies resources for program implementation. Communities that are empowered through organization and active participation in partnerships develop the skills and abilities to solve problems that compromise their health and well-being.

Both national and local community concerns may be the focus of partnerships. Examples of partnerships with national impact are the National Healthy Worksite Program and the Healthways and Partnership for Prevention initiative to advance prevention and well-being improvement policies.

The National Healthy Worksite Program resulted from The Centers for Disease Control and Prevention's (CDC) collaboration with 104 small and mid-size employers in eight counties across the nation. The initiative aimed to reduce chronic disease and to build a healthier, more productive workforce. Begun in 2013, the project, supported through the Affordable Care Act's Prevention and Public Health Fund, designed and offered evidence-based programs at the worksites to reduce chronic diseases. Participating employers receive program and implementation support from a health management firm selected in a competitive process. One of the community selection criteria was the availability of local resources to support a sustainable worksite program including existing health promotion programs and community health care facilities. At the end of the program, best practices and models will be available to all small worksites through various formats. The Healthways and Partnership for Prevention initiative brings together Healthways, a provider of well-being improvement solutions, and Partnership for Prevention, an organization of businesses, nonprofit, and government leaders, whose goal is to create a "prevention culture" in the United States. Formed in 2011, the partnership endeavors to use evidence-based policies and programs to advance nationwide efforts in disease prevention and cost-effective well-being initiatives.

Partnerships organized around community concerns, including adolescent pregnancy, violence, substance abuse, and chronic health problems, highlight the variety of needs in many communities. Examples of partnerships formed to meet these challenging needs are as follows:

1. A community partnership, formed to enhance chronic kidney disease awareness, prevention, and early intervention, included academic leaders, community leaders, clients, caregivers, faith-based organizations, and health care professionals. The members developed shared goals and interventions to achieve an infrastructure, shared objectives, and diverse work groups to reduce the burden of chronic kidney disease (Vargus, Jones, Terry, Nicholas, Kopple, & Forge, 2008).
2. A community partnership was formed among an immigrant-refugee program, a baccalaureate school of nursing, and a community literacy program. Nursing students provided culturally appropriate health promotion and prevention programs to the immigrant population and collaborated with local agencies and businesses to identify health resources for vulnerable populations. Outcomes of the partnership were a cultural awareness learning experience for the students, better access to health care for the refugees, and promoted awareness of a community agency (Sullivan, 2009).

Health partnerships bring greater rationality to health care expenditures by advocating funding, prevention, and health promotion services. Politically active partnerships can redirect public and private health care dollars so that allocations emphasize population-based health care services and clinical preventive services. Key elements for successful community health partnerships are community participation and enlightened health policy. Nurses are potentially significant members of community health partnerships. Their knowledge of health promotion, community health, and community activation, whether as a part of the nurse's job responsibilities or as a member of the community, gives the nurse a place at the table. Nurses are encouraged to seek opportunities to participate and provide leadership in these groups.

THE ROLE OF PARTNERSHIPS IN EDUCATION, RESEARCH, AND PRACTICE

Multidisciplinary education and collaborative practice experiences with community residents help prepare health profession students for the diversity of health care roles they will assume over their careers. As care moves from traditional institutions (except for the critically ill) to the community, knowledge and skills to function in diverse community settings are essential to meet the health needs of individuals, families, and communities. Gaining access to community educational experiences for students and faculty is a win–win situation for both nursing programs and communities.

For example, students in the early stages of baccalaureate nursing education can experience various aspects of the role of community health worker by distributing health education materials in a community, participating in screening programs, helping to organize health fairs, collecting health data from communities, and surveying use of vending machines and fast-food stores to assist in research programs.

Advanced baccalaureate students with a greater understanding of the role of culture and socioeconomic level on health behaviors can provide education classes at schools and work sites, assist community residents in identifying environmental health risks, and provide self-care education to groups of individuals who have similar health-risk profiles (Sullivan, 2009).

Another example involves graduate students including master's and doctoral, faculty, and community member representatives. These groups provide a strong team for training community health workers in underserved communities. To build a successful cohort of community health workers, the following points are essential:

1. Establish rapport with the community.
2. Collaborate with the community to assess health needs.
3. Hire individuals from the community to gain the trust and participation of community residents.
4. Share program ownership and decision making with community health care workers by empowering them to develop program goals and design strategies for greater effectiveness.
5. Facilitate program flexibility so workers are able to adapt to changing needs.
6. Closely link workers with community health and social service agencies so that professional backup is available as necessary.

Community-academic health partnerships are also valuable allies in research. Collaborating with universities throughout all stages of assessing, planning, and conducting health promotion interventions creates a sense of community perspective and ownership and takes advantage of the expertise of university faculty. Community-based participatory research (CBPR) fosters enthusiastic participation, attentiveness to recruitment, thoughtful interpretation of findings, and commitment to dissemination of results to the community (Allen, Culhane-Pera, Perament, & Call, 2011).

Indeed, it is through these strategic partnerships that there has been progress in improving the health of many communities. Community partnerships play a strategic role in creating community capacity to respond to health needs. In addition, partnerships set expectations that the health care system will function as a copartner with other systems in the community in order to shape public policy that will foster healthy living in a safe environment.

Health Promotion in Nurse-Managed Health Centers

Nurse-managed health centers represent an ideal setting for integrating education, practice, and research, offering a spectrum of services, including health promotion and prevention counseling, behavioral interventions to promote healthy lifestyles, and screening to detect health risks. The hallmark of nurse-managed community health centers is primary care delivered by nurses. A focus on "the individual and family" rather than "the presenting illness" has enhanced the appeal of nurse-managed centers to deliver care to a growing segment of the population. Many families prefer health care from nurse practitioners in a setting that is client-friendly and respectful of their unique assets and needs.

Computerized record systems track client outcomes and collect information to evaluate the quality and cost-effectiveness of health services. These data provide evidence needed to document services for both quality and reimbursement purposes. With the increasing emphasis on improving the health-promoting behaviors of individuals, families, and communities and the implementation of the Affordable Health Care Act in 2014, nurse practitioners and nurse-managed centers will play an even more important and visible role in health care.

Nurse-managed centers provide family-oriented, culturally sensitive care to diverse populations. They include direct care services, health education classes, small-support groups, and family and individual counseling, all with a health promotion focus. Many families need assistance with healthy parenting or meeting the health promotion needs of family members. Interventions that engage parent(s), and support parent–child relationships, are more likely to be successful. A collaborative relationship between the nurse practitioner and the parent or adult caregiver facilitates health-promoting behavior in the individual and family unit (Hansen-Turton, Bailey, Torres, & Ritter, 2010).

An example of a successful nurse-managed center is the University of South Carolina Children and Family Healthcare Center. The center opened in 1998 with a limited mission to provide primary health care for children placed in the protective custody of the state because of abuse or potential abuse. The Center expanded to offer comprehensive services to children and families in the surrounding community. Pediatric and family nurse practitioner faculty members provide immunizations, well baby checkups, and health promotion and preventive services for children and adults, as well as 24-hour primary care services. The Center also serves a large population of adolescents who are in foster care. Located in a former strip mall in a low-income area, the Center continues to experience a growing client base. Reimbursement from Medicaid, other third-party reimbursement, private pay, various state and federal programs, and grants and contracts help the Center maintain fiscal stability. Nurse-managed centers are usually located in diverse environments to be accessible to the populations they serve, such as at or near schools to help meet the health needs of children and adolescents in a confidential and developmentally appropriate manner. Nurse-managed centers can also be located in malls, pharmacies, and low-income housing developments to provide access to people where they congregate or spend time when not at school or work. Nurse-managed centers offer care that enhances the health and well-being of all family members, interdisciplinary care, access to social services, and integrated care that covers the life span of families and individuals.

The continued national emphasis on cost containment in health care has made nurse-managed centers appealing as an integral component of the health care system. Most clients are highly satisfied with nurse practitioner services and report that they receive quality health care. Positive client health outcomes and cost-effectiveness are hallmarks of nurse-managed centers (Hansen-Turton, Bailey, Torres, & Ritter, 2010; Pohl, Tanner, Pilon, & Benkert, 2011).

Opportunities to link university nursing programs and nurse-managed centers are particularly attractive as they lead to improved services through the latest evidence-based practice developments. In addition, nurse-managed centers are ideal clinical practice sites for nursing students to observe the care provided by advanced practice nurses and doctors of nursing practice.

Nurse-managed centers are well-positioned to serve as the medical home to a growing, underserved segment of the population, but experience state and national restrictions. Nurses continue to address state and federal legislative impediments that constrain the practice of nurse practitioners, the establishment of nurse-managed centers, and the reimbursement for health promotion and prevention services to individuals and families. Both professional and lay organizations continue concerted efforts to bring nurse-managed community health centers into the mainstream of health-promotion and prevention services (Hansen-Turton, Bailey, Torres, & Ritter, 2010; Pohl, Tanner, Pilon, & Benkert, 2011).

CONSIDERATIONS FOR PRACTICE TO PROMOTE HEALTH IN DIVERSE SETTINGS

Multiple settings offer opportunities to provide health promotion services. Nurses with an understanding of community health issues and problems are ideally suited to provide leadership in the design, development, implementation, and evaluation of health promotion programs in schools, work sites, nursing centers, and other community settings. Today's health problems are best solved by many sectors coming together in partnerships to improve social and environmental conditions that compromise health. Such partnerships offer a way to communicate, collaborate, and empower to achieve solutions not attainable by single groups or organizations. Particularly exciting is the opportunity for nursing programs to join with other health professions' schools, health care provider groups, and communities to build partnerships. These partnerships, designed in a community-sensitive, culturally appropriate manner, will improve prevention and health promotion services provided to diverse populations.

The need has never been greater for nursing programs to take an active role in the development of enduring partnerships. The holistic view of nursing provides the orientation required to work collaboratively with communities to accomplish their health goals. Health care reform and the economic pressures for cost-effective, multidisciplinary, high-quality care places nurses in a unique position to provide leadership in the community.

OPPORTUNITIES FOR RESEARCH IN MULTILEVEL HEALTH PROMOTION SETTINGS

Nurse scientists effectively apply diverse evaluation strategies for families, schools, and communities as units of analysis. Attention to process, as well as outcome evaluation, is needed in order to identify implementation strategies that are most effective in promoting healthy behaviors. Suggested opportunities for research include the following:

1. Describe health promotion and disease prevention beliefs and practices in diverse families and communities as a basis for designing culturally sensitive interventions.
2. Test the synergistic effects of school, family, and community health promotion efforts for adolescents on individual- and community-level health outcomes.
3. Identify facilitators and barriers to increase participation in work site programs.
4. Test community partnership strategies that optimize community and environmental change.
5. Design valid and reliable community-level health outcome indicators.
6. Develop uniform methods and measures to assess health outcomes and cost outcomes across a range of programs and communities.

Evidence suggests that community partnerships make a difference in health practices and the health of the community (Chambers, Pringle, & Juliano-Bult, 2012). However, more study is needed to determine the effectiveness and sustainability of community partnerships, particularly in communities with underserved populations. In addition, intervention research will help to further identify and document the effective components of partnerships. A process-oriented research model outlines three domains—(1) enhanced knowledge, (2) enhanced research skills, and (3) use of information—and offers research partnerships a tool to demonstrate their accountability, improve their operations, and evaluate the impact of research partnerships. Multiple measures are required to assess the behavioral, social, and environmental outcomes of partnership activities.

Summary

Health promotion programs are offered in multiple settings to reach diverse populations. The development and maintenance of healthy lifestyles and healthy environments are critical components of a healthy population. This must be a central goal for families, schools, worksites, and the community.

Community-based programs that are tailored to members' needs enhance cultural buy-in and the likelihood of success. Community partnerships create a network of community members and health care providers that can offer quality health promotion and prevention services.

Learning Activities

1. Identify a community-based health promotion program in your community and assess its effectiveness by interviewing two citizens who live in the community (e.g., the Walk for Life program to promote breast health and cure).
2. Investigate the level of interagency collaboration in a community program. Use the chapter section on creating health partnerships to evaluate your results.
3. Discuss the steps to improve access to immunizations for children in an impoverished community.
4. Identify a worksite health promotion program in your community. Assess its strengths and limitations from the perspectives of the employer, employee, and community.
5. Develop three questions you have about a nurse-managed center. Interview a practitioner and a client, using your questions as a framework.

References

Allen, M., Culhane-Pera, K., Perament, S., & Call, K. (2011). A capacity building program to promote CBPR partnerships between academic researchers and community members. *Clinical Translational Science*, *4*(6), 428–433. doi: 10.1111/j.1752-8062

Baicker, K., Cutler, D., & Song, Z. (2010). Workplace wellness programs can generate savings. *Health Aff (Millwood)*, *29*(2), 304–311. doi: 10.1377/hlthaff.2009.0626

Beets, M. W., Beighle, H. E., & Huberty, J. L. (2009). After-school impact on physical activity and fitness: A meta-analysis. *American Journal of Preventive Medicine*, *36*(6), 527–537.

Bronfenbrenner, U. (1979). *The ecology of human development.* Cambridge, MA: Harvard University Press.

Budin, W., Brewer, C., Chao, Y., & Koyner, C. (2013). Verbal abuse from nurse colleagues and work environment of early career registered nurses. *Journal of Nursing Scholarship*, *45*(3), 308–316.

Cancellere, C., Cassidy, J., Ammendolia, C., & Cote, P. (2011). Are workplace health promotion programs effective at improving presenteeism in workers? A systemic review and best evicence synthesis of the literature. *BMC Public Health*, *11*, 395–406. doi:10,1186/1471-2458-11-395

Centers for Disease Control and Prevention. (2011). *Principles of community engagement* (2nd ed.). NIH Publication No. 11-7782. Retrieved from http://www.atsdr.cdc.gov/communityengagement

Centre for Adolescent Health. (2013). *The Adolescent Health and Social Environments Program.* Retrieved September 4, 2013, from http:www.rch.org.au/cah/research/The Adolescent Health and Social Environments Program

Chambers, D., Pringle, B., & Juliano-Bult, D. (2012). Connecting science and practice in child and adolescent mental health services research. *Administration and Policy in Mental Health, 39*(4), 321–326. doi:10.1007/s10488-011

Chapman, L. (2013). Meta-evaluation of worksite health promotion economic return studies: 2012 update. *The Art of Health Promotion—American Journal of Health Promotion.* doi: 10.4278/ajhp.26.4.taph

Evans, R., Fawole, H., Sheriff, S., Dall, P., Grant, P., & Ryan, C. (2012). Point-of-choice prompts to reduce sitting time at work. *American Journal of Preventive Medicine, 43*(3), 293–297.

Gilson, N .D., et al. (2013). Walk@Work: An automated intervention to increase walking in university employees not achieving 10,000 daily steps. *Preventive Medicine.* Retrieved from http://www.mdlinx.com/internal-medicine/news-article.cfm/4456004/university-employees-and-auto-mated-web-based. doi: 10.1016/j.ypmed.2013.01.022

Hacker, K., Tendulkar, S., Rideout, C., Bhuiya, N., Trinh-Shervrin, C., Savage, C., et al. (2012). Community capacity building and sustainability: Outcome of community-based participatory research. *Programs for Community Health Partnerships, 6*(3), 349–360. doi: 10.1353/cpr.2010

Hansen-Turton, T., Bailey, D., Torres, N., & Ritter, A. (2010). Nurse-managed health centers. *American Journal of Nursing, 110*(9), 23–26. doi:10.1097/01.NAJ0000388257

Inman, D., van Bakergem, K., LaRosa, A., & Garr, D. (2011). Evidence-based health promotion programs for school and communities. *American Journal of Preventive Medicine, 40*(2), 207–219.

Jenerette, C., Funk, M., Ruff, C., Grey, M., Adderley-Kelly, B., & McCorkle, R. (2008). Models of inter-institutional collaboration to build research capacity for reducing health disparities. *Nursing Outlook, 56*(1), 16–24.

Keshavars, N., Nutbeam, D., Rowling, L., & Khavarpour, F. (2010). Schools as social complex adaptive systems: A new way to understand the challenges of introducing the health promotion schools concept. *Social Science & Medicine, 70,* 1467–1474. doi: 10.1016/j.socscimed.2010.01.034

McCullum-Gomez, C., Barroso, C. S., Hoelscher, D. M., Ward, J. L., & Kelder, S. (2006). Factors influencing implementation of the Coordinated Approach to Child Health (CATCH) eat smart school nutrition program in Texas. *Journal of American Dietetic Association, 106,* 2039–2044.

Milkman, K., Beshears, J., Choi, J., Laibson, D., & Madrian, B. (2011). Using implementation intentions prompts to enhance influenza rates. Washington, DC: National Institutes of Health News. Retrieved from http://www.nih.gov/news/health/jun2011

Minkler, M. (2012). *Community organizing and community building for for health.* New Brunswick, NJ: Rutgers University.

Patton, G., Bond, L., Bulter, H., & Glover, S. (2003). Changing schools, changing health? Design and implementation of the gatehouse project. *Journal of Adolescent Health, 33*(4), 231–239.

Pohl, J., Tanner, C., Pilon, B., & Benkert, R. (2011). Comparison of nurse managed centers with federally qualified health centers as safety net providers. *Policy Politics Nursing Practice, 12,* 90–99. doi: 10.1177/15271544114117882

Powell, D. R., & Peet, S. H. (2008). Development and outcomes of a community-based intervention to improve parents' use of inquiry in informal contexts. *Journal of Applied Developmental Psychology, 29*(4), 259–273.

Reed, K., Warburton, D., MacDonald, H., Naylor, P., & McKay, H. (2008). Action Schools! BC: A school based physical activity intervention designed to decrease cardiovascular disease risk factors in children. *Preventive Medicine, 46,* 525–531.

Robroek, S., van Lenthe, F., Empeten, P., & Burdorf, A. (2009). Determinants of participation in worksite health promotion programmes: A systematic review. *International Journal of Behavior Nutrition and Physical Activity.* doi: 10.1186/1479-5868-6-26

Ryan, M. (2011). *Getting employees on board: Factors influencing participation in worksite health promotion programs.* CPH News and Views, Issue #22: The Center for the Promotion of Health in the New England Workplace (CPH-NEW). Retrieved from http://www.uml.edu/Research/Centers/CPH-NEW/emerging-topics/Issue-22.aspx

Saravis, P. (2013). Engaging employees with a healthy nudge. *Training Magazine,* posted February 11, 2013. Retrieved from http://www.trainingmag.com/content/engaging-employees-healthy-nudge

Sullivan, C. H. (2009). Partnering with community agencies to provide nursing students with cultural awareness experiences and refugee health promotion access. *Journal of Nursing Education, 48*(9) 519–522. doi: 10.3928/01484834

Tandon, S., Marshall, B., Templeman, A., & Sonenstein, F. (2008). Health access and status of adolesdents and young adults using youth employment and training programs in an urban environment. *Journal of Adolescent Health, 43*(1), 30–37.

The Incentive Research Foundation Resource Center. (2011). *Energizing workplace wellness programs: The role of incentives and recognition.* St. Louis, MO: Incentive Research Foundation. Retrieved from http://theirf.org/research/content/6078727/energizing-workplace-wellness-programs-the-role-of-incentives

Vargus, R., Jones, L., Terry, C., Nicholas, S., Kopple, S., & Forge, N. (2008). Community-partnered approaches to enhance kidney disease awareness, prevention, and early intervention. *Advances in Chronic Kidney Disease 15*(2), 153–161.

Versey, J., Demarco, R., Gaffney, D. A., & Budin, W. C. (2010). Bullying, harassment, and horizontal violence in the nursing workforce: The state of the science. *Annual Review of Nursing Research, 28*(1), 133–157.

Webber, L. S., Catellier, D. J., Lythe, L. A., Murray, D. M., Pratt, C. A., Young, D. R., et al. (2008). Promoting physical activity in middle school girls: Trial of activity for adolescent girls. *American Journal of Preventive Medicine, 34*(3), 173 184.

World Health Organization. (1996). *Promoting health through schools: The World Health Organization's Global School Health Initiative.* Geneva, Switzerland: World Health Organization.

Witt, L., Olsen, D., & Ablah, E. (2013). Motivating factors for small and midsized businesses to implement worksite health promotion. *Health Promotion Practice, 14*(6), 876–884.

Wright, L. M., & Leahey, M. (2012). *Nurses and families: A guide to family assessment and intervention.* Philadelphia, PA: F. A. Davis Company.

Ziebarth, D., Healy-Haney, N., Gnadt, B., Cronin, L., Jones, B., Jensen, E., & Viscuso, M. (2012). A community-based family intervention program to improve obesity in Hispanic families. *WMJ, 111*(6), 262–266.

Ziebarth, D., Healy-Haney, N., Gnadt, B., Cronin, L., Jones, E., & Viscuso, M. (2012). A community-based family intervention program to improve obesity in Hispanic families. *WMJ, 111*(6), 261–266.

CHAPTER 14

Promoting Health Through Social and Environmental Change

OBJECTIVES

This chapter will enable the reader to:

1. Justify the rationale for describing health as a social goal.
2. Describe the role of public policy in promoting social and environmental change.
3. List common health-damaging factors in the physical environment and their etiologies.
4. Discuss the role of the Patient Protection and Affordable Care Act in addressing health promotion and disease prevention.

Recognition that health is influenced by the social and physical environments in which people live has resulted in new approaches to achieve behavior change. As mentioned throughout previous chapters, large-scale change is best accomplished by altering social and environmental structures that influence health, in addition to changing individual and group behaviors. To effectively promote a healthy society, the dynamic relationships among individuals, families, and their social and environmental contexts are all-important. Health and social policies that fail to directly address inequitable living conditions, such as poverty, abuse, violence, hunger, and unemployment; environmental threats, such as pollutants in work sites and communities; and disparities in access and care will not change the health of individuals and communities. Individual and family efforts to adopt healthy behaviors also are likely to be ineffective in the presence of environmental constraints and policies that do not promote healthy living. The need for a social and environmental focus is not new, as the idea goes back in history as far as Hippocrates. Florence Nightingale also stressed the importance of paying attention to the environment to promote health.

HEALTH AS A SOCIAL GOAL

Health must be identified as a social goal as well as an individual one, because the health status of societies, communities, families, and individuals are integrated and inseparable, as shown in Figure 14–1. Publication of the social determinants of health by the World Health Organization

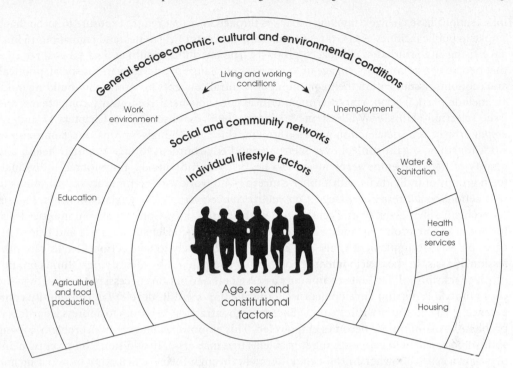

FIGURE 14–1 Social Determinants of Health *Source:* Dahlgren, G., & Whitehead, M. (1993). Tackling inequalities in health: What can we learn from what has been tried? Working paper prepared for the King's Fund International Seminar on Tackling Inequalities in Health, September 1993, Ditchley Park, Oxfordshire. London, The King's Fund, accessible in: Dahlgren, G., & Whitehead, M. (2007). *European strategies for tackling social inequities in health: Levelling up Part 2.* Copenhagen: WHO Regional office for Europe: http://www.euro.who.int/__data/assets/pdf_file/0018/103824/E89384.pdf

(WHO) was a significant milestone, as it documented the social, cultural, economic, and political factors, as well as biological and psychological factors that influence health (WHO, 2008). Health promotion efforts involve working with communities and policy-makers to ameliorate conditions that contribute to poor health, such as inadequate housing, an unsafe water supply, poor nutrition or insufficient food supply, chemical pollutants, poor or absent recreational facilities, inadequate access to care, and lack of economic opportunity. Globally, governments acknowledge that behavior-change strategies must be directed beyond the individual to include community- and policy-level factors.

Health as a social goal requires the integration of theories that address community change (see Chapter 3) with theories that address individual behavior change (see Chapter 2), family change (family stress theory, family development theory, family systems theory), and health care policy. The four perspectives are complementary. When nurses think only in terms of one-to-one relationships, the range and success of intervention possibilities are severely limited.

Health behavior change has been successful when the social context in which the individual lives also is targeted. For example, smoking cessation programs have succeeded, in part, due to addressing individual addictive properties of smoking and the social context in which smoking occurs, including the advertising and sale of cigarettes. Tobacco public policy interventions have changed smoking behaviors through laws that reduce exposure to secondhand smoke in public facilities, excise taxes that increase the costs of cigarettes, and regulations to limit advertising and promotion of tobacco products. The pursuit of health as a social goal requires that people of a community engage in the process of change to address various social, political, and economic issues within their communities. Central concepts in community-building models include participation, empowerment, critical consciousness, community competence, and issue selection (Minkler, Wallerstein, & Wilson, 2008). As discussed in Chapters 11 and 12, *empowerment* is a social action process through which individuals, groups, and communities work together to gain control over their lives and environment to improve their health and quality of life. The empowerment process begins with individuals. Empowered individuals form groups of individuals with similar concerns who work with community organizations to take actions to address their issues. *Community competence,* a closely related concept, focuses on problem-solving ability as a central goal of the community. Competent communities learn to identify their problems and needs, achieve a working consensus on goals and priorities, agree on ways to implement goals, and collaborate effectively to take action. Health care professionals assist in the development of community competence by identifying natural community leaders who will facilitate community assessments and actions necessary to strengthen the community. Leadership development is a critical component in developing community competence. As a community gains competence in negotiating for resources to address a particular problem, the community becomes empowered. This empowerment enhances problem-solving ability and capacity to cope with other problems that may arise. In addition, community members gain a sense of ownership and empowerment through their participation in initiating and promoting change.

Ecological models focus on changing the environmental context, including regulatory changes to support healthy behaviors (see Chapter 3). The *Healthy People 2020* objectives emphasize an ecological approach to health promotion to create health-enhancing social and physical environments (U.S. Department of Health and Human Services, 2013). Social change is generally followed by changes in social norms, or the shared rules and expectations (rules of conduct) that govern everyday life.

When health is considered a social goal as well as an individual one, the health promotion focus includes the community. Individuals can govern their own behavior and should do so. Government formulates broad policies and allocates funding. However, priority decisions and strategies for social change for more complex lifestyle issues can best be made collectively by members of the community. This strategy ensures that programs are relevant and appropriate for these involved and encourages greater buy-in and participation in the planning and implementation process.

HEALTH IN A CHANGING SOCIAL ENVIRONMENT

Comprehensive health reform continues to proceed at a rapid rate in the United States. The U.S. health care system is considered one of the most extravagant and wasteful in the Western world (Editorial, 2009). Excess administrative costs, profits, and costs of prescription drugs have been estimated to exceed the costs of providing health care to all uninsured Americans. Factors responsible for health reform include rising health care costs for consumers (higher premiums, rising deductibles, higher copayments, and escalating out-of-pocket expenses) and lack of access to care for those who are unable to purchase health insurance. Quality and affordable, high-quality health coverage should be available to all Americans. Every community should be able to provide services and monitor the health status of its members and assist its members in accessing health care services.

In addition to health reform, information and communication technology (ICT) has transformed our society to an information- and knowledge-based one in which we are connected globally. ICT has the potential to contribute to reducing health inequities through the delivery of education and access to knowledge resources to improve health. Poverty and illiteracy, costs, and lack of standards challenge the application of ICT. The American Recovery Reinvestment Act of 2009 demonstrates government's commitment to health care technology, by authorizing almost $38 billion over 10 years to support health information technology implementation and adoption. In addition, *Healthy People 2020* emphasizes equitable access to health information and improved health communication. These initiatives are based on evidence that shows improved health knowledge is associated with better lifestyle choices, improved client–provider communication, and greater treatment adherence (Lustria, Smith, & Hinnant, 2011).

Mobile technologies, such as cellular telephones, have rapidly expanded into health promotion and health care. Short messaging service, or text messaging, is used to educate and answer questions about sexual health for teens, send reminders to take medications, enter health data such as food intake or physical activity, and deliver health alerts. An advantage of this technology is the widespread ownership of cell phones by ethnic minorities (Chou, Prestin, Lyons, & Wen, 2013). This technology opens the door to new methods to enhance empowerment through the delivery of health information and care in developed as well as developing nations.

Web 2.0 technologies have shifted the online environment from a passive, unidirectional type of communication to a participative one. Social media sites include social sharing sites, such as YouTube and Flickr; social networking sites, such as Facebook and MySpace; microblogs, including Twitter; virtual worlds, such as Second Life; and text messaging discussion forums or wikis (Bertot, Jaeger, & Hansen, 2012). Social media technologies provide an interactive environment for many individuals to receive and share online information. Such technologies reach a broad audience and can be empowering for individuals, as they are able to obtain health information, solve problems, and gain diverse insights and perspectives through interactions with others who may or may not have expertise. Because multiple opportunities exist for employing this technology, federal agencies now use social media for government purposes, including:

- To foster participatory dialogue, thus providing a voice in discussions of policy development and implementation,
- To improve service quality and delivery by public involvement in design and delivery of government services, and
- To solve large societal issues using public knowledge and talent to develop innovative solutions (Bertot, Jaeger, & Hansen, 2012).

Social media is a central component of e-government. These technologies have become a government priority to increase communication and promote participation in government.

Comprehensive, computerized health assessments can be used to tailor health-promotion programs to the knowledge, beliefs, motivations, and prior health-behavior histories of diverse individuals and families. Health-promotion activities are taking advantage of computer-based technologies such as CD-ROM and the Internet to target audiences, tailor health promotion messages, and promote interactive ongoing exchanges about health. Personal computers in the home and public libraries offer informational resources to answer questions and provide access to support and discussion groups.

Clients and their health care professionals now link electronically as well. Client data has become standardized and communicates with the electronic personal health record (PHR; see Chapter 4). An electronic PHR enables clients to have access to their personal data, act as stewards of their information, and take an active role in their own health. In contrast, an electronic health record (EHR) is managed by health care professionals or institutions. The PHR is a tool to help maintain health and wellness through access to credible information and data, as well as a means to help manage an illness. Technological challenges, organizational barriers, economic and market forces, and individual obstacles have limited the nationwide adoption of both the EHR and PHR. However, adoption is a national priority and is ongoing in the government and private sectors.

The information era has also brought about changes that can empower families. Interactive computer technology enables parents to work at home. They can also obtain health information without visiting a health care provider. The Internet revolution is reshaping health promotion, as individuals now conduct health information searches, share information with their families, and ask informed questions of their health providers.

The information revolution continues to challenge health professionals to think creatively about the delivery of health promotion, new ways to educate health professionals, and the potential consequences of this technology on society. Application of these technologies in ethnically diverse, poor communities remains a major challenge, as skills and access may be lacking. Computer skills need to be taught using strategies that account for health literacy levels, and sites to access computers should be available in communities. Although the digital divide is narrowing, rural communities continue to face technology challenges, including the unavailability of broadband services (Lustria, Smith, & Hinnant, 2011). Public education should be designed for underserved groups that demonstrate how to find health information on the Internet and incorporate the information into daily life.

PROMOTING HEALTH THROUGH PUBLIC POLICY

The importance of shaping healthy policies in the public and private sectors to improve health for populations is widely advocated. Policies set goals and limits and define choices. Personal, social, and political factors all influence the development and implementation of health policy. For example, at the personal level, changes in public sentiment have influenced the development of health policy related to smoking in public places in the United States. At the political level, lobbyists have been successful in maintaining the economic interests of the food industries to prevent changes in food content, such as sugar or salt. On a more positive note, public policy has resulted in removal of cigarette commercials from television.

The idea of developing policies for healthier communities is not new. Historically, local governments provided environmental safeguards against infectious diseases. Social and economic factors, as well as environmental ones, also need attention. Policy formulation to promote health begins at the local level, through identification of problems and development of local ordinances to implement change.

The role of the U.S. government in regulating health behavior is controversial. State and federal policies regulate a range of health behaviors, including alcohol, tobacco, seat belt use, food safety, and drug use. In addition, state and federal governments play a major role in payment for health care services. The *Healthy People 2020* initiative's overarching goals are to achieve health equity and eliminate health disparities, and to create social and physical environments that promote good health for all. These goals challenge local, state, and federal governments, as well as policy-makers, to make policy changes that affect entire populations to address social determinants. For example, local governments can limit youth access to tobacco in local markets and vending machines. Local and state policies also can be developed to target economic development in communities with high unemployment or promote safe housing in poor neighborhoods. Long-term changes occur as a result of modifying the conditions under which people live.

Local and regional policy making can be beneficial for health promotion. It can occur through social service agencies, local transportation authorities, public safety commissions, economic development zones, and professional organizations. Beginning policy making at the local level eliminates the trickle-down time for a policy to have an influence in the community. Community and political leaders, along with the local and state health departments, can advise and advocate large-scale changes to promote health.

Policy making is value driven, dynamic, often chaotic, and is about social influence, as it involves persuasion, attitude change, decision making, and compromise. Facts, or science-based information, are usually used in the early phases of policy development to identify problems and solutions, including the economic costs. However, non–science-based, or less verifiable, information from stakeholders who offer their informed judgments and personal experiences also is used to promote the legitimacy of a proposed policy. Both types of information are needed to gain support for successful policy making. Although scientific knowledge is critical, stakeholders also need to be informed about the political costs, as well as the resources needed to implement the policy. This additional information aids consensus development.

Barriers to public health policy formulation are numerous (Metcalfe & Higgins, 2009):

- Policy-makers may not be committed to the proposed change.
- Scientific evidence substantiating the issue has not been translated in user-friendly language.
- A dominant commercial market, such as the tobacco industry, may hinder policy formulation.
- Timely, relevant information about the issue has not been consistently and personally communicated to policy-makers.

These barriers substantiate the need for political champions, or knowledge brokers—respected persons who are articulate proponents of a particular policy and know how to work with policy-makers to develop policy.

Addressing Obesity with Public Policy

An example of the role of public policy in health promotion and disease prevention is the ongoing development of legislation to target obesity prevention (Graf, Kappagoda, Wooten, McGowan, & Ashe, 2012). The complex factors that promote obesity reinforce the need for policy interventions to target social and environmental conditions that influence lifestyle choice. Lessons learned from successful tobacco control, seatbelt use, and the recycling movements have been incorporated in the obesity prevention movement to promote social change. (See Graf et al., 2012 for a history of the obesity prevention movement.) In addition to local, state, and federal government and concerned citizens, organizations that have played a role in efforts to combat obesity include the Institute of Medicine, the Robert Wood Johnson

Foundation, and The National Alliance for Nutrition and Activity Coalition. In addition, First Lady Michelle Obama drew attention to obesity in 2010 by launching the Let's Move! campaign. Examples of policies and actions that have occurred are the Healthy, Hunger-free Kids Act of 2010, which focuses on healthy lunches and healthy snacks in school vending machines and snack bars; legal action against food markets making misleading claims and marketing sugary food to young children; and the Safe Routes to Schools Program to promote walking.

The overall goal of all of the reports, policies, and campaigns targeting obesity is to change social norms, or the standards of acceptable behavior in a community. Social norm change means indirectly influencing behavior by creating a social climate where the harmful behavior (physical inactivity, unhealthy eating) becomes less desirable, acceptable, and attainable. The change in public acceptance of tobacco smoking in public places is an example of a social norm change. Policies are essential to social norm change, as laws and regulations are instrumental in changing communities in which individuals live and work.

Local and state governments are key players in obesity prevention, as these entities have control over the social and built environments, such as schools, retailers, restaurants, and the transportation system. Examples of state policies and initiatives enacted in cities are banning sugary beverages in schools, limiting fast-food chains in poverty areas, designing transportation with everyone in mind, and attracting healthy retailers to low-income areas, which often are saturated with alcohol retail shops and fast-food chains.

Lessons that are being learned in the obesity prevention movement are applicable to other areas of social policy change. First, policies and programs are not the same. Programs focus on providing services, such as implementing physical activity programs. Policies have broad influence, are longer lasting, and are usually implemented upstream. Last, government can mandate compliance with policies, while programs are voluntary.

Policies need to be legally feasible and financially viable. If a policy does not have a chance of being adopted, time and effort may be wasted; or, the local or state government may not have the authority to enact a policy. Financial viability focuses on the associated costs to implement the policy. If costs are prohibitive, governments may partner with private entities to implement the policy, such as building a recreational facility; or, they may redirect dollars from other programs to implement a policy if it is a priority. Last, policies can be enacted to generate revenues that can be directed to pay for new policies that promote health. For example, a tax on sugary beverages could generate revenue to promote healthy eating. Although opponents of a soft drink use tax argue that the poor would be disproportionately affected, this group suffers the greatest health disparities and diseases that are diet-related. In addition, studies consistently support the relationship between the consumption of sugary beverages and increased body weight, poor nutrition, and risk for obesity (Brownell & Frieden, 2009).

Local and state health departments are positioned to serve as catalysts for institutional and community changes needed to promote healthy lifestyles. Local health departments are usually connected with other community organizations and state agencies to facilitate communication and partnerships across regions. Local and state health policies can support programs in schools, communities, and work sites. Health policies that encourage individuals and communities to place a higher value on health and provide resources needed to implement these policies are a priority for all levels of government. Collaborative partnership models to develop health policy can be implemented and tested to increase access to information and resources. Individuals, communities, local and state governments, as well as the national government are all active partners in this effort.

Promoting Health in All Policies

At the 8th Global Conference on Health Promotion in 2012, consensus was reached on the Helsinki Statement on Health in All Policies (HiAP). The statement defines health in all policies and calls on governments around the world to ensure that health is considered in all policy-making (WHO, 2013). HiAP is a policy approach that takes into account the health implications of policy decisions and avoids making policies with harmful outcomes in order to improve health and eliminate health inequities. Attention to the consequences of public policy-making is considered to be a strategy to increase the accountability of policy-makers for the health impact of their policies (Van den Broucke, 2013). The Helsinki statement is considered a major step toward health promotion and health equity.

Finland's broad approach to policy making to address the health problems of the Finnish people paved the way for the HiAP initiative. Policies targeting nutrition, such as dietary consumption of butter, fat content of milk, maximal salt content of some foods, salt labeling, and changing food subsidies, have led to substantial reductions in blood cholesterol levels and cardiovascular disease mortality rates in the population (Puska & Stahl, 2010). The success of the Finnish policies is considered to be due to basing policy on sound evidence and promoting ethical policies and activities with and by the stakeholders (individuals and communities) to promote the political decision process.

PROMOTING HEALTH BY CHANGING THE PHYSICAL ENVIRONMENT

The quality of the physical environment in which people live is critical to the health of populations. Traditionally, environmental health practices have focused on controlling factors that are beyond the power of most people. However, individuals and communities have control over many external factors that promote healthy environments. Environmental factors that are health-damaging are increasing, such as mold in homes that have been flooded and the health hazards of natural gas production.

Addressing Health-Damaging Features of Environments

LEAD. The harmful effects of toxic substances in the environment continue to be evident in communities. Although there has been a dramatic reduction in the number of children with elevated lead levels, lead paint in older houses remains a childhood environmental disease hazard in the United States (Dixon, Jacobs, Wilson, Akoto, Nevin, & Clark, 2012). About 70 percent of excessive lead exposure is related to houses with lead paint, lead dust, and soil lead. Windows have the highest level of lead paint and lead dust compared to other housing components. Contaminated lead dust settles on floors and window sills and is ingested through normal hand-to-mouth contact. Exposure to high levels of lead can be fatal, but even low exposures can be toxic to the central nervous system, resulting in delayed learning, impaired hearing, and growth deficits. Children under age 6 years are especially vulnerable because their nervous systems are still developing. Regulatory changes, namely the Residential Lead Hazard Reduction Act in 1992, enabled HUD to provide grants to local and state governments to decrease lead content in low-income private homes. Twelve years after window replacement in pre-1975 housing was implemented, a 41% lower lead floor dust level has resulted compared to homes without window replacement.

TOBACCO SMOKE.   Leading indoor air hazards to which many thousands of people are exposed each year are tobacco smoke and radon. Environmental tobacco smoke causes lung cancer in nonsmokers. Children of parents who smoke are more likely to develop lower respiratory tract infections and middle ear infections than are children of parents who do not smoke. Asthma and other respiratory diseases are triggered or worsened by tobacco smoke and other substances in the air. Other indoor hazards include tight building syndrome, which is attributed to recycled air in buildings that may breed fungi and bacteria.

RADON.   The second leading cause of lung cancer, after smoking, is exposure to radon, a well-known carcinogen that is a natural by-product of the breakdown of uranium. When uranium decays in soil and rocks, it can seep up through the ground into ground water and diffuse into the air. It has a tendency to collect in basements or other low places in homes, offices, and schools as it seeps through cracks and holes or diffuses through construction materials (U.S. Environmental Protection Agency, 2009). Radon can dissolve in water and is found in homes that have their own wells. When radon is inhaled, it is deposited in the lungs and damages surrounding lung tissues, laying the foundation for lung cancer. The best way to reduce radon is to educate the public to promote radon testing in homes and buildings to measure its concentration in the air. Since 1996, the EPA has led a campaign recommending that people test their homes and take action when radon concentrations exceed normal, safe levels. Do-it-yourself kits are available in retail stores, or the test can be done by a licensed contractor. Based on the strong evidence between radon exposure, smoking, and lung cancer, programs to test and reduce radon in homes and stop smoking should be priorities to decrease the public health burden (Lanz, Mendez, & Philbert, 2013).

In 2013 HUD unveiled "Advancing Healthy Housing—A Strategy for Action," a plan that aims to make homes healthier. The plan encourages federal agencies to take actions to reduce the number of homes with high levels of radon, damaged paint, water leaks and roofing problems, and pests. This policy is a major step in federal housing efforts to promote healthy housing for vulnerable populations.

OUTDOOR AIR.   Outdoor air quality continues to be a widespread environmental problem nationally and internationally (Laumbach & Kipen, 2012). The effects are noted in premature deaths, cancer, respiratory, and cardiovascular diseases. Motor vehicles account for one fourth of emissions that produce ground-level ozone, the largest problem in air pollution. Although emission controls that were implemented in Europe and North America have decreased ozone precursors to a small degree, concerns remain due to the increased emission of these precursors in rapidly developing areas of the world. Air pollutants other than traffic-related pollution include emissions from domestic fires and burning biomass fuels in less-developed countries.

Employers are now encouraging and rewarding individuals to walk or use public transportation rather than drive their cars. Local and regional governments are designing public transportation systems that are available to outlying communities and streets that facilitate bicyclists and pedestrians. The increasing popularity of hybrid automobiles, which use alternative fuels, is a positive development. Nationally, support must be increased for the development and use of alternative fuels such as ethanol by commercial and private vehicles. Air pollution from traffic is a preventable cause of disease. All health professionals should support campaigns to increase public awareness and advocate for community-level interventions to reduce the health effects of smoke and traffic pollution.

WATER.   Water quality is a major concern because of protozoa and chemical contaminants. Industry and agricultural runoff may contaminate water. For example, the development of intensive animal feeding operations has resulted in the discharge of improperly treated animal wastes into recreational and drinking water. Contaminated run-off may also contaminate the soil. Heavy metals, such as mercury, have been found in water contaminated by mining. Mercury has been found in the breast milk of mothers who live near gold-mining areas and consume fish from contaminated runoff water from the mines. Mercury is used to extract the gold from the ore. Mercury is neurotoxic and a hazard to infant health development. The development of new molecular technologies to detect and monitor water contamination has eliminated the inability to detect parasitic contamination. These new technologies are being implemented to improve water monitoring and surveillance techniques.

NATURAL GAS EXTRACTION.   Technological advances in the production of natural gas have resulted in a boom in an unconventional drilling method to extract natural gas from large underground shale deposits throughout the northeastern and southwestern United States. This method, known as hydraulic fracturing or "fracking," uses a high-volume, high-pressure technique to drill thousands of feet into the earth to reach and fracture hard rocks (shale) to release natural gas. Large volumes of water, sand, and chemicals are used throughout the process to create fractures in the shale. Although the fracking process has been used for over 60 years, horizontal drilling is a recent advance that enables large amounts of natural gas to be extracted. An average of 5.5 million gallons of water is used to fracture a gas well one time, and wells may be repeatedly fractured multiple times over the life of the well. Chemicals are also used throughout the operation to reach and release the gas. When the natural gas is released, anywhere from 30 to 70% of the fracturing solution is returned as backwater, as well as additional chemicals and radioactive material (Finkel, Hays, & Law, 2013).

The disposal and storage of the backwater, the potential contamination of soil and water supplies, and air pollution have become significant public issues because of lack of regulation over the industry (Colborn, Kwiatkowski, Schultz, & Bachran, 2011; Mitka, 2012). The natural gas industry does not have to disclose the chemicals used in the process, based on their exemption from the Toxic Release Inventory of the National Environmental Policy. The lack of disclosure presents a challenge to study the potential health effects. In addition, the federal government has exempted the industry from the Clean Water Act, the Clean Air Act, and the National Environmental Act. These actions have left a void in environmental regulation of the industry, leaving responsibility to the states, which traditionally have not required accountability for wastewater handling and disposal.

The lack of rigorous evidence is a public health issue, as the lack of transparent information and access to data has hindered knowledge of the potential health impact. However, an absence of rigorous data does not imply that no harm is being done. In spite of the limitations, qualitative evidence and case studies as well as other research have documented health risks for humans and animals, contaminated drinking water, contaminated soil, and air pollution (Bamberger & Oswald, 2012; Osborn, Vengosh, Warner, & Jackson, 2011). The potential multiple and serious health and environmental issues should be of concern for health professionals. Nurses need to be advocates for transparency and careful monitoring of water, air, and chemicals as well as the effects of human and animal exposure to chemicals used in extracting the gas. Clients living in areas of gas extraction need education and ongoing monitoring to prevent or reduce exposure to the chemicals to the extent possible, until rigorous research can be conducted.

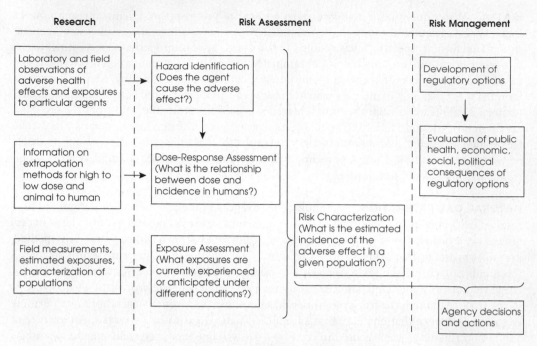

FIGURE 14–2   Elements of Risk Assessment and Risk Management   *Source:* Committee on the Institutional Means for Assessment of Risks to Public Health, Commission on Life Sciences, National Research Council. (1983). *Risk Assessment in the Federal Government: Managing the Process.* Washington, D.C.: National Academy Press. http://www.nap.edu/catalog/366.html

Risk assessment is the means by which currently available information about environmental public health problems can be organized and understood. As noted in Figure 14–2, risk analysis is a process that includes research, risk assessment, and risk management (Sherif, Salama, & Abdel-Wahhab, 2009). *Risk* is the probability of injury, disease, or death due to exposure to hazards, such as chemicals. *Hazards* are a set of circumstances that may cause adverse effects.

Risk analysis is a scientific tool consisting of risk assessment, risk management, and risk communication. *Risk assessment* is an estimate of the likelihood of health risks associated with exposure. All information about the hazard is systematically and objectively evaluated, including identifying and characterizing the hazard, assessing exposure to the hazard, and characterizing the risks. Identifying a hazard is accomplished through analysis of multiple data sources, such as observations and analytical methods. The evidence is evaluated to make a scientific decision concerning the potential adverse effects of being exposed to the hazard. *Risk management* is the process of weighing policy alternatives and developing and implementing controls and regulations, if warranted. *Risk communication* is the discussion of finding about the risk and recommended strategies and regulations for risk management with interested parties, including consumers. The goal of risk analysis is to protect the public from toxic exposures, using state-of-the-art analytic techniques. Risk assessment is not simple and relies on data and resources. The limited knowledge of the potential adverse health effects from gas well extraction is a result of limited access to data as well as lack of resources allocated to study exposure. Comprehensive risk assessments direct attention to the sources of risk that, if reduced, will yield the greatest public health benefits.

The tolerance for risks on the part of individuals and families is based on the characteristics of the risk itself:

1. Voluntarily assumed risks are tolerated better than those imposed by others.
2. Risks over which scientists debate and are uncertain are more feared than those in which there is a scientific consensus.
3. Risks of natural origin are considered to be less threatening than those created by humans.

All of these risk characteristics are applicable to persons who are living in areas of hydraulic fracturing. Responses differ according to the characteristics of the risk being considered, alternating from undue alarm to apathy. To the extent possible, objective information about the nature and extent of various environmental risks should be considered.

Environmental risk reduction objectives should be based on the best available scientific knowledge about the relative risks of various pollutants to health rather than on what is emotionally appealing or politically or economically attractive at a particular point in time. Many major environmental risks require intensive, multifaceted, and often long-term interventions to change attitudes and reallocate resources for their control. Nurses and other health professionals should play a proactive role by focusing on the local community and its work sites, advocating, leading, and facilitating methods to reduce environmental pollutants; safe waste disposal; monitoring and surveillance to ensure good-quality air and water; and worker protection from toxic substances.

Promoting Healthy Social and Built Environments

Where people live makes a difference in their health. The social and built environments are two major factors that need to be addressed in health promotion.

Social capital, an indicator of community capacity, focuses on supportive networks within the community. *Collective efficacy,* the perception of mutual trust and willingness to help each other, is a measure of neighborhood social capital that has been associated with healthy neighborhoods. *Neighborhood cohesion,* another measure of neighborhood social capital, refers to neighborhood residents' sense of shared norms, values, and feelings of belonging within their local area. These measures of social capital need to be assessed prior to building coalitions to identify and tackle issues in the community. Questions might include "How do neighbors help each other?", "How much do you trust your neighbors?", "Do you feel you are a part of the neighborhood?", "Do you and your neighbors agree on similar things such as child rearing?"

Strategies to foster health and well-being in communities in inner cities, at work sites, and in school settings are important for health. For example, community gardens have been shown to facilitate social connections, strengthen neighborhoods, increase leisure-time physical activity, build skills, bridge ethnically and age diverse communities, and improve community nutrition (Teig, Amulya, Bardwell, Buchenau, Marshall, & Litt, 2009). Community gardens have the potential to promote healthy lifestyles through community-based environmental change. They promote health through collective efficacy, a shared willingness to intervene for the good of the community.

Major advances in public health have occurred through improvements in the built environments, such as sanitary reforms and clean water supplies. The *built environment,* defined as

TABLE 14–1   Components of the Built Environment Associated with Health

Built Environment Components	Physical and Mental Health Outcomes
• Air, Water quality	• Physical activity, Walking
• Population density	• Well-being
• Housing density, Quality	• Diet quality
• Land use mix, Zoning	• Asthma, Pulmonary diseases
• Distance to stores, schools, etc.	• Cardiovascular diseases
• Food access, Quality	• Type 2 diabetes
• Street patterns, Lighting	• Restricted elderly mobility
• Sidewalks	• Body Mass Index
• Noise	• Obesity
• Safety (Crime, Traffic)	• Depression
• Public parks, Green space	• Stress
• Recreational facilities	• Alcohol abuse

the way in which communities and neighborhoods are designed, includes buildings, spaces, transportation systems, homes, schools, workplaces, parks, and recreation facilities (Sallis et al., 2009). Table 14–1 provides examples of the components of the built environment associated with health outcomes. These include traffic flow, cleanliness, maintenance of public spaces, zoning and land use mix, presence and conditions of sidewalks, and population density (Renalds, Smith, & Hale, 2010). In other words, the built environment is the place where people live, work, and conduct their leisure activities on a day-to-day basis. The physical characteristics of neighborhoods have been linked to physical activity, obesity, cardiovascular disease, mental health, collective efficacy, and neighborhood cohesiveness.

Built environments have consistently been shown to be associated with physical activity (Sallis, Floyd, Rodriquez, & Saelens, 2013). Factors that support walkability and other physical activity include the presence and conditions of sidewalks and trails, availability of recreational facilities, lighting, land use mix, and perceived safety within the neighborhood. The lack of these factors limits physical activity and is common in low-income and rural communities.

Obesity also has been linked to factors in the built environment, especially for children (Singh, Siahpush, & Kogan, 2010). Physical inactivity is more common in neighborhoods with sidewalks in need of repair and absent or poorly maintained recreation centers and parks. Children who live in unsafe neighborhoods are more likely to stay inside and watch television more than two hours a day compared to children in safe neighborhoods. The availability of local foods is also associated with obesity. In neighborhoods with limited local food stores and higher numbers of fast-food restaurants, the risk for obesity is increased (Black & Macinko, 2010).

Evidence consistently shows that neighborhood characteristics are associated with health-promoting behaviors, and differences in these characteristics exist across neighborhoods and communities. Low-income, ethnically diverse neighborhoods have fewer factors that promote health.

However, all of the adverse conditions are amenable to change through the creation of programs and policies that are aimed at improving the environments in which healthy behaviors are formed and maintained.

Nurses play a pivotal role in promoting healthy community environments. Nurses can help communities define and prioritize issues that need to be addressed and empower its members to advocate with community leaders and policy-makers to obtain needed resources for community infrastructure. Nurses also can engage sectors in the community to support safe living conditions, provide health education, teach family health promotion skills, promote culturally appropriate preventive services, collaborate with schools to develop health promotion curriculum and facilitate physical activity, and promote programs in the workplace.

PROMOTING HEALTH THROUGH LEGISLATION

In a democratic society, it is widely assumed that matters of risk critical to survival and security are subject to regulatory decisions, whereas risks not clearly essential for general health and welfare are issues for personal decision and action. Even essential risks may be left to individual decision, providing that they do not infringe on the rights of others. Controversy over the role of government continues in relation to legislating environmental and behavioral changes that promote good health and increase longevity. If the government uses the means at its disposal to regulate changes in behavior, it may be faced with problems of an ethical nature. However, voluntary, individual approaches may fall short of achieving widespread change in self-damaging behaviors.

Public health policy plays a major role in the regulation of advertising and taxation of harmful products as well as communicable disease control, such as quarantine and surveillance. For example, pandemic influenza preparedness requires health policy. Public policy and laws may make the task of policy-makers easier for large-scale health threats. However, the balance between public good and individual rights is a difficult dilemma. If the state has a moral obligation to protect the right of its citizens, can health measures that benefit the population as a whole be subverted by minority beliefs? The appropriate balance between public good and individual rights is a challenging one.

Government involvement in lifestyle reform is to some extent supported by the long-standing role of the federal government as a health care provider. Although federal regulations might be cost-effective, many individuals view health promotion legislation as unethical or as placing undue intrusion on their individual freedom. Ethical issues, including individual autonomy, must be thoughtfully considered in matters of health.

Personal Choice versus Paternalism

There are two philosophical views of the role of government: individualism, or personal choice, and paternalism (Wiley, Berman, & Blanke, 2013). *Individualism* or *personal choice* is based on the American ideal, in which individuals are given maximum freedom to make their own decisions in the area of health. Health habits are considered personal choices, so outside interventions by governmental policy are not considered to be warranted. Poor health is attributed to individual behaviors; thus, society's responsibility is minimized. *Paternalism,* the counterpoint, holds that experts (professionals and policy-makers) have a moral responsibility to solve health problems because individuals lack the ability to do so. Therefore, interventions, such as laws and public policies, are justified for the health of society. The role of individuals in this model is to adhere to policies. Individuals are not blamed for their problems, as they are viewed as victims of circumstance. Both views have strengths. In the personal control or individualism model, control is in the hands of the individuals, promoting a sense of efficacy and empowerment. Second, diversity of opinions is respected in the individualistic view. The strength of the paternalistic view is that it has the potential to reduce health inequities, also empowering individuals. Health policies are socially responsible as they apply to all segments of the population. In addition, problems over which individuals have no control, such as environmental issues, are recognized and addressed.

Both approaches have limitations as well. An emphasis on personal responsibility for health promotes victim blaming, which becomes problematic, as social and environmental factors also are major determinants of health. However, overemphasis on paternalism or social responsibility may discount individual and group differences and the contributions of individuals to lifestyle behaviors. Public health approaches include individuals and communities, the collective voice, to work together to solve problems.

Deciding whether social changes to enhance health should be voluntary or mandatory is a continuing debate. Are government regulations appropriate? If they are, how and to what extent? Is it coercive to increase cigarette taxes to help defray the cost of smoking-induced disease? Should highly refined sugar products and high-cholesterol foods also be taxed more heavily to pay for the cost of health problems due to obesity? Should taxes on large, high-speed automobiles be proportionately higher than taxes on smaller cars with limited speed and greater fuel economy? Which social changes should be voluntary and which should be mandated through legislation? A balance of voluntary and mandatory action is needed, while continuing to pay close attention to the ethical dimensions of such health-related decisions.

Local, state, and federal governments have been criticized for implementing regulations to change the nutritional content of foods, including sugary beverages, trans-fats, and salt, to address national health problems (Brownell, Kersh, Ludwig, Post, Puhl, Schwartz, & Willett, 2010). Attacks by the food industry have included derogatory labels, such as "nanny state" or "big brother." The attacks are seen as subversive attempts to divert the focus onto government paternalism, rather than the need to address the health problems (Wiley, Berman, & Blanke, 2013). Proponents of healthy food legislation are accused of interfering with the market economy and restricting personal choice. Similar criticisms were voiced by the tobacco industry prior to the passing of smoking restriction legislation. Paternalistic government regulations have been common throughout history to protect and improve the health and safety of the public. Current actions are targeted to decreasing obesity and its long-term health burden. Laws and regulations that promote personal choice and responsibility are possible when authority is used judiciously to address public health problems that are beyond individual control.

The Patient Protection and Affordable Care Act

The Patient Protection and Affordable Care Act (ACA) passed in 2010 is being implemented in phases by the U.S. Department of Health and Human Services. The law is designed to address major problems in the health care system, including access to care and disparities in health and health care. Public confusion about the law is considered to be due, in part, to the ongoing focus on the most controversial parts: the requirement of individuals to have minimal essential health coverage and the expansion of Medicaid (Kimbrough-Melton, 2013).

Both components address access to care. Improved systems of care are addressed by expanding Community Health Centers (CHCs). These centers serve persons who are five times as likely to be poorer and twice as likely to be uninsured compared to the overall population. The act also places a major focus on strengthening primary care through greater reimbursement and new delivery models, such as patient-centered medical homes (Davis, Abrams, & Stemikis, 2011).

Less public attention has been focused on prevention, health promotion, and primary care, major components of the act. However, several provisions address these topics, and the act has been described as a revitalized era for prevention (Koh & Sebelius, 2010). The act provides improved access to clinical preventive services such as screening for cancer, HIV, depression, alcohol misuse, and an annual wellness exam with a health risk assessment and tailored prevention plan. Wellness in the workplace is also promoted; for example, grants for small businesses to implement employee wellness programs. The act has made prevention a national priority through the establishment of a National Prevention, Health Promotion, and Public Health Council that will develop a national strategy for health promotion and prevention. This council will build on the *Healthy People 2020* initiative. Tobacco dependence and obesity are addressed though interventions and counseling for the health risks and coverage of smoking cessation prescriptions. The act has funded demonstration projects for reducing childhood obesity as well as regulations for menu labeling in fast-food chains.

Health disparities are addressed through increasing access to care, prevention and wellness services, and initiatives that are aimed at community-based prevention. The Community Prevention Services Task Force will develop recommendations for improving the social, economic and physical environments of communities with adverse conditions. In addition, a competitive grant program is planned in which the CDC will fund projects to address the community infrastructure and programs to promote healthy lifestyles. Funding is also provided for maternal and child home visits in high-risk communities, oral health, and culturally appropriate education for family planning and prevention of sexually transmitted diseases. Many believe the law does not go far enough in addressing the social determinants of health due to the emphasis on access to health care (Williams, McClellan, & Rivin, 2010). However, access to care is the first step in enabling individuals to learn how to prevent diseases and promote a healthy lifestyle. Access to care and preventive services in partnership with initiatives to address issues in the social and physical environments will reduce health disparities and promote equity in health.

The dependence of the American people on diagnosis and treatment of disease to improve health and increase longevity is economically and socially rooted in our culture. Until recently, Americans were willing to spend escalating proportions of both personal and public dollars on an increasing array of medical services, hoping for "magic bullets" to cure all ills. However, the availability of health care technology and medical interventions has exceeded society's ability to afford them. In addition, medical care is considered to account for only 10 to 15% of the declines in premature death in the twentieth century; factors that help prevent illness have been responsible for the remaining decline. The need for transformation of the health care system has never been greater. The Affordable Care Act is seen by many to be a step in this direction.

All evidence to date has shown that, without health care reform to make health insurance more accessible and affordable, the United States will continue to face accelerating costs for individuals, employers, and government. The rate of health care costs will continue to increase along with the numbers of uninsured. The ACA changes who bears the burden of financing the health care system and how the burden is shared. Although the law is complex and expensive, it is projected to ultimately improve both the health and financial security of Americans.

CONSIDERATIONS FOR PRACTICE TO PROMOTE SOCIAL AND ENVIRONMENTAL CHANGE

Nurses' role in health care and health care reform has been recognized in the Affordable Care Act, as funds have been allocated to increase the primary care workforce. In 2012, a four-year, $200 million investment was awarded in nursing education to increase the number of advanced practice nurses. The increase in the number of advanced practice nurses will help transform health care and provide leaders in primary care. The role of nurses in health reform was also emphasized in the Institute of Medicine Report on the Future of Nursing (Mahoney & Jones, 2013). This report underscores the need for professional nursing to be transformed by addressing education and practice. The report calls for higher levels of education and training in an improved education system, the ability to practice to the full extent of one's certification and training, and full partnership with physicians and other health professionals in redesigning health care. The IOM report and the ACA introduce major opportunities for advanced practice and public health nurses to lead new care delivery models and health-promoting and preventive services.

As mentioned through the text, health promotion and prevention interventions can no longer focus exclusively on the individual to achieve large-scale behavior change. The comprehensive view of health promotion emphasizes the need for collaboration and partnership with other health professionals, health care organizations, and policy-makers at the local, state, and national levels. Advanced practice nurses will be in positions to provide leadership to build healthy communities by designing and implementing interventions that develop community competence and empowerment, and to participate with communities to identify resources, problems, and opportunities. Advanced practice nurses will know how to employ strategies to involve community members and teach leadership skills, so that community leaders will be able to play an influential role in changing their communities.

Because of the multiple factors involved in behavior change that go beyond the individual, advanced practice nurses can also become advocates for health policies to decrease social and environmental risks. This can be accomplished by working with local health departments and state legislatures to make change as well as participating in lobbying efforts to increase funds and services. Health promotion in the 21st century brings many changes and challenges due to the rapid, ongoing changes in the population, workforce, technology, and health care environment. However, these challenges bring new opportunities for nurses, who, with other members of an interdisciplinary team, can create innovative health plans and programs to improve health.

OPPORTUNITIES FOR RESEARCH IN SOCIAL AND ENVIRONMENTAL CHANGE

Social and environmental approaches to promote health and health care reform offer many opportunities for research. New health care and prevention programs as well as new advanced nursing programs and interprofessional models need rigorous evaluation and replication. Underserved populations and racial/ethnic groups should be included in all studies. Community-based partici-patory research to promote partnerships with communities should be emphasized. Additional directions for nursing and interdisciplinary research efforts include the following:

1. Test the effects of community health promotion interventions on altering health-related social norms among children and adolescents.
2. Design observational studies to describe the effects of chemicals used in hydraulic fractur-ing on humans and animals, as well as the air and water supply in affected areas.
3. Design studies to evaluate both short-term and long-term effects of policy change on the health of individuals in low-income communities.
4. Identify factors in the built environment that facilitate physical activity in adolescents and the elderly, and design and test the effects of eliminating the barriers on physical activity long term.
5. Evaluate the effectiveness of policy changes that eliminate environmental barriers to healthy food choices and active lifestyles on obesity.

The study of human and environmental factors in health and disease is complex and requires research collaboration, multilevel models, and multiple methods to address the many gaps in knowledge that exist.

Summary

This chapter focuses on society as a collective and the impact of public policy and social and physical environments on the health status of individuals, families, and communities. Attempt-ing to promote healthy lifestyles without chang-ing the environments in which people live results in frustration and failure of health promotion efforts. A balanced approach to disease preven-tion and health promotion requires attention to (1) quality of the social and physical environ-ments, (2) inequities in health-promoting options available for all, and (3) changes in health policy to create healthier communities. Because health is no longer viewed as an aim in itself, but as a resource for personal and social development as well as a product of social condi-tions, changes in public policies should become part of any effort to promote health.

Learning Activities

1. Conduct a home or work site assessment to identify a health-damaging environmental factor. Describe the history of the problem, its effects on the health of the family or workers, barriers to solving the problem, resources needed to solve the problem, and strategies to obtain resources, if they are not available to solve the problem.
2. Develop three community strategies to solve the problem identified in Learning Activity 1, and out-line an evaluation plan of your possible solutions.

3. Write a letter to your state legislators voicing your concerns about the environmental problem identi-fied in Learning Activity 1 and recommend poten-tial solutions.
4. Describe the steps and strategies you would imple-ment to empower and mobilize individuals who have expressed a concern about the lack of recre-ational facilities for their children and families in their community.

References

Bamberger, M., & Oswald, R. E. (2012). Impacts of gas drilling on human and animal health. *New Solutions, 22*, 51–77.

Bertot, J. C., Jaeger, P. T., & Hansen, R. (2012). The impact of policies on government social media usage: Issues, challenges, and recommendations. *Government Information Quality, 29*, 30–40.

Black, J. L., & Macinko, J. (2010). The changing distribution of determinants of obesity in the neighborhoods of New York City, 2003–2007. *American Journal of Epidemiology, 171*, 765–775.

Brownell, K. D., & Frieden, T. R. (2009). Ounces of prevention—The public policy case for taxes on sugared beverages. *New England of Medicine, 360*, 1805–1807.

Brownell, K. D., Kersh, R., Ludwig, D. S., Post, R. C., Puhl, R. M., Schwartz, M. B., & Willett, W. C. (2010). Personal responsibility and obesity: A constructive approach to a controversial issue. *Health Affairs, 29*, 379–387.

Chou, W., Prestin, A., Lyons, C., & Wen, K. (2013). Web 2.0 for health promotion: Reviewing the current evidence. *American Journal of Public Health, 103*, e9–e18.

Colborn, T., Kwiatkowski, C., Schultz, K., & Bachran, M. (2011). Natural gas operations form a public health perspective. *Human & Ecological Risk Assessment, 17*, 1039–1056.

Davis, K., Abrams, M., & Stemikis, K. (2011). How the affordable care act will strengthen the nation's primary care foundation. *Journal of General Internal Medicine, 26*, 1201–1203.

Dixon, S. L., Jacobs, D. E., Wilson, J. W., Akoto, J. Y., Nevin, R., & Clark, C. S. (2012). Window replacement and residential lead paint hazard control 12 years later. *Environmental Research, 113*, 14–20.

Editorial. (2009). What price health? *Nature, 458*(7234), 7 (published online 4 March 2009). Retrieved from http://www.nature.com/nature/journal/v458/n7234/pdf/458007a.pdf

Finkel, M., Hays, J., & Law, A. (2013). The shale gas boom and the need for rational policy. *American Journal of Public Health, 103*(7): 1161–1163.

Graf, S. K., Kappagoda, M., Wooten, H. M., McGowan, A. K., & Ashe, M. (2012). Policies for healthier communities: Historical, legal, and practical elements of the Obesity Prevention Movement. *Annual Review of Public Health, 33*, 307–324.

Kimbrough-Melton, R. J. (2013). Health for all: The promise of the Affordable Care Health Act for racially and ethnically diverse populations. *American Journal of Orthopsychiatry, 83*, 352–358.

Koh, H. K., & Sebelius, K. G. (2010). Promoting prevention through the Affordable Care Act. *The New England Journal of Medicine, 363*, 1296–1299.

Lanz, P. M., Mendez, D., & Philbert, M. A. (2013). Radon, smoking, and lung cancer: The need to refocus radon control policy. *American Journal of Public Health, 103*, 443–447.

Laumbach, R. J., & Kipen, H. M. (2012). Respiratory health effects of air pollution: Update on biomass smoke and traffic pollution. *Journal of Allergy and Clinical Immunology, 129*, 3–11.

Lustria, M. L., Smith, S. A., & Hinnant, C. C. (2011). Exploring the digital divide: An examination of eHealth technology use in health information seeking, communication, and personal health information management in the USA. *Health Informatics Journal, 17*, 224–243.

Mahoney, D., & Jones, E. J. (2013). Social determinants of health in nursing education, research, and health policy. *Nursing Science Quarterly, 26*, 280–284.

Metcalfe, G., & Higgins, C. (2009). Health public policy: Is health impact assessment the cornerstone? *Public Health, 123*, 296–310.

Minkler, M., Wallerstein, N., & Wilson, N. (2008). Improving health through community organization and community building. In K. Glanz, B. K. Rimer, & K. Viswanath (Eds.), *Health behavior and health education* (4th ed., pp. 287–309). San Francisco, CA: Jossey-Bass Publishers.

Mitka, M. (2012). Rigorous evidence slim for determining health risks from natural gas fracking. *Journal of the American Medical Association (JAMA), 307*, 2135–2136.

Osborn, S. G., Vengosh, A., Warner, N. R., & Jackson, R. B. (2011). Methane contamination of drinking water accompanying gas-well drilling and hydraulic fracturing. *PNAS, 108*, 8172–8176.

Puska, P., & Stahl, T. (2010). Health in all policies—the Finnish Initiative: Background, principles, and current issues. *Annual Review of Public Health, 31*, 315–328.

Renalds, A., Smith, T. H., & Hale, P. J. (2010). A systematic review of built environment and health. *Family and Community Health, 33*, 68–78.

Sallis, J. F., Floyd, M. K., Rodriquez, D. A., & Saelens, B. E. (2013). Role of built environments in physical activity, obesity, and cardiovascular disease. *Circulation, 125*, 729–737.

Sallis, J. F., Saelens, B. E., Frank, L. D., Conway, T. L., Slymen, D. J., Cain, K. L., et al. (2009). Neighborhood built environment and income: Examining multiple health outcomes. *Social Science & Medicine, 68*, 1285–1293.

Sherif, S., Salama, E. E., & Abdel-Wahhab, M. A. (2009). Mycotoxins and child health: The need for health risk assessment. *International Journal of Hygiene and Environmental Health, 212*, 347–368.

Singh, G. K., Siahpush, M., & Kogan, M. D. (2010). Rising social inequities in US childhood obesity, 2003–2007. *Annals of Epidemiology, 20*, 40–52.

Teig, E., Amulya, J., Bardwell, L., Buchenau, M., Marshall, J. A., & Litt, J. S. (2009). Collective efficacy in Denver, Colorado: Strengthening neighborhoods and health through community gardens. *Health & Place, 15*, 1115–1122.

U.S. Department of Health and Human Services. (2013). *Healthy People 2020*. Retrieved from http://www.healthypeople2020.gov

U.S. Environmental Protection Agency. (2009). *Radon,* Retrieved from http://www.epa.gov/radiatoin/radionuclides/radon.htm

Van den Broucke, S. (2013). Implementing health in all policies post Helsinki 2013: Why, what, who, and how. *Health Promotion International, 28*, 281–284.

Wiley, W. F., Berman, M. L., & Blanke, D. (2013). Who's your nanny? Choice, paternalism and public health in the age of personal responsibility. *Journal of Law, Medicine, & Ethics, 41*, 88–91.

Williams, D. R., McClellan, M. B., & Rivin, A. M. (2010). Beyond the Affordable Care Act: Achieving real improvements in American's health. *Health Affairs, 29*, 1481–1488.

World Health Organization (WHO). (2008). *Closing the gap in a generation*. Geneva, Switzerland: WHO. Retrieved from http://who.int/social determinants/the commission/final report/en/index.htm

World Health Organization (WHO). (2013). Helsinki statement on health in all policies. *Eighth Global Conference on Health Promotion*. Retrieved from: http://www.who.int/healthpromotion/conferences/8gchp/8gchp_helsinki_statement.pdf

INDEX